Delivering CBT for Inso
in Psychosis

Individuals with psychiatric disorders such as schizophrenia, bipolar disorder, and post-traumatic stress disorder often report Insomnia and difficulties sleeping, which can significantly impede recovery, worsen symptoms, and reduce quality of life. This volume presents a detailed theoretical rationale and session-by-session outline for delivering Cognitive Behaviour Therapy for Insomnia to people with these mental health disorders. The treatment has been developed in close collaboration with people living with mental illness, as well as sleep specialists and psychosis experts. Information regarding the efficacy of the programme is presented, along with resources offering information on complicating factors, avoiding relapse, managing stress, and restoring lifestyle balance.

Flavie Waters, PhD, is a leading expert in psychosis at the University of Western Australia and North Metro Health Service Mental Health, Western Australia.

Melissa J. Ree, PhD, is a clinical psychologist and CBT Insomnia expert at the Marian Centre and Sleep Matters, Western Australia.

Vivian Chiu, BPsych (Hons), is a research psychologist at the University of Western Australia and North Metro Health Service Mental Health, Western Australia.

Practical Clinical Guidebooks Series

Exposure Treatments for Anxiety Disorders
A Practitioner's Guide to Concepts, Methods, and Evidence-Based Practice
Rosqvist

Treating Sexual Offenders
An Integrated Approach
Marshall, Marshall, Serran, and Fernandez

Evidence-Based Treatments for Alcohol and Drug Abuse
A Practitioner's Guide to Theory, Methods, and Practice
Emmelkamp and Vede

Cognitive-Behavioral Treatment for Generalized Anxiety Disorder
From Science to Practice
Dugas and Robichaud

Cognitive Behavior Therapy for Smoking Cessation
A Practical Guidebook to the Most Effective Treatments
Perkins, Conklin, and Levine

Cognitive Behavioral Therapy for Adult ADHD
An Integrative Psychosocial and Medical Approach
Ramsay and Rostain

Cognitive Behavioral Therapy for Social Anxiety Disorder
Evidence-Based and Disorder-Specific Treatment Techniques
Hofmann and Otto

Compulsive Buying
Clinical Foundations and Treatment
Muller and Mitchell

Contextual Anger Regulation Therapy
A Mindfulness and Acceptance-Based Approach
Gardner and Moore

Specialized Cognitive Behavior Therapy for Obsessive Compulsive Disorder
An Expert Clinician Guidebook
Sookman

Delivering CBT for Insomnia in Psychosis
A Clinical Guide
Waters, Ree, and Chiu

Delivering CBT for Insomnia in Psychosis

A Clinical Guide

Flavie Waters, Melissa J. Ree, and Vivian Chiu

Routledge
Taylor & Francis Group
NEW YORK AND LONDON

First published 2017
by Routledge
711 Third Avenue, New York, NY 10017

and by Routledge
2 Park Square, Milton Park, Abingdon, Oxon, OX14 4RN

Routledge is an imprint of the Taylor & Francis Group, an informa business

Library of Congress Cataloging in Publication Data
Names: Waters, Flavie, author. | Ree, Melissa J., author. | Chiu, Vivian, author.
Title: Delivering CBT for Insomnia in psychosis : a clinical guide / By Flavie Waters, Melissa J. Ree, and Vivian Chiu.
Description: New York, NY : Routledge, 2017. Includes bibliographical references and index.
Identifiers: LCCN 2016045646| ISBN 9781138186514 (hbk : alk. paper) | ISBN 9781138186521 (pbk : alk. paper) | ISBN 9781315643793 (ebk)
Subjects: | MESH: Sleep Initiation and Maintenance Disorders—therapy | Cognitive Therapy—methods | Psychotic Disorders—therapy
Classification: LCC RC548 NLM WM 188 DDC 616.8/49820651—dc23
LC record available at https://lccn.loc.gov/2016045646

ISBN: 978-1-138-18651-4 (hbk)
ISBN: 978-1-138-18652-1 (pbk)
ISBN: 978-1-315-64379-3 (ebk)

Typeset in Baskerville
by Florence Production Ltd, Stoodleigh, Devon, UK

Contents

Figures, Tables, and Text Boxes

Figures

Tables

Text Boxes

Preface

There is such solid evidence with regards to the pivotal role that sleep plays in mental health. Poor sleep is not just an epiphenomenon of a psychiatric condition, but rather it is both a cause and a consequence of poorer mental health. It is clear that treatment of sleep problems in their own right ought to be the standard for everyone reporting mental health problems and sleep difficulties.

In the case of psychotic disorders, we know that, when sleep improves, psychiatric symptoms and daytime function also improve. Evidence is accumulating that even those with severe mental illness can benefit from psychological and behavioural approaches to poor sleep. Although the field of CBT for Insomnia (CBT-I) in the context of psychotic disorders is relatively new, it has reached a stage where dissemination of CBT-I treatment details may facilitate clinical outcomes and personal recovery. This book is intended to provide a concise description of both the treatment rationale and treatment delivery particulars. It also provides a CBT-I Therapist Manual and take-home client resources to address Insomnia and related sleep problems in people with chronic psychotic disorders whose levels of functioning and psychopathology are at the severe end of the continuum, and who have previously been considered too low functioning for traditional CBT-I treatment options.

We hope that this book may serve as a step towards better awareness regarding the effectiveness of CBT-I and greater opportunities for training in behavioural sleep medicine in the psychiatric sector so that the ideal of routine sleep treatment can become a reality.

Acknowledgements

We would like to express our deepest appreciation to all the participants who contributed to the development and evaluation of the CBT-I manual, and to the mental health staff from different mental health organisations across Perth who supported our efforts to make sleep intervention an integral part of patient care and treatment.

In addition, we would like to thank the following family members, friends, mentors, and colleagues who provided inspiration, knowledge, and support in the writing of this book:

Flavie Waters: I am forever thankful for my Mother, Diana Laurie, who tirelessly helped to support me and edit chapters; Keira James, who is always up for a challenge; Daniel Rock and Patrick Marwick, for supporting clinical research activities within mental health services; and Michael Waters, for always saying yes.

Melissa Ree: My past supervision from Professor Allison Harvey has heavily influenced my understanding and thinking about Insomnia and its treatment, and this certainly comes through in this book. Further, a heartfelt thank you to my husband and fellow clinical psychologist, Paul Jeffery, for his insightful reviews of chapters and manual sessions. Finally, to clinician friends and colleagues who edited chapters—thank you, Gayle Maloney and Hanedy Catalan.

Vivian Chiu: Aleksandar Janca for his support and kindness; Alan and Jessica Chiu for feeding me; my friends and partner for encouraging me and keeping me away from the TV.

Abbreviations

5HT	Serotonin
ACh	Acetylcholine
BzRA	Benzodiazepine receptor agonistic modulator
CBT	Cognitive Behaviour Therapy
CBT-I	Cognitive Behaviour Therapy for Insomnia
CBTp	Cognitive Behaviour Therapy for psychosis
CPAP	Continuous positive airway pressure
CT	Cognitive therapy
DASS	Depression Anxiety Stress Scales
DBAS	Dysfunctional Beliefs About Sleep scale
DBAS-16	Dysfunctional Beliefs and Attitudes about Sleep Scale—16-item version
DLMO	Dim light melatonin onset
DSM-V	*Diagnostic and Statistical Manual of Mental Disorders* (fifth edition)
EEG	Electroencephalogram
ESS	Epworth Sleepiness Scale
GABA	Gamma-aminobutyric acid
GOOBICS	Get out of bed if you can't sleep
HPA	Hypothalamic–pituitary–adrenal
ICSD-3	*International Classification of Sleep Disorders* (3rd edition)
ISI	Insomnia Severity Index
MAOI	Monoamine oxidase inhibitor
MEQ	Morningness–Eveningness Questionnaire
MINI	Mini International Neuropsychiatric Interview
MINI psychosis	Mini International Neuropsychiatric Interview Psychotic Disorders module
MSLT	Multiple Sleep Latency Test
N1	Stage 1 NREM sleep
N2	Stage 2 NREM sleep
N3	Stage 3 NREM sleep
N4	Stage 4 NREM sleep
NGO	Non-governmental organisation
NREM	Non-rapid eye movement
OCD	Obsessive–compulsive disorder
OSA	Obstructive sleep apnoea
PHQ-4	Patient Health Questionnaire for Anxiety and Depression
PLMD	Periodic limb movement disorder
PSG	Polysomnography

PSQI	Pittsburgh Sleep Quality Index
PTSD	Post-traumatic stress disorder
REM	Rapid eye movement
RLS	Restless legs syndrome
SAMI	Sleep Associated Monitoring Index
SHiK	Sleep Hygiene Knowledge Scale
SHiK-B	Sleep Hygiene Behaviours Scale
SNRI	Serotonin-norepinephrine-reuptake inhibitors
SSRI	Selective serotonin-reuptake inhibitors
TAU	Treatment as usual
TCQI-R	Thought Control Questionnaire for Insomnia-Revised
TNID	Turning nightmares into dreams
Z-drugs	Benzodiazepine receptor agonistic modulators

1 Introduction

The term 'psychosis' refers to a constellation of clinical symptoms such as hallucinations, delusions, and disorganised thinking, alongside negative symptoms such as reduced motivation and social withdrawal. People living with psychotic symptoms often suffer from disorders such as schizophrenia, schizoaffective disorder, bipolar disorder, substance-induced psychosis, and even major depression or post-traumatic stress disorder (PTSD).

Approximately half of these individuals have other co-occurring difficulties such as cognitive impairments, social and occupational difficulties, and other physical health concerns, many of which persist between psychotic episodes. There is increasing evidence that almost all individuals with psychotic disorders also experience difficulties with their sleep. Approximately half meet the criteria for Insomnia Disorder (from hereon in, also referred to as Insomnia) and/or co-morbid sleep complaints such as hypersomnia, circadian rhythm disturbances, and nightmares.

These disorders of sleep are often distressing and can directly impact on clinical symptoms and the clinical course of an individual's mental health disorder, as well as their physical health, cognition, and quality of life (see Figure 1.1). Consequently, so that the health and functional recovery of people with psychotic disorders can be optimised, there is a critical need to address and provide effective treatment options for their disturbed sleep. To this end, cognitive behavioural therapy for Insomnia (CBT-I) offers great promise, and this book outlines the theory, evidence, and a detailed description of CBT-I for use in the context of psychotic disorders.

The Psychological Treatment of Psychotic Disorders

There is now robust evidence that psychological treatments can assist in the recovery of individuals with psychotic disorders. Clinical practice guidelines recommend that psychological interventions, such as cognitive behavioural therapy (CBT), should be routinely offered alongside antipsychotic medications as a first-line treatment option (e.g. National Collaborating Centre for Mental Health, 2014).

The use of CBT, in particular, has a 20-year history of treating symptoms of psychotic disorders, with more than 50 randomised controlled trials. Typically, effect sizes are robust, with reports ranging between 0.3 and 0.5 (e.g. Beck and Rector, 2000; Wykes et al., 2008; Grant et al., 2012). Furthermore, CBT has been found to promote a recovery-oriented approach to mental health practice (Bellack, 2006) and is a treatment option that people with psychosis express a desire to engage in (e.g. Kilbride et al., 2013; Waters et al., 2015).

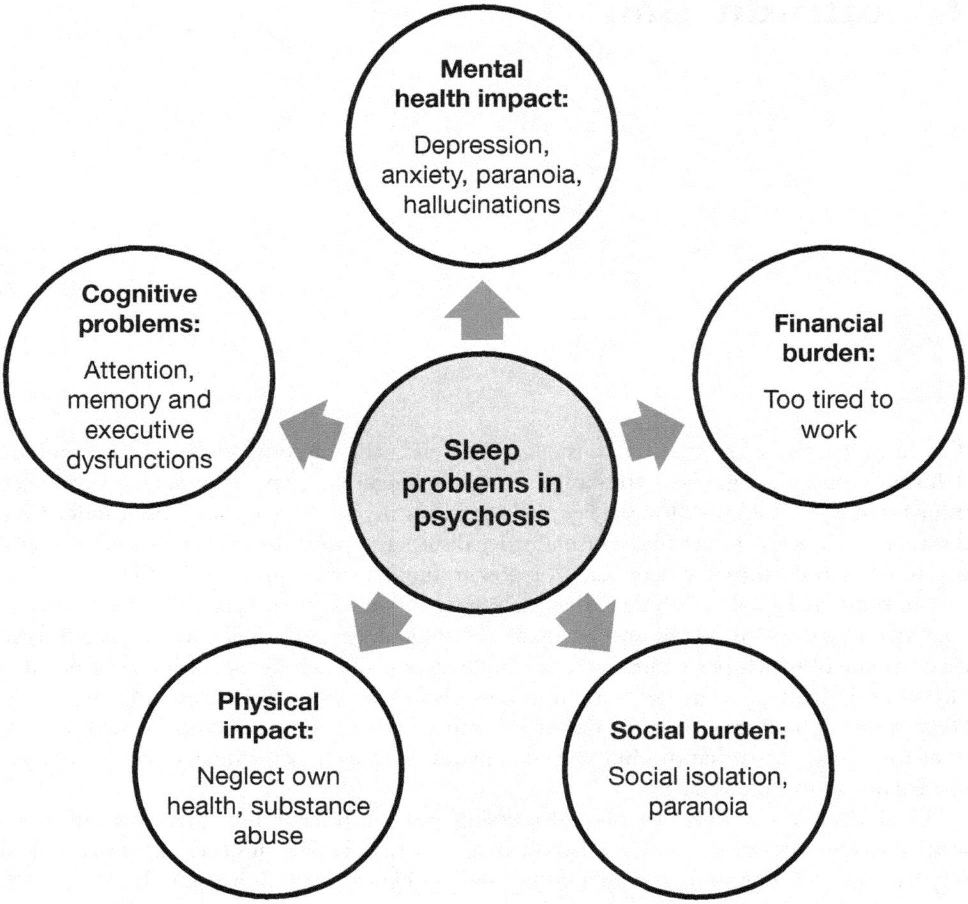

Figure 1.1 Impact of Sleep Problems in Psychotic Disorders

The Treatment of Insomnia and Other Sleep Disturbances Using CBT-I

There is extremely robust evidence for the effectiveness of CBT in addressing sleep disturbances in the general population (CBT-I). Findings show that CBT-I produces longer-lasting effects than pharmacological interventions alone and should be promoted as a first-line treatment option (Jacobs et al., 2004; Qaseem et al., 2016; Schutte-Rodin et al., 2008).

More recently, CBT-I alongside usual treatment (i.e. pharmacological) has emerged as an intervention that has the potential to provide long-term solutions for sleep problems in people with a psychotic disorder (e.g. Freeman et al., 2015; Harvey et al., 2015). Despite the benefits of evidence-based psychological interventions, however, people living with severe and persistent psychotic symptoms often have limited access to these treatment options. This is partly because standard CBT-I programmes need to be adapted to address the additional challenges and circumstances of people with psychotic disorders. When they are adapted appropriately, there is emerging evidence that such programmes can be highly effective for this population.

The aim of this book is to provide a CBT-I framework for clinicians working to address and treat the disorders of sleep in individuals with a psychotic illness. In particular, the manual provides strategies to address Insomnia and related sleep problems in people with chronic psychotic disorders whose levels of functioning and psychopathology are at the severe end of the continuum, and who have previously been considered too low-functioning for traditional CBT-I treatment options. We hope that this book presents a strong argument that clinically meaningful gains can be made with a CBT-I approach for individuals with psychosis.

The development of the manual

We have developed and evaluated a manualised, four-session CBT-I intervention that specifically addresses sleep complaints and related daytime sleepiness in low-functioning individuals with psychotic disorders. Client resource packs and additional materials are also provided to assist the therapeutic process and to encourage clients to self-manage their difficulties. The intervention manual can be administered in either a group or individual format.

The development of this manual and its resources arose from close collaboration with people living with psychotic disorders and Insomnia. Between 2011 and 2014, surveys and focus groups were conducted with representatives from this clinical group to elicit detailed information regarding their personal experience of sleep problems, antecedent factors, and the subsequent impact of these difficulties (Waters et al., 2011, 2012, 2013; Chiu et al., 2016). This preliminary research also identified the knowledge gaps and cognitive styles of these individuals (Chiu et al., 2015), as well as the symptoms they most wanted treated and their preferred method of treatment (Waters et al., 2015).

These findings, together with in-depth enquiries during the development and piloting of the intervention, have ensured that the manual and its resources meet the needs and particular treatment challenges of people with psychotic disorders. Our research indicated that adaptations to standard CBT-I were required so that the specific challenges faced by those with a psychotic disorder were addressed.

Adaptations to CBT-I in this population should ideally accommodate:

- hypersomnia, circadian (sleep–wake) rhythm disruptions, and nightmares because these commonly co-occur with Insomnia;
- the intrusive thoughts, hallucinations, and paranoia that contribute to difficulties in falling asleep and night-time arousal;
- the common use of nicotine, caffeine, alcohol, illicit drugs, and psychotropic medications that impact on sleep onset and quality;
- the lack of daytime structure (e.g. due to low mood, avoidance, unemployment, social isolation) that disrupts sleep routines and circadian rhythms;
- the presence of learning difficulties and other cognitive deficits in domains such as attention and concentration;
- negative symptoms (see Box 2.1), low mood and anxiety;
- low motivation and low self-efficacy.

It is extremely encouraging to see that independent international research appears to be converging on a similar set of adaptations to standard CBT-I for use in individuals with a psychotic disorder. In particular, the work of Freeman and colleagues, in the UK, and Harvey and colleagues, in the USA, have suggested consistent adaptations in their CBT-I protocols.

The specific objectives for our adapted CBT-I intervention for psychosis ensure that it:

1. can be delivered to clients with complex needs, varied capacity, and multiple comorbidities;
2. provides content that encourages choice and action and that stimulates motivation in order to promote enduring changes in sleep and daytime function;
3. is sufficiently practical to be delivered in different clinical settings (inpatient, forensic, community, private);
4. can be delivered either in small groups, to facilitate empowerment through peer learning and sharing and to maximise cost-effectiveness, or in an individual format when this is more appropriate;
5. is suitable for various health practitioners, including front-line clinicians who have (a) some prior experience in delivering psychological therapies, and (b) a basic understanding of sleep and its regulation (see Chapter 5);
6. is based on empirical evidence of beneficial effects on sleep, symptoms, and daytime functioning, and is sufficiently detailed to be independently researched under controlled conditions.

The efficacy of this intervention was evaluated in 72 individuals diagnosed with a psychotic disorder, who presented with a range of psychopathology and functional capacity. Participants received outpatient sessions of adapted CBT-I plus usual treatment or usual treatment alone. Analyses demonstrated significant improvements in sleep and daytime sleepiness, as well as reductions in psychotic symptom severity and psychological distress. None of these benefits was reported by control individuals who received their usual treatment alone (see Chapter 9 for further detail). One of our participants described her experience of CBT-I as follows:

> I gave it all I have, because I've grown to understand that I have to break the bad sleeping habits really. Psychological therapies probably work better in the long term than medications, I think, because what you learn stays with you.

The collective evidence demonstrates that individuals across the spectrum of psychopathology are capable of engaging with modified CBT-I interventions to make the behavioural and cognitive changes required to improve their sleep and daytime functioning.

What Is and Isn't Covered in this Book

Our CBT-I Therapist Manual has been designed to treat Insomnia in the context of psychotic disorders. Although the primary treatment focus is Insomnia, we also touch on other sleep disorders that commonly co-occur with Insomnia in psychotic disorders and have demonstrated capacity to be improved by CBT interventions, namely hypersomnia, nightmares, and circadian rhythm dysfunction. We also specifically address low motivation and low self-efficacy, as these are common difficulties reported in those with psychosis.

The CBT-I intervention is not, however, designed to treat sleep disorders that require specialised assessment and treatment by a sleep physician or sleep technologist—for example, obstructive sleep apnoea (OSA) or narcolepsy. In these cases, treatments will be guided primarily by medical or mechanical therapies, although CBT is a useful adjunct (Luyster et al., 2010, Wickwire et al., 2010).

Book Contents

This book comprises four parts. The first part describes psychotic disorders and Insomnia and provides a rationale for, and a description of, CBT-I and its psychosis-specific adaptations. The second and third parts present the modified CBT-I Therapist Manual for the clinician and take-home resources for clients that relate to each session. The final part consists of 17 appendices.

Part I: Conceptual Frameworks and Evidence Base

This part contains the following:

- an overview of psychotic disorders, including their causes and treatment options (Chapter 2);
- descriptive and epidemiological features of Insomnia Disorder and co-occurring disturbances of sleep (Chapter 3);
- a description of the clinical features of Insomnia Disorder and other sleep disturbance in psychotic disorders (Chapter 4);
- a detailed description of sleep, its regulation, and barriers to good sleep (Chapter 5);
- understanding disturbances of sleep in psychotic disorders: predisposing, precipitating, and perpetuating factors (Chapter 6);
- theoretical framework and description of CBT-I (Chapter 7);
- methods of sleep assessment (Chapter 8);
- evidence base for CBT-I in psychotic disorders (Chapter 9);
- clinical case studies (Chapter 10).

Part II: Therapist Manual

This contains:

- tips and instructions to the therapist (Chapter 11);
- Therapist Manual (Chapters 12–15).

Part III: Client Resource Packs

Part III has resource packs for clients, including sleep diaries, charts, and activity material (Chapters 16–19).

Part IV: Appendices

The appendices have additional resources for clinicians and clients.

Summary

The aims of this book are to (a) provide a brief orientation to both psychotic disorders and Insomnia, and the bidirectional influence that these have on each other; (b) describe the theoretical orientation of CBT as a treatment approach for Insomnia; and (c) present a detailed description of, and therapist manual for, an adapted CBT-I protocol for use in psychotic disorders.

A recurrent theme throughout the book is the importance of paying specific attention to the identification and treatment of Insomnia and sleep problems as conditions distinct from psychosis, rather than sleep problems being seen as merely epiphenomena of a psychotic disorder.

We hope that any clinician who picks up this book will come to be mindful of sleep and its potential to bring about clinical changes for the patient in front of them. This book should assist clinicians in feeling more knowledgeable and confident in treating sleep problems in their clients with psychotic disorders. Finally, we hope that the interventions outlined in this book will benefit many people living with a severe mental illness.

References

Beck, A. T., and Rector, N. A. (2000) "Cognitive therapy of schizophrenia: A new therapy for the new millennium", *American Journal of Psychotherapy*, 54(3), p. 291.

Bellack, A. S. (2006) "Scientific and consumer models of recovery in schizophrenia: Concordance, contrasts, and implications", *Schizophrenia Bulletin*, 32(3), pp. 432–442.

Chiu, V. W., Harvey, R. H., Sloan, N. B., Ree, M., Lin, A., Janca, A., and Waters, F. (2015) "Cognitive and behavioral factors associated with insomnia in inpatients with schizophrenia and related psychoses", *The Journal of Nervous and Mental Disease*, 203(10), pp. 798–803.

Chiu, V. W., Ree, M., Janca, A., and Waters, F. (2016) "Sleep in schizophrenia: Exploring subjective experiences of sleep problems, and implications for treatment", *Psychiatric Quarterly*, 87(4), pp. 633–648.

Freeman, D., Waite, F., Startup, H., Myers, E., Lister, R., McInerney, J., Harvey, A. G., Geddes, J., Zaiwalla, Z., Luengo-Fernandez, R., Foster, R., Clifton, L., and Yu, L.-M. (2015) "Efficacy of cognitive behavioural therapy for sleep improvement in patients with persistent delusions and hallucinations (BEST): A prospective, assessor-blind, randomised controlled pilot trial", *The Lancet Psychiatry*, 2(11), pp. 975–983.

Grant, P. M., Huh, G. A., Perivoliotis, D., Stolar, N. M., and Beck, A. T. (2012) "Randomized trial to evaluate the efficacy of cognitive therapy for low-functioning patients with schizophrenia", *Archives of General Psychiatry*, 69(2), pp. 121–127.

Harvey, A. G., Soehner, A. M., Kaplan, K. A., Hein, K., Lee, J., Kanady, J., Li, D., Rabe-Hesketh, S., Ketter, T. A., Neylan, T. C., and Buysse, D. J. (2015) "Treating insomnia improves mood state, sleep, and functioning in bipolar disorder: A pilot randomized controlled trial", *Journal of Consulting & Clinical Psychology*, 83(3), pp. 564–577.

Jacobs, G. D., Pace-Schott, E. F., Stickgold, R., and Otto, M. W. (2004) "Cognitive behavior therapy and pharmacotherapy for insomnia: A randomized controlled trial and direct comparison", *Archives of Internal Medicine*, 164(17), pp. 1888–1896.

Kilbride, M., Byrne, R., Price, J., Wood, L., Barratt, S., Welford, M., and Morrison, A. P. (2013) "Exploring service users' perceptions of cognitive behavioural therapy for psychosis: A user led study", *Behavioural & Cognitive Psychotherapy*, 41(1), pp. 89–102.

Luyster, F. S., Buysse, D. J., and Strollo, P. J. (2010) "Comorbid insomnia and obstructive sleep apnea: Challenges for clinical practice and research", *Journal of Clinical Sleep Medicine: Official Publication of the American Academy of Sleep Medicine*, 6(2), pp. 196–204.

National Collaborating Centre for Mental Health (2014) *Psychosis and schizophrenia in adults: Treatment and management.* NICE Clinical Guideline 178. London: NICE.

Qaseem, A., Kansagara, D., Forciea, M. A., Cooke, M., Denberg, T. D., for the Clinical Guidelines Committee of the American College of Physicians. (2016) "Management of Chronic Insomnia Disorder in Adults: A Clinical Practice Guideline From the American College of Physicians", *Annals of Internal Medicine,* 165, pp. 125–133. doi: 10.7326/M15-2175

Schutte-Rodin, S., Broch, L., Buysse, D., Dorsey, C., and Sateia, M. (2008) "Clinical guideline for the evaluation and management of chronic insomnia in adults", *Journal of Clinical Sleep Medicine: Official Publication of the American Academy of Sleep Medicine*, 4(5), pp. 487–504.

Waters, F., Chiu, V., Janca, S., Atkinson, A., and Ree, M. (2015) "Preferences for different insomnia treatment options in people with schizophrenia and related psychoses: A qualitative study", *Frontiers in Psychology*, 14(6), p. 990.

Waters, F., Faulkner, D., Naik, N., and Rock, D. (2012) "Effects of polypharmacy on sleep in psychiatric inpatients", *Schizophrenia Research*, 139, pp. 225–228.

Waters, F., Naik, N., and Rock, D. (2013) "Sleep, fatigue, and functional health in psychotic patients", *Schizophrenia Research & Treatment*, 2013, article ID 425826.

Waters, F., Sinclair, C., Rock, D., Jablensky, A., Foster, R. G., and Wulff, K. (2011) "Daily variations in sleep–wake patterns and severity of psychopathology: A pilot study in community-dwelling individuals with chronic schizophrenia", *Psychiatry Research*, 187(1), pp. 304–306.

Wickwire, E. M., Smith, M. T., Birnbaum, S., and Collop, N. A. (2010) "Sleep maintenance insomnia complaints predict poor CPAP adherence: A clinical case series", *Sleep Medicine*, 11(8), pp. 772–776.

Wykes, T., Steel, C., Everitt, B., and Tarrier, N. (2008) "Cognitive behavior therapy for schizophrenia: Effect sizes, clinical models, and methodological rigor", *Schizophrenia Bulletin*, 34(3), pp. 523–537.

Part I

Conceptual Frameworks and Evidence Base

2 Psychotic Disorders

An Overview of Clinical Features and Treatment Approaches

The term 'psychosis' was first coined in the nineteenth century to denote a range of mental changes occurring in the context of a serious mental illness. It remains a broad, non-specific term that does not, in itself, reflect a clinical disorder. Instead, it is used to represent a neurobiological condition associated with various clinical symptoms. These symptoms include hallucinations, delusions, formal thought disorders, negative symptoms, and physical changes—which are described in Text Box 2.1 (American Psychiatric Association, 2013). It is now widely appreciated that the individual experience of psychosis is unique: some people might experience only some of these symptoms, whereas others might experience all of them. A common feature, however, is a distorted perception of reality that is associated with confusion and/or inappropriate or erratic behaviour.

Text Box 2.1 Clinical Symptoms Commonly Associated with Psychosis

Hallucinations: Hearing voices speaking, sounds, or music when there is no one there or nothing that can account for it; seeing, feeling, or smelling things that others do not.

Delusions: Strong beliefs that others would not share and that lead to the misinterpretation of situations. Suspicious, paranoid thoughts are common symptoms in psychosis.

Formal thought disorder: Difficulties thinking and concentrating. Sometimes, everyday thoughts can become jumbled and confused, making speech unclear or hard to understand. Thoughts can seem to speed up or slow down.

Negative symptoms: Negative symptoms reflect a reduction in, or loss of, normal function. Examples include restricted displays of emotion, monotone speech, reduced eye contact, slow movements, low motivation, lethargy, inability to feel pleasure, and lack of spontaneity.

Affective disturbances: Strong emotions and feelings, such as worry, fear, anxiety, and depression.

Physical changes: These include Insomnia, agitation, and poor hygiene.

Who Experiences Psychotic Symptoms?

Some people experience an episode of psychosis only once in their lives (often at a time of stress), whereas others have recurrent episodes of psychosis, with periods of full or partial remission and varying degrees of residual symptoms and impairments.

Symptoms of psychosis occur in several psychiatric disorders, as well as in the wider general population. Isolated symptoms of hallucinations, unusual sensory experiences, or delusional ideations have been reported in the absence of other co-occurring psychotic features in otherwise healthy individuals (Larøi et al., 2012). In this group, symptoms are typically transient and sporadic and are not a cause for significant distress, impairment, or help-seeking behaviour.

Other people might experience isolated symptoms of psychosis in the context of a neurological disorder such as stroke, epilepsy, tumours, or different dementias (such as Parkinson's Disease). Further, those under the influence of alcohol or illicit substances, or withdrawal from them, may also experience symptoms of psychosis. In all of these latter cases, the psychotic symptoms are attributed to other conditions or disorders.

Symptoms of psychosis also occur in the following psychiatric disorders:

- **Schizophrenia-spectrum disorders:** Psychotic symptoms are a diagnostic feature of these disorders, together with impaired social and occupational functioning. This diagnostic grouping includes conditions such as schizophrenia, schizoaffective disorder, schizotypal personality disorder, as well as psychosis associated with substance use or a medical condition (American Psychiatric Association, 2013). Symptoms may include delusions, multiple modalities of hallucinations, disorganised thoughts, and lack of insight causing distress and substantial interference with daytime functions.
- **Mood disorders:** Mood disorders describe emotional difficulties consisting of prolonged periods of excessive sadness or excessive joyousness, or alternation between both. Mood disorders are categorised as 'depressive' or 'bipolar' type. Psychotic symptoms such as hallucinations and/or delusions are found in approximately 14 per cent of people diagnosed with **major depression**, termed psychotic depression subtype (Johnson et al., 1991). **Bipolar disorders** are characterised by episodes of mania (excessive joyousness) and episodes of depression (excessive sadness). More than half of people diagnosed with bipolar disorder will report psychotic symptoms during a manic episode (Dunayevich and Keck, 2000), particularly persecutory or grandiose delusions, formal thought disorders, hallucinations, or reduced insight. These symptoms may be so severe that individuals cannot maintain their usual daytime occupation or activities.
- **Personality disorders:** Personality disorders are characterised by patterns of maladaptive perceptions, reactions, and relations with others that cause significant distress or functional impairment. Some personality disorders, such as the borderline subtype, are associated with psychotic symptoms in 25–50 per cent of cases (Slotema et al., 2012).
- **Trauma- and stress-related disorders:** These refer to a mental disorder that occurs after an overwhelming traumatic event. In PTSD, thoughts and memories associated with trauma are experienced as recurrent and intrusive. Auditory and visual hallucinations and paranoid delusions may occur in up to 15–65 per cent of individuals with PTSD (Gaudiano and Zimmerman, 2010).

As the focus of this book is on psychosis for which the primary cause is a psychotic disorder, the remainder of this section will focus on schizophrenia-spectrum disorders and mood disorders with psychotic features.

Causes of Psychotic Disorders

The causes of psychotic disorders are complex and not well understood. It is likely that a combination of genetic, neurobiological, and environmental factors all contribute to the onset and progression of these disorders.

The notion of a biological underpinning is supported by evidence showing a higher incidence of relatives with a severe psychiatric disorder within a family compared with the general population. Moreover, where there is a family history of severe mental illness, the risk of developing psychosis increases with the number of affected relatives and degree of relatedness (Gershon et al., 1982; Kendler et al., 1993). Together, such evidence points to the important influence of genetic factors in the emergence of psychotic disorders.

Neurobiological causes of psychotic disorders also propose a role for changes in the brain. For example, the abnormal production of different neurotransmitters, such as dopamine, glutamate, and serotonin, have been observed (Howes et al., 2015). The dopamine dysregulation hypothesis, in particular, is a popular theory for schizophrenia-spectrum disorders, because pharmacological treatments that block dopamine release have been found to be effective in reducing symptoms. Furthermore, symptoms that resemble psychosis have been observed subsequent to the use of drugs such as amphetamines that act to increase dopamine transmission (Howes and Kapur, 2009). Dysregulation of the neurotransmitter serotonin, which affects mood, is believed to play a role in mood disorders such as bipolar disorder.

However, neurobiological explanations alone have been criticised in recent years as being overly simplistic and dismissive of the important role that the *environment* has on the onset of psychotic disorders. Factors such as trauma and an individual's social upbringing, combined with psychological traits, are now believed to play a key role in how an individual's genes are expressed in relation to the onset and relapse of psychosis (van Os et al., 2010). According to this view, events that are traumatic or highly stressful cause an enduring vulnerability in an individual's risk of developing psychotic disorders (Read et al., 2005).

Support for this view comes from research highlighting the importance of trauma-related environmental factors in increasing future risk of psychosis (e.g. Dean and Murray, 2005). Research shows that, in schizophrenia-spectrum disorders, these factors include 'first hit' events occurring during the prenatal period of an individual's life (such as maternal malnutrition and obstetric complications), as well as during childhood (such as trauma and other adverse events). A genetic vulnerability, combined with such adverse events in early life, can produce a long-term vulnerability for psychotic disorders (Read et al., 2005). 'Second hit' events (such as drug abuse, social isolation, trauma, and adversity) typically occur in late adolescence and early adulthood. When coupled with the biological changes that occur during this phase of human development, such events can trigger the onset of a psychotic disorder (Rapoport et al., 2012). Stressful life events have also been linked to the onset of mood disorders and PTSD.

The period of time immediately preceding the onset of a psychotic disorder is often characterised by a drop in functioning, and reports of changed perceptions, unusual beliefs, cognitive disorganisation, sleep disturbance, and anxiety/mood fluctuations. The onset of anxiety and depression also plays a key role in precipitating the transition into psychotic disorders.

Treatment Options for Psychotic Disorders

Treatments vary, depending on the severity of the symptoms and whether people are experiencing distress. In schizophrenia-spectrum disorders, medications that are efficacious for reducing the symptoms of psychosis include antipsychotics (first and second generation), mood stabilisers, and antidepressants. In bipolar disorders, medications often include lithium, sodium valproate, and antipsychotic medications. Psychotic symptoms in psychotic major depression may be treated with a combination of antidepressant and antipsychotic medications or electroconvulsive therapy.

Antipsychotic medications are the cornerstone of treatment and lifesaving in some instances, although two main limitations exist. First, there are many unwanted side effects, including drowsiness, tremors, muscle contractions, metabolic changes, significant weight gain, and an increased risk of diabetes (Leucht et al., 1999; American Diabetes Association, 2004). Many people feel these side effects to be unacceptable, resulting in a discontinuation of their medications and risking relapse.

The second problem is that, all too often, people with a psychotic disorder are prescribed medications for symptoms of psychosis, but are not also offered other therapies. Clinical guidelines for the treatment of psychotic disorders recommend that a combination of antipsychotic medications, together with psychological therapies and social support, provides the best possible outcome (Dixon et al., 2010). In fact, psychological therapies are suggested as a first-line treatment alongside medication (National Collaborating Centre for Mental Health, 2014). In practice, however, they are more often offered as a second-line treatment for those who do not respond well to antipsychotic medications.

The most common psychological therapy for psychotic disorders is CBT for psychosis (CBTp). It involves assisting the person to develop an adaptive understanding of their experiences, helping them to restructure appraisals in relation to distress and personal challenges, and changing the person's relationship with their internal experiences. A strong emphasis is placed on the therapeutic relationship, active engagement, and an individualised formulation approach (Morrison and Barratt, 2010). There are several types of CBTp intervention, with varied emphasis and approaches to symptoms, crisis and trauma, motivational enhancement, coping strategies, behavioural activation, social integration, and occupational support.

Often, CBTp is delivered at the same time as medications and other support services. Randomised controlled trials show good evidence for beneficial effects when it is used as an adjunct to antipsychotic medications, in comparison with treatment as usual (for a meta-analytic review, see Sarin et al., 2011). The evidence shows that CBTp reduces psychotic symptoms over the course of treatment, particularly by reducing negative symptoms and the distress and disruption caused by persistent hallucinations and delusions (Pfammatter et al., 2006; Thomas et al., 2015). Other effects that have been reported include improved medication adherence and functioning (Pilling et al., 2002; Thomas et al., 2015). Positive improvements following CBTp have been demonstrated for as long as 9–12 months (Pilling et al., 2002), as well as in individuals who are low functioning (Grant et al., 2012). To our knowledge, however, the effect of CBTp on sleep has not yet been investigated (Pilling et al., 2002; Thomas et al., 2015).

Although good empirical evidence exists for CBTp, these interventions are rarely offered systematically in clinical practice. Difficulties include implementation issues, lack of specialist staff, and transfer of knowledge from rigorous experimental settings to everyday clinical settings (Prytys et al., 2011). Interventions that remain accessible to clients with a mixed range of clinical presentations, and in a variety of settings, are therefore critical.

Working with Distressing Hallucinations and Other Psychotic Symptoms

There are many comprehensive cognitive models and written resources on cognitive therapy in schizophrenia and psychosis (such as Morrison et al., 2004; Kingdon and Turkington, 2005). Some have specifically focused on hallucinations and other psychotic symptoms

(Morrison and Barratt, 2010; Thomas et al., 2015). The model of Chadwick and Birchwood (1994) has been influential in the development of a cognitive understanding of hallucinations. With respect to auditory hallucinations, it suggests that beliefs about power and intent (such as omnipotence, malevolence, and benevolence) play a key role in determining emotional and behavioural reactions. Identifying and challenging such beliefs has been shown to be effective. Appraisals and beliefs regarding *visual* hallucinations also influence the level of distress and thus should be a target for treatment (Collerton and Dudley, 2004).

Cognitive therapy for hallucinations may involve helping clients make the distinction between the experience they are having (the facts) and the beliefs associated with this experience concerning purpose, meaning, control, and power (Morrison et al., 2004; Byrne et al., 2006). The emphasis is that it is not necessarily the hallucination itself that is distressing, but the feelings and thoughts that result from it. There is, indeed, much evidence suggesting that discussion of the client's experience of hallucinations reduces anxiety and depression (Wykes et al., 1999; Casstevens et al., 2006).

Normalising the experience can also be immensely helpful. Although Western society, for the most part, tends to consider hallucinations abnormal, there is evidence that 'normalising' and accepting the experience can be useful in clinical settings. A review by Beavan and colleagues (2011) shows that 5–15 per cent of the general adult population (i.e. about one in ten people) have had the experience of hearing voices at some point in their lives. This may be used to provide some alternative perspective on the experience of these symptoms, so that individuals feel that their hallucinations are not so abnormal in themselves.

In addition to hallucinations being 'normalised', restructuring these experiences as meaningful, rather than abnormal, can have beneficial effects (Corstens et al., 2008; Romme et al., 2009). For example, the personalisation of a hallucination in the form of a significant individual in the person's life can be used as a way to increase coping and reduce distress. The person is asked to talk to and engage with the voice/hallucination, negotiate what they want, and treat the experience as they would another person. If the experience is treated as real and meaningful, rather than abnormal, the experience becomes less distressing and becomes weaker over time.

Summary

- The focus of this book is on psychosis, the primary causes of which are schizophrenia-spectrum disorders and mood disorders with psychotic features, although the book's contents and manual are relevant to any psychiatric disorder with psychotic symptoms that cause distress and interference with daytime function.
- It is likely that a combination of genetic, neurobiological, and environmental factors contribute to the onset of psychotic disorders.
- Best-practice guidelines for the treatment of psychotic disorders suggest that a combination of medications, together with psychological therapies, provides the best outcome.
- A strong evidence base exists for CBT in psychosis, with an emphasis on therapeutic relationships, personalised formulation, and motivational enhancement.

References

American Diabetes Association (2004) "Consensus Development Conference on Antipsychotic Drugs and Obesity and Diabetes", *Diabetes Care*, 27(2), pp. 596–601.

American Psychiatric Association (2013) *Diagnostic and statistical manual of mental disorders* (5th ed.). Arlington, VA: American Psychiatric Association.

Beavan, V., Read, J., and Cartwright, C. (2011) "The prevalence of voice-hearers in the general population: A literature review", *Journal of Mental Health*, 20(3), pp. 281–292.

Byrne, S., Birchwood, M., Trower, P. E., and Meaden, A. (2006) *A casebook of cognitive behaviour therapy for command hallucinations: A social rank theory approach.* New York: Routledge.

Casstevens, W. J., Cohen, D., Newman, F. L., and Dumaine, M. (2006) "Evaluation of a mentored self-help intervention for the management of psychotic symptoms", *International Journal of Psychosocial Rehabilitation*, 11(1), pp. 37–49.

Chadwick, P., and Birchwood, M. (1994) "The omnipotence of voices: A cognitive approach to auditory hallucinations", *British Journal of Psychiatry*, 164(2), pp. 190–201.

Collerton, D., and Dudley, R. (2004) "A cognitive behavioural framework for the treatment of distressing visual hallucinations in older people", *Behavioural & Cognitive Psychotherapy*, 32(4), pp. 443–455.

Corstens, D., Escher, S., and Romme, M. (2008) "Accepting and working with voices: The Maastricht approach", in Moskowitz, A., Schafer, I., and Dorahy, M. J. (Eds.) *Psychosis, trauma and dissociation: Emerging perspectives on severe psychopathology*. Chicester, UK: Wiley-Blackwell, pp. 319–332.

Dean, K., and Murray, R. M. (2005) "Environmental risk factors for psychosis", *Dialogues in Clinical Neuroscience*, 7(1), pp. 69–80.

Dixon, L. B., Dickerson, F., Bellack, A. S., Bennett, M., Dickinson, D., Goldberg, R. W., Lehman, A., Tenhula, W. N., Calmes, C., Pasillas, R. M., Peer, J., and Kreyenbuhl, J. (2010) "The 2009 Schizophrenia PORT Psychosocial Treatment Recommendations and Summary Statements", *Schizophrenia Bulletin*, 36(1), pp. 48–70.

Dunayevich, E., and Keck, P. E. (2000) "Prevalence and description of psychotic features in bipolar mania", *Current Psychiatry Reports*, 2(4), pp. 286–290.

Gaudiano, B. A., and Zimmerman, M. (2010) "Evaluation of evidence for the psychotic subtyping of post-traumatic stress disorder", *British Journal of Psychiatry*, 197(4), pp. 326–327.

Gershon, E. S., Hamovit, J., Guroff, J. J., Dibble, E., Leckman, J. F., Sceery, W., Targum, S. D., Nurnberger, J. I., Goldin, L. R., and Bunney, W. E. (1982) "A family study of schizoaffective, bipolar I, bipolar II, unipolar, and normal control probands", *Archives of General Psychiatry*, 39(10), pp. 1157–1167.

Grant, P. M., Huh, G. A., Perivoliotis, D., Stolar, N. M., and Beck, A. T. (2012) "Randomized trial to evaluate the efficacy of cognitive therapy for low-functioning patients with schizophrenia", *Archives of General Psychiatry*, 69(2), pp. 121–127.

Howes, O., and Kapur, S. (2009) "The Dopamine hypothesis of schizophrenia: Version III—the final common pathway", *Schizophrenia Bulletin*, 35(3), pp. 549–562.

Howes, O., McCutcheon, R., and Stone, J. (2015) "Glutamate and dopamine in schizophrenia: An update for the 21st century", *Journal of Psychopharmacology*, 29(2), pp. 97–115.

Johnson, J., Horwath, E., and Weissman, M. M. (1991) "The validity of major depression with psychotic features based on a community study", *Archives of General Psychiatry*, 48(12), pp. 1075–1081.

Kendler, K. S., McGuire, M., Gruenberg, A. M., O'Hare, A., Spellman, M., and Walsh, D. (1993) "The Roscommon family study: I. Methods, diagnosis of probands, and risk of schizophrenia in relatives", *Archives of General Psychiatry*, 50(7), pp. 527–540.

Kingdon, D. G., and Turkington, D. (2005) *Cognitive-behavioral therapy of schizophrenia.* New York: Guilford Press.

Larøi, F., Sommer, I. E., Blom, J. D., Fernyhough, C., Ffytche, D. H., Hugdahl, K., Johns, L. C., McCarthy-Jones, S., Preti, A., Raballo, A., Slotema, C. W., Stephane, M., and Waters, F. (2012) "The characteristic features of auditory verbal hallucinations in clinical and nonclinical groups: State-of-the-art overview and future directions", *Schizophrenia Bulletin*, 38(4), pp. 724–733.

Leucht, S., Pitschel-Walz, G., Abraham, D., and Kissling, W. (1999) "Efficacy and extrapyramidal side-effects of the new antipsychotics olanzapine, quetiapine, risperidone, and sertindole compared to conventional antipsychotics and placebo: A meta-analysis of randomized controlled trials", *Schizophrenia Research*, 35(1), pp. 51–68.

Morrison, A. P., and Barratt, S. (2010) "What are the components of CBT for psychosis? A Delphi study", *Schizophrenia Bulletin*, 36(1), pp. 136–142.

Morrison, A., Renton, J., Dunn, H., Williams, S., and Bentall, R. (2004). *Cognitive therapy for psychosis: A formulation-based approach.* Hove, UK: Routledge.

National Collaborating Centre for Mental Health (2014) *Psychosis and schizophrenia in adults: Treatment and management.* NICE Clinical Guideline 178. London: NICE.

Pfammatter, M., Junghan, U. M., and Brenner, H. D. (2006) "Efficacy of psychological therapy in schizophrenia: Conclusions from meta-analyses", *Schizophrenia Bulletin*, 32(Suppl. 1), pp. S64–S80.

Pilling, S., Bebbington, P., Kuipers, E., Garety, P., Geddes, J., Orbach, G., and Morgan, C. (2002) "Psychological treatments in schizophrenia: I. Meta-analysis of family intervention and cognitive behaviour therapy", *Psychological Medicine*, 32(5), pp. 763–782.

Prytys, M., Garety, P. A., Jolley, S., Onwumere, J., and Craig, T. (2011) "Implementing the NICE guideline for schizophrenia recommendations for psychological therapies: A qualitative analysis of the attitudes of CMHT staff", *Clinical Psychology & Psychotherapy*, 18(1), pp. 48–59.

Rapoport, J. L., Giedd, J. N., and Gogtay, N. (2012) "Neurodevelopmental model of schizophrenia: Update 2012", *Molecular Psychiatry*, 17(12), pp. 1228–1238.

Read, J., van Os, J., Morrison, A. P., and Ross, C. A. (2005) "Childhood trauma, psychosis and schizophrenia: A literature review with theoretical and clinical implications", *Acta Psychiatrica Scandinavica*, 112(5), pp. 330–350.

Romme, M., Escher, S., Dillon, J., Corstens, D., and Morris, M. (2009) *Living with voices: 50 stories of recovery*. Ross-on-Wye, UK: PCCS Books.

Sarin, F., Wallin, L., and Widerlöv, B. (2011) "Cognitive behavior therapy for schizophrenia: A meta-analytical review of randomized controlled trials", *Nordic Journal of Psychiatry*, 65(3), pp. 162–174.

Slotema, C. W., Daalman, K., Blom, J. D., Diederen, K. M., Hoek, H. W., and Sommer, I. E. C. (2012) "Auditory verbal hallucinations in patients with borderline personality disorder are similar to those in schizophrenia", *Psychological Medicine*, 42(9), pp. 1873–1878.

Thomas, N., Farhall, J., and Shawyer, F. (2015) "Beliefs about voices and schemas about self and others in psychosis", *Behavioural & Cognitive Psychotherapy*, 43(2), pp. 209–223.

van Os, J., Kenis, G., and Rutten, B. P. F. (2010) "The environment and schizophrenia", *Nature*, 468(7321), pp. 203–212.

Wykes, T., Parr, A. M., and Landau, S. (1999) "Group treatment of auditory hallucinations: Exploratory study of effectiveness", *British Journal of Psychiatry*, 175(2), pp. 180–185.

3 Insomnia Disorder and Other Sleep Disturbances

An Overview

The experience of poor sleep in relation to stressful life events or illness is almost universal across humans. Usually, sleep improves once the stress has resolved and/or once the person has gained an understanding as to why their sleep had deteriorated, enabling them to modify the factors causing the disturbance. The term *Insomnia* is often used informally in the media and popular culture to describe an undefined period of sleeplessness, or short bouts of poor sleep. These episodes are, however, distinct from Insomnia Disorder, which is a diagnosable condition that has unique clinical features and requires active management. Insomnia Disorder occurs chronically for several nights a week, remains despite the resolution of identifiable precipitating triggers, can feel out of control, and is associated with negative long-term mental health outcomes.

This chapter will outline the diagnostic features, prevalence rates, and clinical course of Insomnia Disorder and will review the consequences and burden of this condition. The relationship between Insomnia and psychosis will be addressed. Finally, as Insomnia often co-occurs with other sleep disorders, this chapter will also describe sleep disorders for which there are efficacious evidence-based psychological behavioural interventions. These include hypersomnia, circadian rhythm disorders, and nightmares.

Insomnia Disorder

In clinical practice, Insomnia is characterised by subjective complaints of:

(a) difficulties getting to sleep at the start of the sleep period ('sleep onset Insomnia'), typically defined as taking longer than 30 minutes to fall asleep;
(b) waking during the sleep period ('sleep maintenance Insomnia'), typically characterised by spending more than 30 minutes awake during the night;
(c) early waking, that is, waking appproximately 30 minutes or more before desired waking time in the morning and struggling to get back to sleep; and/or
(d) unrefreshing sleep.

To meet diagnosis for Insomnia using formal classification systems, such as the *Diagnostic and Statistical Manual of Mental Disorders* (fifth edition, *DSM-V*; American Psychiatric Association, 2013) and the *International Classification of Sleep Disorders* (3rd edition, *ICSD-3*; American Academy of Sleep Medicine, 2014), additional specific criteria must also be met (see Text Box 3.1).

Text Box 3.1 Diagnostic Classification Criteria for Insomnia Disorder

Diagnostic Statistical Manual (DSM-V)

- Long-standing (more than 3 months) subjective difficulty initiating sleep (more than 20–30 minutes to fall asleep) or maintaining sleep (more than 20–30 minutes awake in the night), or waking too early (more than 30 minutes prior to desired wake time and resulting in less than 6.5 hours sleep).
- Clinically significant distress or impairment in social, occupational, educational, or behavioural areas of functioning.
- The difficulty with sleep occurs at least three nights per week and occurs despite adequate opportunity for sleep.
- Five Insomnia subtypes:

  1. sleep initiation Insomnia (initial Insomnia);
  2. sleep maintenance Insomnia (middle Insomnia);
  3. early morning awakening Insomnia (late Insomnia);
  4. combination of subtypes 1, 2, and 3;
  5. non-restorative sleep (not feeling rested despite adequate sleep duration).

International Classification of Sleep Disorders (ICSD-3)

- Sleep initiation or maintenance problems, in combination with adequate opportunity and circumstances to sleep, and daytime consequences.
- The disturbance must have been at least three nights per week, and for a minimum of 3 months.
- Three categories of Insomnia:

  1. chronic Insomnia Disorder (more than 3 months);
  2. short-term Insomnia Disorder (less than 3 months);
  3. other Insomnia.

These criteria include sleep symptoms that:

- are especially prominent or prolonged (3 or more months);
- occur despite adequate opportunity for sleep;
- are not fully explained by another sleep or mental disorder; and
- are accompanied by distress and/or impairment in daily functioning; common complaints might include fatigue, anxiety about sleep, low mood, irritability, social withdrawal, reduced motivation and productivity, impaired memory and concentration, and physical symptoms such as headaches and tension;
- are present for at least three nights of the week; for many sufferers, however, symptoms occur on a nightly basis.

Commonly, individuals with Insomnia complain of feeling tired and fatigued. It is less common for individuals to feel *sleepy* (i.e. being able to fall asleep quickly). The distinction between sleepiness and fatigue is an important one. Whereas sleepiness is defined as a person's propensity to fall asleep quickly and easily if given the opportunity, fatigue is the experience of exhaustion and decreased capacity for physical and mental work. People with fatigue, as opposed to sleepiness, cannot fall asleep given adequate opportunity.

The diagnostic features of Insomnia can be assessed through a clinical interview (see Chapter 8 and Appendix 1) and, preferably, a sleep diary (Appendix 2). It is important to note that the diagnosis of Insomnia is based on subjective complaints of poor sleep. In other words, the person's description of symptoms, rather than objective assessment of sleep parameters (such as total sleep duration), is used to make the diagnosis. This is partly owing to the fact that large variations in the need for sleep exist across individuals. Where one person may function well and be satisfied by a sleep duration of 6 hours, another person might sleep an average of 8 hours a night but still report fatigue and unrefreshing sleep. In support, only 50 per cent of individuals diagnosed with Insomnia actually display objective short sleep durations of less than 6 hours per night (Vgontzas et al., 2010).

The Obsolete Primary and Secondary Insomnia Distinction

Historically, Insomnia was often overlooked in people living with a psychiatric disorder as being 'just another symptom' of the person's condition. This notion was in accordance with a previous diagnostic distinction that had been made between *Primary* and *Secondary* Insomnia. Primary Insomnia was viewed as a sleep disorder, whereas Secondary Insomnia was seen as a symptom of another condition (psychiatric disorder, pain, etc.). Unfortunately, this view led to significant barriers to people accessing treatment for Insomnia, as it assumed that the mental condition was responsible for the Insomnia, and that treatment of the 'primary' condition would be sufficient to resolve the Insomnia (National Institutes of Health, 2005).

There is now, however, much evidence to suggest that Insomnia does not always resolve upon successful treatment of a comorbid condition (e.g. Carney et al., 2007). Indeed, we know that unhelpful thoughts and behaviours exist in both stand-alone and comorbid Insomnia, and that these should be specifically addressed in order to optimise treatment outcomes. It is important to emphasise that, whereas Insomnia onset may be linked to an event or illness, chronic Insomnia is maintained by specific (psychological and behavioural) factors that are not addressed by treating the other condition.

Prevalence Rates

Insomnia is the most prevalent of all sleep disorders and is one of the most common reasons people present to their primary care physician. Population-based studies across various countries suggest that approximately 30 per cent of adults report one or more of the following symptoms of Insomnia: (a) difficulty initiating sleep, (b) difficulty maintaining sleep, (c) waking up too early, and (d) non-restorative or poor quality of sleep. The number of people meeting criteria for a formal diagnosis of Insomnia Disorder is approximately 10 per cent (for reviews, see Roth, 2007; Ohayon and Reynolds, 2009; Morgan, 2012).

With regards to risk factors, as discussed more fully in Chapter 4, the prevalence of Insomnia is higher in women and increases as people get older. In addition, Insomnia commonly co-occurs with medical and psychiatric illness (Katz and McHorney, 1998; Sateia, 2014). In particular, Insomnia is commonly concurrent in people with the following:

- psychiatric disorders: It is estimated that between 40 per cent and 50 per cent of all patients with Insomnia have a coexisting psychiatric condition (Ford and Kamerow, 1989; American Psychiatric Association, 2013), and that almost all individuals with psychotic disorders complain of one or more symptoms of Insomnia;
- other sleep disorders, notably, OSA, periodic limb movement disorder (PLMD), and parasomnias such as nightmare disorder;
- medical comorbidities, such as chronic pain, high blood pressure, gastrointestinal problems, respiratory problems, heart disease, urinary problems, and neurologic disease (Taylor et al., 2007), as well as alcohol and drug abuse.

Course

Insomnia may be acute (lasting less than 1 month), sub-acute (1–3 months), or chronic (lasting more than 3 months). Insomnia is classified as recurrent if two or more episodes occur within 12 months. Although many cases of Insomnia resolve spontaneously, it becomes chronic in at least 50 per cent of cases (American Psychiatric Association, 2013). Morin et al. (2009) found that 75 per cent of individuals diagnosed with Insomnia continue to report symptoms 1 year later. Furthermore, nearly 50 per cent continued to have Insomnia at three further annual assessment points. That is, a diagnosis of Insomnia was strongly predictive of ongoing Insomnia up to 4 years after an initial diagnosis. Thus, Insomnia is best viewed as a chronic disorder requiring a long-term treatment approach. Psychological and behavioural treatment approaches, as opposed to pharmacotherapy, are potentially better suited for long-term management, as the self-management skills that are taught continue to treat the disorder after the active treatment phase is over. Additionally, pharmacological treatments for Insomnia are not recommended for long-term use owing to issues with side effects, dependence, and tolerance.

The course of Insomnia over time can provide useful clinical information. As a general rule, for individuals experiencing distinct, acute episodes of Insomnia that remit over time, *or* for those experiencing less frequent symptoms (e.g. fewer than 3 nights/days a week), the role of social, environmental, and mood factors are generally considered instrumental in driving the Insomnia. In this case, the Insomnia may be considered situational. For individuals experiencing a more persistent course of Insomnia (with fewer significant periods of remission), and with more consistent symptoms (5 or more nights/days per week), the maintaining factors more often include unhelpful sleep-related cognitions (e.g. worry about sleep) and behaviours (e.g. daytime napping) that act to perpetuate disturbed sleep.

Consequences

Almost everyone can identify with the negative consequences of poor sleep, which include tiredness, irritability, and reduced resilience. If the sleep disruption persists (such as in Insomnia), these consequences are often intensified as worries about sleep develop, thereby intensifying the problem and reducing mood. Academic interest regarding the impact of Insomnia on health and well-being has seen a significant increase in research output over the last decade. We understand clearly now that Insomnia is a condition with a high disease burden. It is associated with poorer physical health, mental health, and quality of life, as well as substantial economic costs. It has also become clear that Insomnia can function as both a cause and consequence of coexisting medical and psychiatric conditions, and often has bidirectional effects, each impacting the other and potentially affecting their respective treatments, outcomes, and recoveries.

With respect to *physical health* consequences, a chronically tired body is more susceptible to illness, is less able to ward off infection and disease, and inflammatory conditions, such as arthritis, and chronic pain may worsen. The tired body is also more susceptible to stress and hypertension (American Psychiatric Association, 2013). Consequently, people with Insomnia use more health-care services, have more frequent sick days, and take more medications, leading to large personal and societal economic burdens (Daley et al., 2009).

The *mental health* consequences of Insomnia include increased risk of developing depression, mania, anxiety, and substance misuse problems in individuals without a pre-existing psychiatric condition (Breslau et al., 1996; Baglioni et al., 2011). Although the relationship between Insomnia and mental health conditions is bidirectional, there is increased awareness that Insomnia more often precedes rather than follows the development of a mood disorder. Ohayon and Roth (2003), for example, showed that an episode of Insomnia preceded the onset of depression in 69 per cent of cases.

Moreover, viewing Insomnia as a prodromal symptom of psychiatric illnesses may have preventative benefits. Eaton et al. (1995) hypothesised that 47 per cent of the incidence of depression at 1-year follow-up could have been prevented if the existing Insomnia had been addressed at baseline. Similarly, longitudinal studies of individuals with mood disorders, such as depression, show that patients who experience improvements in their sleep have a more rapid response to antidepressant medication, (Manber et al, 2008) and that those patients whose Insomnia persists tend to relapse sooner (Perlis et al., 1997).

Overall, Insomnia can function as both a cause and consequence of coexisting medical and psychiatric conditions and can have bidirectional effects, each impacting the other and potentially affecting the treatment course, outcome, and recovery.

In terms of *quality of life*, studies consistently show that individuals with Insomnia have reduced quality of life in domains such as physical functioning, role functioning, bodily pain, general health, vitality, and social functioning (Roth, 2007). In individuals with pre-existing mental or physical health problems, including psychosis, the effects of Insomnia can be severe (see Chapter 4).

Co-occurring Sleep Dysfunction

As described above, Insomnia is highly prevalent in psychotic disorders, and, as such, the relationship between Insomnia and psychosis is described in detail in Chapter 4. In this section, we bring attention to hypersomnia, circadian rhythm disturbances, and nightmares, as they frequently co-occur with Insomnia in individuals with psychosis. Furthermore, there is emerging evidence to suggest that specifically modified CBT-I interventions can be effective in the treatment of these co-occurring sleep dysfunctions (see Chapter 9).

Hypersomnia

Hypersomnia describes difficulties with excessive daytime fatigue and sleepiness despite adequate sleep. The average total sleep time in individuals suffering hypersomnia may be more than 9 hours across a 24-hour period. However, for many individuals, total sleep time can be much higher (as much as 18 hours). Whereas people suffering from Insomnia often report being 'tired but wired' during the day, those with hypersomnia feel sleepy and find it difficult to stay awake and alert during the major waking hours of the day. It is possible for an individual to have Insomnia and also have features of hypersomnia—for example, spending a lot of time sleeping during the day and then having difficulty with sleep onset and maintenance at night.

Hypersomnia occurring independently of a medical or psychiatric disorder is thought to be rare, although, to date, no prevalence studies have provided solid evidence to confirm or dispute this fact (Morin and Espie, 2012). In psychosis, hypersomnia comorbid with Insomnia is more common than previously thought, perhaps occurring in 25 per cent of these patients. In many cases, hypersomnia is thought to be accounted for, to a large extent, by medication side effects. Regardless, it warrants further independent clinical attention (American Psychiatric Association, 2013).

Some recent CBT-I protocols have included strategies for managing excessive daytime sleepiness comorbid with Insomnia and have demonstrated positive outcomes (Harvey et al., 2007, 2014, 2015; Manber and Carney, 2015). These research outcomes suggest that cognitive and behavioural approaches may be an effective way to address this condition.

There are many possible causes of excessive daytime sleepiness, including lifestyle factors (e.g. stress, substance use), psychiatric conditions, and medical causes, including sleep disorders such as:

- circadian rhythm disorders (discussed below);
- OSA, where breathing repeatedly stops and starts during sleep because the muscles in the throat relax and block the upper airway;
- restless legs syndrome (RLS), which refers to unpleasant sensations in the legs and the urge to move the legs for relief, usually experienced when trying to initiate sleep;
- PLMD, where limbs move involuntarily during sleep causing disruption;
- narcolepsy, which is experienced as irresistible periods of sleep during the day ('sleep attacks'), even in unlikely circumstances such as in the middle of a conversation or during a meal. It can be associated with either cataplexy (sudden, brief loss of muscle tone usually associated with intense emotion), sleep paralysis, and/or hallucinations at the beginning or end of the sleep attack.

The last four conditions discussed above (OSA, RLS, PLMD, and narcolepsy) will not be addressed further in this book, as first-line treatments recommend either mechanical interventions—such as continuous positive airway pressure (CPAP), mandibular advancement splint—or pharmacological intervention. Differential diagnoses, however, are addressed in Chapter 8, which describes clinical assessment.

Circadian Rhythm Disturbances

Circadian rhythm disturbances refer to sleep disruptions due to a misalignment between the internal circadian rhythm (the 'body clock') and the sleep–wake schedule required by an individual's physical environment or social or professional schedule (American Psychiatric Association, 2013). These sleep disruptions tend to result in excessive sleepiness (hypersomnia; see above), Insomnia, or both.

The body clock responds strongly to light exposure. Humans usually sleep when it is dark and are awake during daylight hours. Circadian rhythm disturbances occur when there are abnormalities in the timing or duration of the sleep–wake cycle relative to the day–night cycle (in Chapter 5, we describe how circadian rhythms regulate sleep). Circadian rhythm disturbance can cause significant distress or impairment, and diagnosis requires careful attention to the person's exposure to natural light and other daily routines over a period of at least 1 or 2 weeks.

Different subtypes of circadian rhythm disorder exist:

- **Delayed sleep phase** is characterised by difficulty falling asleep until late at night or the early hours of the morning and so can appear similar to sleep onset Insomnia. Once asleep, however, the individual can usually sleep until late morning or the middle of the day. The timing of sleep is usually later than the person would like. Delayed sleep phase is more common in teenagers and young adults.
- **Advanced sleep phase** is characterised by falling asleep early in the evening and waking in the early hours of the morning. Advanced sleep phase is more common in the elderly. People with psychosis often retire to bed early owing to boredom, anxiety, or depression, and this needs to be distinguished from a true advanced sleep phase (where sleep onset will be rapid on retiring to bed in the early evening).
- **Irregular sleep–wake disorder** is characterised by highly disorganised patterns of sleep and wake, where there is no clear sleep or wake pattern. Instead of one long period of sleep, multiple naps occur over a 24-hour period. During the day, sufferers may appear sleepy because they nap so much. During the night, they may appear to have Insomnia because they are awake for long periods of time.
- **Non-24-hour sleep–wake disorder**, also known as free-running type, is characterised by the person falling asleep a little later each day. Generally, the delay is an hour or two, corresponding to a circadian cycle of 25–26 hours. It is most commonly seen in people who are totally blind. The daily delay in sleep onset causes the patient to gradually 'cycle around the clock', sometimes sleeping during the day and, at other times of the month, sleeping at night. In extreme cases, as may be observed in psychosis, day–night reversal may occur, where the person has a strong propensity to sleep during the day and be awake during the night.

Misaligned circadian patterns of sleep are a prominent symptom of psychotic disorders (Mansour et al., 2005; Harvey, 2008), especially delayed sleep phase, followed by irregular sleep–wake disorder, and non-24-hour sleep–wake disorders.

Common treatment approaches for delayed sleep phase include the use of oral melatonin in the evening and exposure to bright light in the morning, with either sunlight or artificial bright light therapy (see Morgenthaler et al., 2007). Light sends a signal to the brain to stop producing melatonin and to produce alertness-promoting hormones, such as cortisol. Delayed or irregular sleep phase disorders can therefore be helped with exposure to bright light in the morning, as this switches melatonin production off. By contrast, evening's darkness tells the brain to produce melatonin and therefore promotes sedation. This can be artificially induced with the use of melatonin tablets. Artificial light at night can delay melatonin production and the onset of sleep, intensifying a delayed sleep phase pattern (in the case of treating advanced sleep phase, evening bright light is beneficial (e.g. Lack and Wright, 1993), but in the case of delayed sleep phase it is unhelpful).

CBT-I can also be helpful in realigning sleep patterns to the 24-hour cycle, a practice also known as 'entrainment', by encouraging good sleep hygiene (e.g. careful timing of the use of stimulants and light exposure) and the establishment of more conducive day and night routines (e.g. regular rising time, morning exposure to sunlight, timing of meals and medications).

Nightmares

Nightmares are vivid dreams (often including threats to survival, security, or self-esteem) that cause feelings of fear or terror. They often occur during the second half of the sleep period (American Psychiatric Association, 2013). Usually, the person having a nightmare suddenly wakes from REM sleep oriented and alert, and has a clear, detailed memory of the dream content. The onset of sleep following a nightmare is often prolonged owing to the cognitive and physiological arousal that it produces. Nightmare disorder, in which nightmares occur three or more times a week and cause significant distress, affects about 4 per cent of the general adult population (the proportion is higher in children and teens). Rates are significantly higher in those with psychosis, with estimated prevalence rates as high as 50 per cent (Mume, 2009; Swart et al., 2013; Sheaves et al., 2015).

Risk factors for nightmares include physical and mental illness, anxiety, trauma, stress, and substance use (including medication side effects). In turn, the presence of nightmares predicts poorer outcomes for disorders such as PTSD, depression, and anxiety (e.g. Sjöström et al., 2009). In people with psychosis, nightmares and other vivid dreams can lead to pathological fears about going to sleep and, therefore, sleep deprivation. If sleep deprivation occurs, this unfortunately makes nightmares more likely and more intense. See Aurora et al. (2010) and Nadorff et al. (2014) for further reading about nightmare disorder.

Imagery rehearsal therapy draws from cognitive therapy principles and is recommended as a first-line intervention for nightmares (Aurora et al., 2010). This intervention asks clients to write their nightmare down, imagine a change to the nightmare (for example, imagine a more positive outcome), and then rehearse the 'new dream' while awake, on a daily basis. This is described in more detail in Chapter 7.

Summary

- Insomnia is a high-prevalence disorder associated with a high disease burden.
- Existing research emphasises the high frequency of psychiatric illness and psychological distress in Insomnia, and vice versa.
- Insomnia comorbid with a psychiatric disorder can worsen the prognosis of the comorbid disorder.
- Insomnia is often a chronic condition that requires long-term treatment approaches that upskill patients in self-management.
- Insomnia is a disorder in its own right that requires independent clinical attention, even when it is comorbid with other conditions.
- Hypersomnia, circadian rhythm disorders, and nightmares are other sleep disorders that co-occur with Insomnia in psychosis and should be considered in CBT-I interventions.

References

American Academy of Sleep Medicine (2014) *International classification of sleep disorders* (3rd ed.). Westchester, IL: American Academy of Sleep Medicine.

American Psychiatric Association (2013) *Diagnostic and statistical manual of mental disorders* (5th ed.). Arlington, VA: American Psychiatric Association.

Aurora, R. N., Zak, R. S., Auerbach, S. H., Casey, K. R., Chowdhuri, S., Karippot, A., Maganti, R. K., Ramar, K., Kristo, D. A., Bista, S. R., Lamm, C. I., Morgenthaler, T. I., and Standards of Practice Committee (2010) "Best practice guide for the treatment of nightmare disorder in adults", *Journal of Clinical Sleep Medicine: Official Publication of the American Academy of Sleep Medicine*, 6(4), pp. 389–401.

Baglioni, C., Battagliese, G., Feige, B., Spiegelhalder, K., Nissen, C., Voderholzer, U., Lombardo, C., and Riemann, D. (2011) "Insomnia as a predictor of depression: A meta-analytic evaluation of longitudinal epidemiological studies", *Journal of Affective Disorders*, 135(1–3), pp. 10–19.

Breslau, N., Roth, T., Rosenthal, L., and Andreski, P. (1996) "Sleep disturbance and psychiatric disorders: A longitudinal epidemiological study of young Adults", *Biological Psychiatry*, 39(6), pp. 411–418.

Carney, C. E., Segal, Z. V., Edinger, J. D., Krystal, A. D. (2007) "A comparison of rates of residual insomnia symptoms following pharmacotherapy or cognitive-behavioral therapy for major depressive disorder", *Journal of Clinical Psychiatry*, 68, pp. 254–260.

Daley, M., Morin, C. M., Leblanc, M., Grègoire, J. P., Savard, J., and Baillargeon, L. (2009) "Insomnia and its relationship to health-care utilization, work absenteeism, productivity and accidents", *Sleep Medicine*, 10, pp. 427–438.

Eaton, W. W., Badawi, M., and Melton, B. (1995) "Prodromes and precursors: Epidemiologic data for primary prevention of disorders with slow onset", *American Journal of Psychiatry*, 152(7), pp. 967–972.

Ford, D. E., and Kamerow, D. B. (1989) "Epidemiologic study of sleep disturbances and psychiatric disorders: An opportunity for prevention?", *JAMA*, 262(11), pp. 1479–1484.

Harvey, A. G. (2008) "Sleep and circadian rhythms in bipolar disorder: Seeking synchrony, harmony, and regulation", *American Journal of Psychiatry*, 165(7), pp. 820–829.

Harvey, A. G., Bélanger, L., Talbot, L., Eidelman, P., Beaulieu-Bonneau, S., Fortier-Brochu, É., Ivers, H., Lamy, M., Hein, K., Soehner, A. M., Mérette, C., and Morin, C. M. (2014) "Comparative efficacy of behavior therapy, cognitive therapy, and cognitive behavior therapy for chronic insomnia: A randomized controlled trial", *Journal of Consulting & Clinical Psychology*, 82(4), pp. 670–683.

Harvey, A. G., Sharpley, A. L., Ree, M. J., Stinson, K., and Clark, D. M. (2007) "An open trial of cognitive therapy for chronic insomnia", *Behaviour Research & Therapy*, 45(10), pp. 2491–2501.

Harvey, A. G., Soehner, A. M., Kaplan, K. A., Hein, K., Lee, J., Kanady, J., Li, D., Rabe-Hesketh, S., Ketter, T. A., Neylan, T. C., and Buysse, D. J. (2015) "Treating insomnia improves mood state, sleep, and functioning in bipolar disorder: A pilot randomized controlled trial", *Journal of Consulting & Clinical Psychology*, 83(3), pp. 564–577.

Katz, D. A., and McHorney, C. A. (1998) "Clinical correlates of insomnia in patients with chronic illness", *Archives of Internal Medicine*, 158(10), pp. 1099–1107.

Lack, L., and Wright, H. (1993) "The effect of evening bright light in delaying the circadian rhythms and lengthening the sleep of early morning awakening insomniacs", *Sleep*, 16(5), pp. 436–443.

Manber, R., Edinger, J. D., Gress, J. L., San Pedro-Salcedo, M. G., Kuo, T. F., & Kalista, T. (2008) "Cognitive Behavioral Therapy for Insomnia Enhances Depression Outcome in Patients with Comorbid Major Depressive Disorder and Insomnia", *Sleep*, 31(4), pp. 489–495.

Manber, R., and Carney, C. E. (2015) *Treatment plans and interventions for Insomnia: A case formulation approach.* New York: Guilford Press.

Mansour, H. A., Wood, J., Chowdari, K. V., Dayal, M., Thase, M. E., Kupfer, D. J., Monk, T. H., Devlin, B., and Nimgaonkar, V. L. (2005) "Circadian phase variation in bipolar I disorder", *Chronobiology International*, 22(3), pp. 571–584.

Morgan, K. (2012) "The epidemiology of sleep", in Morin, C. M., and Espie, C. A. (Eds.) *The Oxford handbook of sleep and sleep disorders.* New York: Oxford University Press, pp. 303–323.

Morgenthaler, T., Alessi, C., Friedman, L., Owens, J., Kapur, V., Boehlecke, B., Brown, T., Chesson Jr, A., Coleman, J., Lee-Chiong, T., Pancer, J., and Swick, T. J. (2007) "Practice parameters for the use of actigraphy in the assessment of sleep and sleep disorders: An update for 2007", *Sleep*, 30(4), pp. 519–529.

Morin, C. M., Bélanger, L., LeBlanc, M., Ivers, H., Savard, J., Espie, C. A., Mérette, C., Baillargeon, L., and Grégoire, J. P. (2009) "The natural history of insomnia: A population-based 3-year longitudinal study", *Archives of Internal Medicine*, 169(5), pp. 447–453.

Morin, C. M., and Espie, C. A. (2012) *The Oxford handbook of sleep and sleep disorders.* New York: Oxford University Press.

Mume, C. O. (2009) "Nightmare in schizophrenic and depressed patients", *The European Journal of Psychiatry*, 23(3), pp. 177–183.

Nadorff, M. R., Lambdin, K. K., and Germain, A. (2014) "Pharmacological and non-pharmacological treatments for nightmare disorder", *International Review of Psychiatry*, 26(2), pp. 225–236.

National Institutes of Health (2005) "National Institutes of Health State of the Science Conference statement on manifestations and management of chronic insomnia in adults, June 13–15, 2005", *Sleep*, 28(9), pp. 1049–1057.

Ohayon, M. M., and Reynolds, C. F. (2009) "Epidemiological and clinical relevance of insomnia diagnosis algorithms according to the DSM-IV and the International Classification of Sleep Disorders (ICSD)", *Sleep Medicine*, 10(9), pp. 952–960.

Ohayon, M. M., and Roth, T. (2003) "Place of chronic insomnia in the course of depressive and anxiety disorders", *Journal of Psychiatric Research*, 37(1), pp. 9–15.

Perlis, M. L., Giles, D. E., Buysse, D. J., Tu, X., and Kupfer, D. J. (1997) "Self-reported sleep disturbance as a prodromal symptom in recurrent depression", *Journal of Affective Disorders*, 42(2–3), pp. 209–212.

Roth, T. (2007) "Insomnia: Definition, prevalence, etiology, and consequences", *Journal of Clinical Sleep Medicine: Official Publication of the American Academy of Sleep Medicine*, 3(5 Suppl.), pp. S7–S10.

Sateia, M. J. (2014) "International classification of sleep disorders—third edition: Highlights and modifications", *Chest*, 146(5), pp. 1387–1394.

Sheaves, B., Onwumere, J., Keen, N., Stahl, D., and Kuipers, E. (2015) "Nightmares in patients with psychosis: The relation with sleep, psychotic, affective, and cognitive symptoms", *The Canadian Journal of Psychiatry*, 60(8), pp. 354–361.

Sjöström, N., Hetta, J., and Waern, M. (2009) "Persistent nightmares are associated with repeat suicide attempt: A prospective study", *Psychiatry Research*, 170(2–3), pp. 208–211.

Swart, M. L., van Schagen, A. M., Lancee, J., and van den Bout, J. (2013) "Prevalence of nightmare disorder in psychiatric outpatients", *Psychotherapy & Psychosomatics*, 82(4), pp. 267–268.

Taylor, D. J., Mallory, L. J., Lichstein, K. L., Durrence, H. H., Riedel, B. W., and Bush, A. J. (2007) "Comorbidity of chronic insomnia with medical problems", *Sleep*, 30(2), pp. 213–218.

Vgontzas, A. N., Liao, D., Pejovic, S., Calhoun, S., Karataraki, M., Basta, M., Fernández-Mendoza, J., and Bixler, E. O. (2010) "Insomnia with short sleep duration and mortality: The Penn State cohort", *Sleep*, 33(9), pp. 1159–1164.

4 Characteristics of Insomnia and Other Sleep Disturbances in Psychotic Disorders

Sleep disturbance is reported in almost all individuals with psychotic disorders. This includes pronounced symptoms of Insomnia, prolonged time to fall asleep, and repeated and prolonged bouts of night-time waking. Insomnia frequently co-occurs with other disturbances, such as hypersomnia, circadian rhythm disruptions, and nightmare disorder. There is also a higher prevalence of OSA within this population, although this is not a focus of this book. Sleep problems can be highly disruptive and distressing, causing an exacerbation of psychiatric symptoms, reduced mood, as well as poorer coping and quality of life. In this chapter, we present an overview of Insomnia and other sleep disturbance in people diagnosed with psychotic disorders, and we explain the relationship between sleep and psychosis.

Prevalence and Course

Estimated rates of Insomnia and other sleep problems vary considerably between studies, depending on the method of assessing sleep (self-reports, polysomnography, or actigraphy) and the criteria used to define sleep dysfunction. Differences in findings can also be attributed to the duration of illness; whether the person is in an acute state, between episode, or in remission; and the types of medication and other substances they are taking.

In schizophrenia-spectrum disorders, estimated rates of Insomnia and other sleep problems range from 40 to 80 per cent (Cohrs, 2008). These rates may be even higher in mood disorders, ranging from 65 to 90 per cent (Harvey et al., 2009; Gruber et al., 2011). Estimated rates of Insomnia are also very high in other psychiatric disorders that present with psychotic symptoms, such as borderline personality disorders (72–90 per cent; Plante et al., 2013), anxiety, and PTSD (both 30–50 per cent; Ohayon and Shapiro, 2000; Soehner and Harvey, 2012).

People with psychotic disorders report that their sleep difficulties fluctuate over time. In particular, sleep tends to worsen when psychiatric symptoms become more severe, when a mental health relapse is imminent, and when they are in an acute psychotic or manic state. This may be accompanied by a sudden change from usual sleep patterns, alongside disturbing nightmares and hypnagogic hallucinations. Sleep problems tend not to go away during remission. In support, studies show that sleep complaints remain pervasive in 65–70 per cent of individuals who are clinically stable and between psychotic episodes (Gruber et al., 2009; Plante et al., 2013).

Characteristics of Insomnia and Other Sleep Problems in Psychotic Disorders

In addition to published empirical evidence, here we present some findings from a recent survey of 136 individuals receiving care and treatment for a psychotic disorder (living in the community or psychiatric hospital) to illustrate in greater detail the characteristics of sleep disturbances within this population. Survey participants were aged 18–64 years of age, were medicated, and had diagnoses of schizophrenia, schizoaffective disorder, bipolar disorder, and major depression with psychotic features.

Sleep Latency

Sleep latency (also referred to as sleep onset latency: SOL) refers to the length of time that it takes to fall asleep. Typical SOL in the general community is 10–30 minutes. It is a well-replicated finding that sleep latency is significantly prolonged in approximately 50–60 per cent of individuals with bipolar disorder (Casper et al., 1985) and schizophrenia (Lauer et al., 1997; Poulin et al., 2003).

Among our survey participants, the average time taken to fall asleep was 38 minutes, with a standard deviation of 39 minutes. More than one third of participants (37%) took 45 minutes or longer to fall asleep (some took up to 3 or 4 hours; see Figure 4.1).

Sleep Efficiency and Wakings

Sleep efficiency is the percentage of time that a person in bed is actually asleep. It is assessed by calculating time spent in bed divided by time actually asleep. It is a common measure of sleep health, and information from sleep diaries is often used to calculate this parameter. The higher the number, the better sleep efficiency is estimated to be. A sleep efficiency below 85 per cent is considered low, and a sleep efficiency below 80 per cent is usually taken to indicate clinically significant sleep disturbance. Low sleep efficiency may be due to difficulties reaching a state of persistent sleep (remaining asleep for more than 10 minutes) and multiple, and/or prolonged periods of waking.

Reduced sleep efficiency is characteristic of psychotic disorders (Benson and Zarcone, 2005; Cohrs, 2008). In our survey, 70 per cent of respondents reported night-time awakenings occurring several times a week, with difficulties getting back to sleep lasting several hours.

Early morning awakening tends to be more indicative of mood disorders and has been noted in 27–77 per cent of individuals with bipolar disorder (Casper et al., 1985).

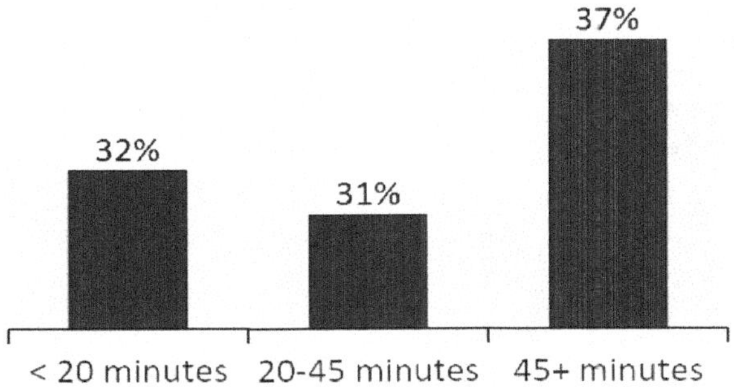

Figure 4.1 Sleep Latency in Psychotic Disorders

Sleep Duration

The recommended sleep duration for adults is 7–9 hours, with 6–10 hours being appropriate for some individuals (Hirshkowitz et al., 2015). A large-scale study with more than 1 million participants found that the average self-reported sleep duration is 6.5 hours (Spurgeon, 2002). The same study also suggested that sleeping too little or too much may both have negative consequences. Disturbed sleep duration is widely reported in individuals with psychotic disorders. There is, however, much intra- and interindividual variability regarding sleep duration in psychosis, as seen in Figure 4.2, with some people sleeping too little (Loudon et al., 1977; Krystal, 2006) and others sleeping too much (Harvey et al., 2009; Kaplan et al., 2011).

Sleeping too Little

A substantial number of people with psychotic disorders sleep below the recommended duration of 7 hours per night. In our survey, one-quarter (26 per cent) reported sleeping for less than 6 hours a night. Figure 4.2 shows that 10 per cent slept for only 3–4 hours per night, and another 16 per cent slept for 5–6 hours.

Typically, short sleepers with psychosis fall into three categories:

1. People in the first group would like to sleep more, but are in a state of **hyperarousal**. Cognitive and somatic hyperarousal is a common clinical feature of Insomnia and is associated with rumination, distress associated with hallucinations and paranoia, problem-solving efforts, and worry. In this chronic state of anxiety and alertness, individuals have difficulty initiating and maintaining sleep and become exhausted from lack of sleep. Many people respond to such sleep difficulties with compensatory behaviours such as spending extra time in bed and reducing daytime activities. Reducing this state of hyperarousal is a key mechanism of action in CBT-I.
2. The second group comprises individuals in a **manic/hypomanic phase**, or in a state of psychotic agitation. This state is characterised by a decreased need for sleep, and in some cases total sleeplessness, which might last for several days. This reduced need for sleep is a clinical feature of a manic episode, occurring in 70–95 per cent of affected patients (Krystal, 2006). In this phase, individuals report very short sleep durations and feel rested after only 3 hours of sleep in a 24-hour sleep–wake cycle. These episodes are often accompanied by heightened mood or euphoria, and are not experienced as distressing or disturbing. However, the longer the duration of sleeplessness, the harder it is to treat, and hospitalisation may be required.

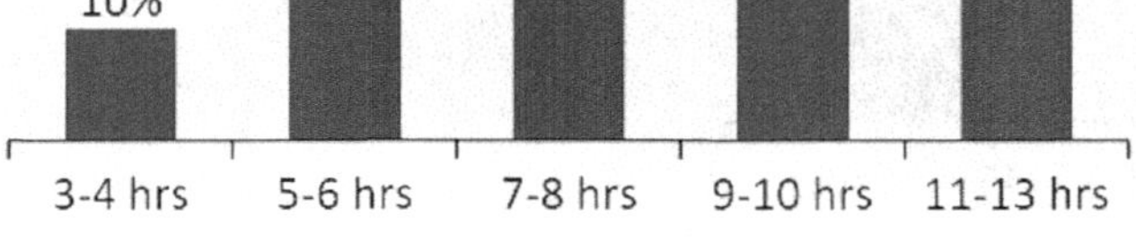

Figure 4.2 Total Sleep Duration in Psychotic Disorders

3. Members of the third group are sleeping little at night but are **compensating** for this during the day. Three to four hours of night-time sleep might be balanced by another 3–4 (or more) hours daytime sleep. So, although members of this group may be meeting their sleep requirements, it may be happening in a haphazard way that interferes with daily functioning.

Sleeping too Much (Hypersomnia)

Excessive daytime sleepiness is referred to as hypersomnia, or sometimes hypersomnolence. This is characterised by extended periods of time in bed, with more than 9 hours of sleep over the 24-hour period, difficulties remaining awake during the day, together with subjective reports of inadequate or unrefreshing sleep (see Chapter 3).

Hypersomnia may be particularly common in mood disorders (as high as 10–20 per cent) and in people with psychotic disorders taking antipsychotics, benzodiazepines, and tricyclic antidepressants (McWhirter et al., 2007). A National Institute of Mental Health population-based study showed that 46.5 per cent of patients diagnosed with hypersomnia were also diagnosed with a psychiatric illness (Ford and Kamerow, 1989).

Empirical studies of hypersomnia have so far only been reported in bipolar disorder, and they show prevalence rates ranging between 23 and 78 per cent (Harvey et al., 2009; Kaplan et al., 2011). High rates of hypersomnia were also found in our survey participants. Figure 4.2 shows that 43 per cent reported sleeping more than 9 hours overnight, including 14 per cent sleeping between 11 and 13 hours.

Hypersomnia can occur concurrently with Insomnia. Our survey and other studies show that these conditions co-occur in approximately 25 per cent of individuals with a psychotic disorder, and they are associated with a greater psychopathological profile than when Insomnia occurs alone (Ohayon and Schatzberg, 2002; Soehner et al., 2014).

Circadian Rhythm Disturbance

Irregular sleep–wake rhythms occur more commonly in people with psychotic disorders than in healthy adults (Wulff et al., 2012) and are associated with subjective complaints of poor sleep quality (Hofstetter et al., 2005). Irregular sleep–wake rhythms are most often reported in the initial phases of a psychotic episode (Castro et al., 2015) and may be more common in people with predominantly positive symptoms (64 per cent), compared with people with predominantly negative symptoms (33 per cent; Afonso et al., 2011).

The different types of circadian rhythm disturbance are reviewed in Chapter 3. In psychotic disorders, sleep–wake disruptions commonly manifest as:

(a) *severely delayed sleep phase (delayed bedtime)*, in which individuals are not sleepy until very late (e.g. 2 a.m.) and can sleep until late morning or the middle of the day;
(b) *irregular or non-24-hour (free-running)* sleep–wake cycle disorder, whereby sleep patterns do not differentiate between night and day or conform to the 24-hour cycle;
(c) *sleep–wake reversal*, where individuals are awake at night and sleep during daytime hours.

In our survey, five participants (3.7 per cent) reported complete sleep–wake reversals, and a further 30 per cent presented with delayed sleep phase. This finding supports empirical studies that report a prevalence rate of irregular sleep–wake rhythms in 40 per cent of individuals with schizophrenia (Wulff et al., 2012) and in 10 per cent of individuals with bipolar disorder (Murray and Harvey, 2010).

It is important to make a distinction between *chronic* and *acute* sleep–wake dysregulation. For many individuals, sleep–wake dysregulation may be ongoing for years, and it continues during a period of remission from psychosis (Seleem et al., 2015). In such chronic cases, it does not represent an immediate, discernible clinical risk, although it still affects quality of life and functional capacity. For others, however, a change in the sleep–wake pattern occurs abruptly and for no discernible reason. In this case, acute sleep–wake dysregulation may represent an indication of an oncoming psychotic episode. In this case, medications are often prescribed to help with sleep onset and maintenance, together with CBT-I strategies to help normalise sleep patterns.

Nightmares and Night-time Hallucinations

Repeated awakenings might occur in the context of dysphoric and well-remembered frightening dreams. Studies using questionnaires report a 50 per cent prevalence rate of nightmare disorder in psychiatric populations (Semiz et al., 2008). Nightmares and night terrors are particularly common in these groups because childhood trauma and adverse events are common in psychotic disorders, causing disruptions to sleep that persist for many years after the initial trauma. In many individuals with schizophrenia, bipolar disorder, PTSD, and borderline personality disorders, nightmares might occur several times per week or, in some cases, several times per night.

In psychosis, it may be difficult to differentiate between frightening dreams and disturbing hallucination-like experiences that occur during the transition between wakefulness and sleep (hypnagogic hallucinations) or the transition from sleep to wakefulness (hypnopompic hallucinations). These experiences comprise vivid visual or auditory impressions and can be accompanied by intensely frightening sensations of flying and out-of-body experiences. They can be perceived as vividly real and interpreted as occult or metaphysical events, contributing to awakenings and panic attacks at night and prolonged periods of wakefulness. They may also become incorporated into the person's delusions and hallucinations.

The Relationship between Sleep and Symptoms of Psychosis

For a long time, disturbances of sleep were perceived as purely a by-product or 'another symptom' of psychotic disorders. They are now, however, recognised as disorders in their own right, with their own underlying mechanisms and independent perpetuating factors (American Academy of Sleep Medicine, 2005). Furthermore, sleep disturbance is associated with a range of negative health and functional consequences, including increased severity of psychopathology.

The evidence highlighting the close relationship between sleep dysfunction and psychotic symptoms suggests that it is both complex and bidirectional:

- *Sleep dysfunctions may predate the onset of mental illness*, occurring months or sometimes years before illness onset. In interviews with 145 individuals with schizophrenia and their family members, 70 per cent reported that changes in sleep were the first symptoms signalling that the person was becoming unwell (Herz and Melville, 1980).
- *Sleep dysfunctions correlate with levels of negative mood and psychotic symptoms.* Short sleep duration and poor sleep efficiency correlate with increased levels of depression and suicidality in people with both mood and schizophrenia-spectrum disorders (Gershon et al., 2012). Abnormalities in sleep electroencephalogram (EEG) are also linked to increased levels

of psychotic symptom ratings and negative mood (Lauer et al., 1997; Zarcone and Benson, 1997). Dysfunctions of sleep can precede mood change by as little as 1 day, with short sleep durations associated with a next-day increase in negative mood and psychotic symptom ratings (Bauer et al., 2006; Waters et al., 2011). Insomnia and hypersomnia also correlate with future depressive symptoms in individuals with mood disorders (Perlman et al., 2006).

- *Sleeplessness, or a sudden change in sleep–wake pattern, is a marker of potential relapse.* Prolonged periods of sleeplessness or an abrupt change in sleep patterns may be a warning sign of impending psychotic breakdown in remitted individuals (Heinrichs and Carpenter, 1985). In bipolar disorder, a change from previous sleep patterns of more than 3 hours suggests that a significant disturbance of mood is imminent (Bauer et al., 2006). Sleep deprivation also represents a risk factor in the onset of psychotic symptoms (Koranyi and Lehmann, 1960).
- *Mental health symptoms are risk factors for sleep problems.* It is well documented that low mood and anxiety impact on subsequent sleep and the ability to fall asleep (Espie, 2002; Ohayon and Roth, 2003). A core mechanism through which symptoms impact on sleep is their effect on arousal. For example, a first episode of anxiety and depression predicts the onset of Insomnia by several weeks or months (Sivertsen et al., 2012).

Together, the above studies show evidence that dysfunctions of sleep can trigger or aggravate mood and psychotic symptoms, but also that this relationship is bidirectional.

The Impact of Sleep Problems on Daytime Function

The functional consequences of Insomnia and sleep disturbance include tiredness, social isolation/withdrawal, impairments in occupational functioning, substance use, and barriers to recovery. Disturbances of sleep have been estimated to account for 25 per cent of the variance of reduced quality of life in people with schizophrenia (Hofstetter et al., 2005), even after controlling for depression and medication side effects (Cohrs, 2008). In other words, one-quarter of life satisfaction problems in people with schizophrenia may be explained by sleep difficulties alone.

Sleep problems contribute to reduced quality of life in the context of psychiatric disorders in many different ways.

Tiredness

Excessive daytime tiredness is a symptom and consequence of Insomnia and other sleep disturbance. It impacts on motivation, mood, self-care, and the ability to cope with life and difficulties as they arise (Hofstetter et al., 2005; Chiu et al., 2015). Excessive daytime tiredness can also act to maintain sleep problems through excessive napping, sleeping in late, and reduced daytime activity.

Social Isolation

Insomnia and inappropriate timing of sleep impact on the ability to join community, family, social, and occupational activities. Loneliness and isolation have been reported in those who are awake at night (Goldsmith et al., 2006). Avoidance of sleeping away from home (e.g. on holiday or staying with friends) may occur because the individual finds it even harder to sleep in those situations.

Reduced Work/Study Capacity

Many people with psychotic disorders have difficulties completing studies and maintaining regular employment and have reduced capacity to access opportunities in the workforce. Although there are several factors that contribute to this situation, the contributions of disabling daytime tiredness and disrupted sleep are particularly important. For example, poor sleep has been found to be associated with poor work performance in those with bipolar disorder, causing increased risk of unemployment and of being made redundant (Boland et al., 2015).

Physical Health and Substance Abuse

Sleep dysfunction contributes to reduced daytime physical activity, as well as unhealthy lifestyle habits, including an increased reliance on alcohol, sedatives, and other drugs to get to sleep (Strine and Chapman, 2005). There is also often a reliance on stimulants to stay awake during the day, as well as excessive caffeine intake and smoking to compensate for daytime tiredness, all of which can exacerbate other health complications (e.g. respiratory problems, gastrointestinal reflux, tremor).

Cognitive and Emotional Difficulties

It is common for people to report that, when tired, they have difficulties reading and performing tasks requiring attention or working memory. In both psychotic and mood disorders, reduced social cognition, visual learning, and working memory have all been linked to sleep disruptions (Russo et al., 2015). Studies conducted with overnight polysomnography confirm that poor sleepers have reduced daytime cognitive capacity. For example, electrical brain activity during sleep (particularly slow waves in the deep sleep stage) correlates with performance on tests of attention and vigilance in schizophrenia (Forest et al., 2007). By contrast, people with psychotic disorders and normal sleep patterns show better cognitive performance than those with disturbed sleep (Bromundt et al., 2011).

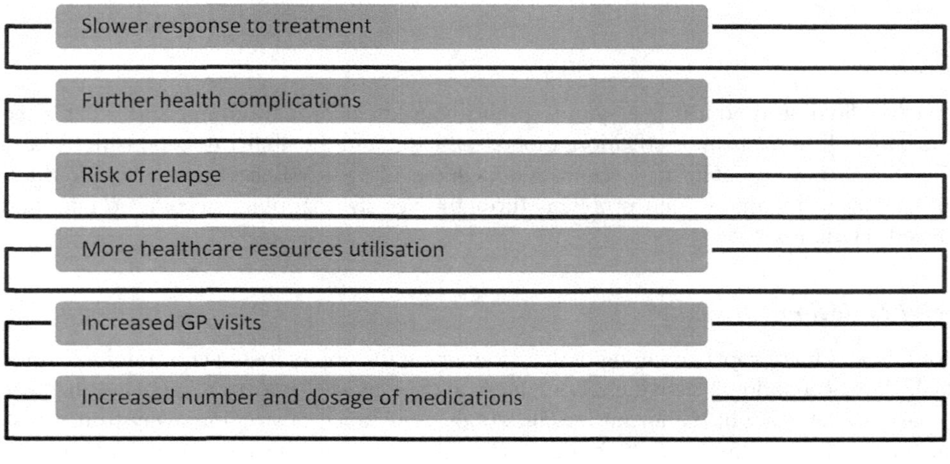

Figure 4.3 Negative Impact of Sleep Dysfunctions on Recovery in Psychiatric Disorders

Recovery

Sleep dysfunction puts people at a higher risk of relapse of their psychiatric condition (Harvey et al., 2015; Cretu et al., 2016), depression (Ohayon and Roth, 2003), and alcohol and drug addictions (Brower and Perron, 2010). It causes significant interference with treatment and functional outcome because of missed appointments, inappropriately timed intake of medication, and withdrawal from supportive social networks. Sleep dysfunction also impacts on progress with recovery goals, greater use of medication, and higher financial disadvantage. Finally, sleep dysfunctions are associated with a slower response to treatment and an increase in health-care utilisation compared with individuals without a sleep disorder (Manocchia et al., 2001; Léger et al., 2002; see Figure 4.3). Further, longitudinal studies show that patients who experience improvements in their sleep have a more rapid response to antidepressant medication, and that those patients whose Insomnia persists tend to relapse sooner (Perlis et al., 1997).

Summary

- Sleep disturbance is one of the most common complaint in people living with a psychiatric illness. These individuals often experience significantly prolonged time to fall asleep (sleep latency) and low sleep efficiency, and they may either sleep too little (less than 6 hours) or sleep too much (more than 9 hours).
- Insomnia in psychotic disorders can co-occur with other sleep problems, such as hypersomnia (excessive daytime sleepiness), circadian sleep–wake rhythm disturbance (delayed sleep phase, irregular cycle, or sleep–wake reversal), and nightmares.
- There is a close relationship between sleep disturbance and psychiatric symptoms, daytime tiredness, social isolation, reduced capacity for work and study, physical health, substance abuse, cognitive deficits, and capacity for recovery.
- Sleep disturbance may precede psychotic relapse and may be considered a prodromal factor.
- Treating disturbed sleep may protect against relapse.

References

Afonso, P., Brissos, S., Figueira, M. L., and Paiva, T. (2011) "Schizophrenia patients with predominantly positive symptoms have more disturbed sleep–wake cycles measured by actigraphy", *Psychiatry Research*, 189, pp. 62–66.

American Academy of Sleep Medicine (2005) *The international classification of sleep disorders: Diagnostic and coding manual.* Westchester, IL: American Academy of Sleep Medicine.

Bauer, M., Grof, P., Rasgon, N., Bschor, T., Glenn, T., and Whybrow, P. C. (2006) "Temporal relation between sleep and mood in patients with bipolar disorder", *Bipolar Disorders*, 8(2), pp. 160–167.

Benson, K. L., and Zarcone, V. P. (2005) "Schizophrenia", in Kryger, M. H., Roth, T., and Dement, W. C. (Eds.) *Principles and practice of sleep medicine* (4th ed.). Philadelphia, PA: Elsevier Saunders, pp. 1327–1336.

Boland, E. M., Stange, J. P., Molz Adams, A., LaBelle, D. R., Ong, M.-L., Hamilton, J. L., Connolly, S. L., Black, C. L., Cedeño, A. B., and Alloy, L. B. (2015) "Associations between sleep disturbance, cognitive functioning and work disability in Bipolar Disorder", *Psychiatry Research*, 230(2), pp. 567–574.

Bromundt, V., Köster, M., Georgiev-Kill, A., Opwis, K., Wirz-Justice, A., Stoppe, G., and Cajochen, C. (2011) "Sleep–wake cycles and cognitive functioning in schizophrenia", *British Journal of Psychiatry*, 198, pp. 269–276.

Brower, K. J., and Perron, B. E. (2010) "Sleep disturbance as a universal risk factor for relapse in addictions to psychoactive substances", *Medical Hypotheses*, 74(5), pp. 928–933.

Casper, R. C., Redmond Jr, D., Katz, M. M., Schaffer, C. B., Davis, J. M., and Koslow, S. H. (1985) "Somatic symptoms in primary affective disorder: Presence and relationship to the classification of depression", *Archives of General Psychiatry*, 42(11), pp. 1098–1104.

Castro, J., Zanini, M., Gonçalves, B. d. S. B., Coelho, F. M. S., Bressan, R., Bittencourt, L., Gadelha, A., Brietzke, E., and Tufik, S. (2015) "Circadian rest–activity rhythm in individuals at risk for psychosis and bipolar disorder", *Schizophrenia Research*, 168(1), pp. 50–55.

Chiu, V. W., Ree, M., Janca, A., and Waters, F. (2015) "Sleep in schizophrenia: Exploring subjective experiences of sleep problems, and implications for treatment", *Psychiatric Quarterly*, 87(4), pp. 633–648.

Cohrs, S. (2008) "Sleep disturbances in patients with schizophrenia: Impact and effect of antipsychotics", *CNS Drugs*, 22(11), pp. 939–962.

Cretu, J. B., Culver, J. L., Goffin, K. C., Shah, S., and Ketter, T. A. (2016) "Sleep, residual mood symptoms, and time to relapse in recovered patients with bipolar disorder", *Journal of Affective Disorders*, 190, pp. 162–166.

Espie, C. A. (2002) "Insomnia: Conceptual issues in the development, persistence, and treatment of sleep disorder in adults", *Annual Review of Psychology*, 53, pp. 215–243.

Ford, D. E., and Kamerow, D. B. (1989) "Epidemiologic study of sleep disturbances and psychiatric disorders: An opportunity for prevention?", *JAMA*, 262(11), pp. 1479–1484.

Forest, G., Poulin, J., Daoust, A.-M., Lussier, I., Stip, E., and Godbout, R. (2007) "Attention and non-REM sleep in neuroleptic-naive persons with schizophrenia and control participants", *Psychiatry Research*, 149(1–3), pp. 33–40.

Gershon, A., Thompson, W. K., Eidelman, P., McGlinchey, E. L., Kaplan, K. A., and Harvey, A. G. (2012) "Restless pillow, ruffled mind: Sleep and affect coupling in interepisode bipolar disorder", *Journal of Abnormal Psychology*, 121(4), pp. 863–873.

Goldsmith, R. J., Casola, P., and Varenbut, M. (2006) "Sleep complications in depression, anxiety, and psychotic disorders and their treatment", *Psychiatric Annals*, 36(12).

Gruber, J., Harvey, A. G., Wang, P. W., Brooks Iii, J. O., Thase, M. E., Sachs, G. S., and Ketter, T. A. (2009) "Sleep functioning in relation to mood, function, and quality of life at entry to the Systematic Treatment Enhancement Program for Bipolar Disorder (STEP-BD)", *Journal of Affective Disorders*, 114(1–3), pp. 41–49.

Gruber, J., Miklowitz, D. J., Harvey, A. G., Frank, E., Kupfer, D., Thase, M. E., Sachs, G. S., and Ketter, T. A. (2011) "Sleep matters: Sleep functioning and course of illness in bipolar disorder", *Journal of Affective Disorders*, 134(1–3), pp. 416–420.

Harvey, A. G., Soehner, A. M., Kaplan, K. A., Hein, K., Lee, J., Kanady, J., Li, D., Rabe-Hesketh, S., Ketter, T. A., Neylan, T. C., and Buysse, D. J. (2015) "Treating insomnia improves mood state, sleep, and functioning in bipolar disorder: A pilot randomized controlled trial", *Journal of Consulting & Clinical Psychology*, 83(3), pp. 564–577.

Harvey, A. G., Talbot, L. S., and Gershon, A. (2009) "Sleep disturbance in bipolar disorder across the lifespan", *Clinical Psychology: Science & Practice*, 16(2), pp. 256–277.

Heinrichs, D. W., and Carpenter, W. T. (1985) "Prospective study of prodromal symptoms in schizophrenic relapse", *American Journal of Psychiatry*, 142(3), pp. 371–373.

Herz, M. I., and Melville, C. (1980) "Relapse in schizophrenia", *American Journal of Psychiatry*, 137(7), pp. 801–805.

Hirshkowitz, M., Whiton, K., Albert, S. M., Alessi, C., Bruni, O., DonCarlos, L., Hazen, N., Herman, J., Katz, E. S., Kheirandish-Gozal, L., and Neubauer, D. N. (2015) "National Sleep Foundation's sleep time duration recommendations: Methodology and results summary", *Sleep Health*, 1(1), pp. 40–43.

Hofstetter, J. R., Lysaker, P. H., and Mayeda, A. R. (2005) "Quality of sleep in patients with schizophrenia is associated with quality of life and coping", *BMC Psychiatry*, 5, pp. 13–17.

Kaplan, K. A., Gruber, J., Eidelman, P., Talbot, L. S., and Harvey, A. G. (2011) "Hypersomnia in inter-episode bipolar disorder: Does it have prognostic significance?", *Journal of Affective Disorders*, 132(3), pp. 438–444.

Koranyi, E. K., and Lehmann, H. E. (1960) "Experimental sleep deprivation in schizophrenic patients", *AMA Archives of General Psychiatry*, 2, pp. 534–544.

Krystal, A. D. (2006) "Sleep and psychiatric disorders: Future directions", *Psychiatric Clinics of North America*, 29(4), pp. 1115–1130.

Lauer, C. J., Schreiber, W., Pollmächer, T., Holsboer, F., and Krieg, J.-C. (1997) "Sleep in schizophrenia: A polysomnographic study on drug-naive patients", *Neuropsychopharmacology*, 16(1), pp. 51–60.

Léger, D., Guilleminault, C., Bader, G., Lévy, E., and Paillard, M. (2002) "Medical and socio-professional impact of insomnia", *Sleep*, 25(6), pp. 625–629.

Loudon, J. B., Ashworth, C. M., and Blackburn, I. M. (1977) "A study of the symptomatology and course of manic illness using a new scale", *Psychological Medicine*, 7(04), pp. 723–729.

Manocchia, M., Keller, S., and Ware, J. E. (2001) "Sleep problems, health-related quality of life, work functioning and health care utilization among the chronically ill", *Quality of Life Research*, 10(4), pp. 331–345.

McWhirter, D., Bae, C., and Budur, K. (2007) "The assessment, diagnosis, and treatment of excessive sleepiness: Practical considerations for the psychiatrist", *Psychiatry (Edgmont)*, 4(9), pp. 26–35.

Murray, G., and Harvey, A. (2010) "Circadian rhythms and sleep in bipolar disorder", *Bipolar Disorders*, 12(5), pp. 459–472.

Ohayon, M. M., and Roth, T. (2003) "Place of chronic insomnia in the course of depressive and anxiety disorders", *Journal of Psychiatric Research*, 37(1), pp. 9–15.

Ohayon, M. M., and Schatzberg, A. F. (2002) "Prevalence of depressive episodes with psychotic features in the general population", *American Journal of Psychiatry*, 159(11), pp. 1855–1861.

Ohayon, M. M., and Shapiro, C. M. (2000) "Sleep disturbances and psychiatric disorders associated with posttraumatic stress disorder in the general population", *Comprehensive Psychiatry*, 41(6), pp. 469–478.

Perlis, M. L., Giles, D. E., Buysse, D. J., Tu, X., and Kupfer, D. J. (1997) "Self-reported sleep disturbance as a prodromal symptom in recurrent depression", *Journal of Affective Disorders*, 42(2–3), pp. 209–212.

Perlman, C. A., Johnson, S. L., and Mellman, T. A. (2006) "The prospective impact of sleep duration on depression and mania", *Bipolar Disorders*, 8(3), pp. 271–274.

Plante, D. T., Frankenburg, F. R., Fitzmaurice, G. M., and Zanarini, M. C. (2013) "Relationship between sleep disturbance and recovery in patients with borderline personality disorder", *Journal of Psychosomatic Research*, 74(4), pp. 278–282.

Poulin, J., Daoust, A.-M., Forest, G., Stip, E., and Godbout, R. (2003) "Sleep architecture and its clinical correlates in first episode and neuroleptic-naive patients with schizophrenia", *Schizophrenia Research*, 62(1–2), pp. 147–153.

Russo, M., Mahon, K., Shanahan, M., Ramjas, E., Solon, C., Purcell, S. M., and Burdick, K. E. (2015) "The relationship between sleep quality and neurocognition in bipolar disorder", *Journal of Affective Disorders*, 187, pp. 156–162.

Seleem, M. A., Merranko, J. A., Goldstein, T. R., Goldstein, B. I., Axelson, D. A., Brent, D. A., Nimgaonkar, V. L., Diler, R. S., Sakolsky, D. J., Kupfer, D. J., and Birmaher, B. (2015) "The longitudinal course of sleep timing and circadian preferences in adults with bipolar disorder", *Bipolar Disorders*, 17(4), pp. 392–402.

Semiz, U. B., Basoglu, C., Ebrinc, S., and Cetin, M. (2008) "Nightmare disorder, dream anxiety, and subjective sleep quality in patients with borderline personality disorder", *Psychiatry & Clinical Neurosciences*, 62(1), pp. 48–55.

Sivertsen, B., Salo, P., Mykletun, A., Hysing, M., Pallesen, S., Krokstad, S., Nordhus, I. H., and Øverland, S. (2012) "The bidirectional association between depression and insomnia: The HUNT study", *Psychosomatic Medicine*, 74(7), pp. 758–765.

Soehner, A. M., and Harvey, A. G. (2012) "Prevalence and functional consequences of severe insomnia symptoms in mood and anxiety disorders: Results from a nationally representative sample", *Sleep*, 35(10), pp. 1367–1375.

Soehner, A. M., Kaplan, K. A., and Harvey, A. G. (2014) "Prevalence and clinical correlates of co-occurring insomnia and hypersomnia symptoms in depression", *Journal of Affective Disorders*, 167, pp. 93–97.

Spurgeon, D. (2002) "People who sleep for seven hours a night live longest", *BMJ*, 324(7335), p. 446.

Strine, T. W., and Chapman, D. P. (2005) "Associations of frequent sleep insufficiency with health-related quality of life and health behaviors", *Sleep Medicine*, 6(1), pp. 23–27.

Waters, F., Sinclair, C., Rock, D., Jablensky, A., Foster, R. G., and Wulff, K. (2011) "Daily variations in sleep–wake patterns and severity of psychopathology: A pilot study in community-dwelling individuals with chronic schizophrenia", *Psychiatry Research*, 187(1), pp. 304–306.

Wulff, K., Dijk, D. J., Middleton, B., Foster, R. G., and Joyce, E. (2012) "Sleep and circadian rhythm disruption in schizophrenia", *British Journal of Psychiatry*, 200, pp. 308–316.

Zarcone, V. P., and Benson, K. L. (1997) "BPRS symptom factors and sleep variables in schizophrenia", *Psychiatry Research*, 66, pp. 111–120.

5 Sleep, its Regulation, and Barriers to Good Sleep

In this chapter, we introduce some basic facts about sleep and how it is regulated in healthy adults. This background knowledge is important, because a comprehensive understanding of the features of a healthy night of sleep, and how it is achieved, is needed to deliver the CBT-I intervention. It is also important that the clinician administering the CBT-I intervention does not hold common faulty beliefs about sleep, which are often perpetuated in the media (for example, that everyone needs 8 hours sleep).

What Is Sleep?

Sleep is a state characterised by changes in brainwave activity, breathing, heart rate, body temperature, and several other physiological functions. It is a state of reduced consciousness, and typically there is little memory of the hours that passed during sleep. Sleep is not a passive, dormant part of daily life; it is a time when parts of the brain may be more active than during wakefulness.

Humans cannot live without sleep, and there is strong evidence that good sleep serves to support health and well-being. Although scientists are unsure exactly why people sleep, there exists evidence that sleep restores brain energy, is involved in the cleansing and maintenance of metabolic functions, and is responsible for promoting cell synthesis and repair (Kunz and Herrmann, 2000; Bellesi et al., 2013; Xie et al., 2013).

Sleep Stages

Sleep architecture refers to the way that sleep is structured across the night. Briefly, sleep architecture comprises four stages and two states—non-rapid eye movement (NREM: N1, N2, and N3) and rapid eye movement (REM) sleep—which alternate cyclically. These sleep stages are characterised by different patterns of brain activity that can be assessed with an EEG. Sleep architecture can be represented by a graph called a hypnogram.

A healthy night of sleep will have four or five cycles (see Figure 5.1 for a visual representation of a hypogram depicting a healthy night of sleep). In any given sleep cycle, the sleeper will start in light sleep (stage N1–N2) and then progress to deeper sleep (stage N3), before finishing the cycle with light sleep and, often, a period of vivid dreaming (REM; see Table 5.1). Note that, in sleep classification systems, deep sleep formerly also comprised a fourth stage (stage N4). In 2007, however, the American Academy of Sleep Medicine updated its methods of analysing sleep by merging stages N3 and N4 sleep together (i.e. NREM stage 'N3' now represents deep sleep; Iber et al., 2007; Schulz, 2008).

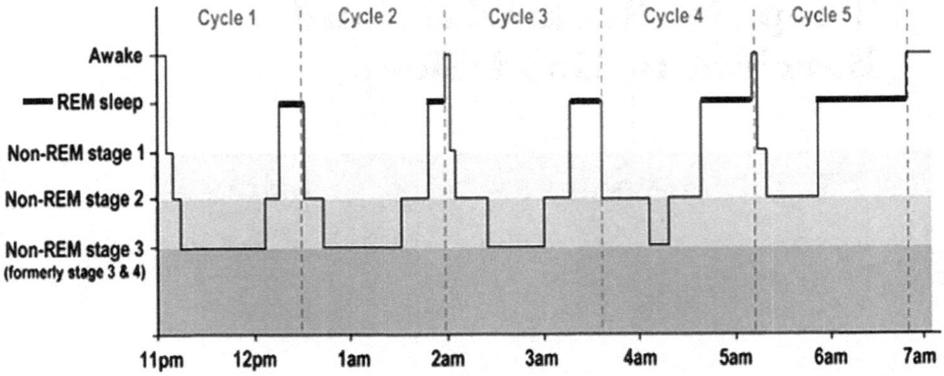

Figure 5.1 Transition between Sleep Stages (Hypnogram)

Table 5.1 Sleep Stages: Brief Description and Time Spent in Each Stage

Stage	*Description*	*Amount of Time Spent in Each Stage per Night*
Awake in bed	Conscious and aware Time awake in bed increases through adulthood	5% age 20 12% age 40 18% age 70
REM	Vivid dreaming Eyes closed but moving fast and 'shaking' side to side Easily roused Brief waking may occur after REM Breathing and heart rate increases	25%
Stage 1	Light sleep, dozing Easily roused Breathing slows, and heart rate becomes more regular	5%
Stage 2	Brain starts to emit larger waves Metabolism slows	47%
Stage 3 (also known as slow wave sleep)	Deep sleep; difficult to rouse Sleeper will feel groggy or disoriented if woken Brain emits large, slow waves Time in deep sleep reduces through adulthood	20% age 20 15% age 40 9% age 70

Source: Statistics from Ohayon et al., 2004

Some Important Facts about Healthy Sleep

- Healthy sleep is not characterised by hours of uninterrupted deep sleep. Rather, healthy sleep is more like riding ocean waves, cycling through peaks and troughs of lighter and deeper sleep throughout the night.
- As the night progresses, sleep cycles contain less deep sleep and more REM. So, there is more deep sleep in the first half of the night, but more vivid dreams in the second half of the night. In fact, nearly all deep sleep occurs in the first 4 hours of the sleep

period. This suggests that a person who sleeps only 4 hours has likely had the same amount of deep sleep as someone who slept a full 7 hours. This doesn't mean that our body only needs 4 hours of sleep, because light sleep and REM sleep are also important, but it can be reassuring to know that deep sleep requirements can usually be met with even a short night of sleep.

- A normal, healthy night of sleep usually contains a small number (two to five) of brief (less than 5 minutes) awakenings, which may reflect the transition from one cycle ('wave') of sleep to the next.
- Further, it is important to be aware that the amount of time people spend in each stage of sleep varies across adulthood; see Table 5.1 for details.

In many psychiatric disorders, including psychotic disorders, there are characteristic changes in sleep architecture compared with that of healthy people. These changes may both be a marker of specific disorders and help to explain some of the observable symptoms. These changes in the case of psychotic disorders are outlined in Chapter 6.

Sleep Requirements

Large-scale studies (with more than 1 million participants) have found that the average sleep duration of adults in the general population is 6.5–7 hours (e.g. Kripke et al., 2002). This research also suggested that more sleep is not necessarily better, with people sleeping on average more than 8 hours a night having poor health outcomes similar to those who routinely sleep less than 5 hours a night. Interestingly, the best health outcomes were for those sleeping about 7 hours a night.

The USA National Sleep Foundation recommendations for sleep duration are displayed in Table 5.2, along with the average time spent awake in bed by people in different age groups (Hirshkowitz et al., 2015). It is important to emphasise that there is a range of healthy sleep duration for adults, and that sleep duration is not 'one size fits all'. Like food, too much or too little sleep is not good for health. Table 5.2 also emphasises that sleep architecture changes throughout adulthood.

In psychotic disorders, sleep hours may be too few or too many. There may be many reasons for this, including an acute psychotic state (e.g. hallucinations, paranoia, confusion), drugs and substances (prescribed and illicit), lack of regular daytime and sleep routine, low mood, and anxiety.

Table 5.2 Recommendations for Sleep Duration for Adults

Age Group	*Suggested Sleep Duration*	*May Be Appropriate*	*Not Recommended*	*Time Awake in Bed*
Young adults, 18–25 years	7–9 hours	6 hours 10 to 11 hours	Less than 6 hours More than 11 hours	5%
Adults, 26–64 years	7–9 hours	6 hours 10 hours	Less than 6 hours More than 10 hours	12%
Older adults, ≥ 65 years	7–8 hours	5–6 hours 9 hours	Less than 5 hours More than 9 hours	20%

Sources: Ohayon et al., 2004; Hirshkowitz et al., 2015

Biological Regulation of Sleep: The Two Process Model

Understanding of how sleep is regulated is critical for treating Insomnia, as it assists clinicians in understanding and explaining the rationale behind treatment components, providing psychoeducation, and selecting relevant treatment components. We present a brief overview that will serve as a minimum requirement for effective delivery of CBT-I. Further details can be obtained from several good sources (e.g. Morin and Espie, 2004).

Healthy sleep is regulated by biological drives. Just as going without food produces sensations of hunger, going without sleep produces feelings of fatigue and sleepiness. The hunger drives us to eat, and we feel better. Sleepiness drives us to sleep, and we feel better.

Two important biological processes that regulate sleep are the homeostatic sleep drive and the body clock. Alexander Borbély (1982) tied these two processes together in his 'two process' model of sleep regulation.

Homeostatic Sleep Drive

Homeostasis refers to the drive to sleep that accumulates with time spent awake. With every hour of being awake, the homeostatic sleep drive increases. After a person has been awake for a long period of time, the sleep drive indicates that the need for sleep is increasing, and that it is time to sleep. For sound sleep, an individual needs to retire to bed when their sleep drive is strong (i.e. only after they have been awake for a sufficiently long time for their sleep drive to have built).

Being awake for longer increases sleep drive, and the opposite is also true. Behaviours such as sleeping in, going to bed early, reduced daytime activity levels, and napping will reduce sleep drive at night. Excessive and/or late caffeine intake will also reduce sleep drive. These behaviours are common in psychotic disorders and are targets for change in CBT-I.

If the sleep drive system operated alone, it would mean that sleepiness was at its lowest in the morning after an adequate night of sleep, and would increase steadily throughout the day for as long as the individual was awake. Instead of this steady increase in sleep drive with time spent awake, sleepiness and fatigue levels actually rise and fall somewhat through the day. This is owing, in part, to the body clock.

Body Clock

Also called the circadian clock or circadian rhythm, this process is operated by an internal (or 'master') clock that is regulated by the suprachiasmatic nucleus in the hypothalamus. Circadian rhythms refer to the internal, regular timing of physiological and behavioural activities. These occur in a fixed cycle of roughly 24 hours, ensuring that sleep is synchronised by environmental cues such as natural light and the regular timing of meals.

The body clock controls the release of certain hormones, including melatonin and cortisol, at different times during the day. This regulated release acts to influence feelings of sleepiness and alertness, which ebb and flow through the day, instead of changing in a linear fashion with increasing time awake. It is, therefore, normal to have rises and dips in energy across the day.

Alertness is typically best mid-to-late morning and early evening. Tiredness is usually highest in the early morning and late evening (just before bed), and also after lunch (the 'post-lunch dip' in energy). The post-lunch dip is a normal increase in sleepiness and explains why millions of people in the world have a siesta after lunch.

Sleep difficulties related to the body clock have been linked to the abnormal timing of melatonin production. Melatonin, also known as the 'sleep' hormone, helps the body to fall and stay asleep. Melatonin levels increase roughly 2 hours before bedtime, peak in the middle of sleep (around 2 a.m. to 4 a.m.), and then decline before waking up (Scheer et al., 2005). Abnormal timing of melatonin secretion is linked to changes in sleep phase, including delayed sleep phase and non-24-hour sleep–wake disorders, which occur more commonly in people with psychotic disorders than in the general population (to be discussed further in Chapter 6).

The timing of melatonin production is strongly influenced by exposure to light, with bright light exposure acting to switch off melatonin production. Exposure to bright light in the evening, therefore, can delay sleep onset. Bright light in the morning can assist in increasing daytime energy. We come back to this later, as light exposure (or avoidance of light) can be a very useful tool in helping people to improve their sleep and energy levels. Now, we turn to a third factor in the regulation of sleep, namely, arousal.

The Role of Physiological and Cognitive Arousal

Sound sleep is facilitated by a strong sleep drive and a sleep–wake schedule that is congruent with the body clock. If sleep is disturbed despite adequate sleep drive and body clock alignment with night and day, this suggests that elevated arousal may be at play. This may be in the form of *cognitive* arousal (worry, rumination, planning, problem-solving, mind flitting), *emotional* arousal (anxiety, fear, upset, anger, excitement), and/or *physiological* arousal (increased heart rate and breathing rate, muscle tension arousal).

One type of arousal frequently leads to the other two, creating a feedback loop. A worrisome thought, for example, can lead to elevated heart rate and anxiety, which can generate further negative thoughts. Increased arousal may help to account for poor night-time sleep, as well as reduced ability to nap during the day, in people with Insomnia. Skills to reduce arousal during the day, prior to bedtime, and during nocturnal wakings are often important for resolving Insomnia.

Much research has highlighted the role of increased arousal in Insomnia. In terms of physiological arousal, there is evidence that people with Insomnia have elevated basal metabolic rate and core body temperature, both day and night (Bonnet and Arand, 1995; Lushington et al., 2000). Physiological arousal may also be elevated at bedtime owing to anxiety. Arousal may also be increased by caffeinated or sugary drinks, stimulant medication or illicit drugs, foods with high sugar content, and cigarettes, during the day and before bed. Commonly, physiological arousal may also be caused by excessive cognitive activity (Harvey, 2002), which can lead to the 'tired but wired' state that many people with Insomnia describe.

Cognitive arousal may arise from sleep-related or non-sleep-related cognitions:

- Non-sleep-related cognitive arousal is common in people who are under stress, anxious, depressed, or experiencing symptoms of psychosis. These are examples of situations in which Insomnia is due to an underlying source of stress. Worries, rumination, fear, and catastrophic or paranoid thinking are potent examples of cognitive arousal that can interfere with sleep. Difficulties with distancing from worries or challenging them and unwinding at the end of the day will increase the likelihood that cognitive arousal will interfere with sleep.
- Sleep-related cognitive arousal, on the other hand, refers to thoughts and cognitive processes that occur in response to a prolonged or severe period of poor sleep. This

is often in the form of worries about the impact of sleep loss on daytime functioning and health.

Each of the above examples of cognitive arousal will typically lead to increased physiological arousal and delayed sleep onset. The delayed sleep onset then creates additional worry, frustration, anxiety, and tension, delaying sleep even further (see Lundh, 2005).

Unhelpful Thoughts and Cognitions

In addition to cognitive arousal associated with stress, anxiety, or low mood, Harvey (2002) described several cognitive characteristics associated with Insomnia. Examples of these are shown in Table 5.3 (also see Figure 5.2).

Table 5.3 Unhelpful Cognitive Characteristics about Sleep that Lead to Arousal

Cognitive Characteristics	*Examples*
Worries about sleeping poorly	Worry about sleep can perpetuate Insomnia. Common worries include: – 'I won't cope tomorrow' – 'I can't stand being awake like this' – 'I should be able to control my sleep' – 'What if I don't sleep at all tonight?' – 'Poor sleep is going to do me harm'
Unhelpful beliefs drive about sleep[1]	Unhelpful beliefs about sleep have been widely studied and are thought to worry about sleep (Morin et al., 1993; Harvey, 2002). Examples of unhelpful beliefs include: – 'I need 8 hours of sleep every night to feel refreshed' – 'If I don't sleep well at night I know I cannot function well the following day' – 'Insomnia is a result of a chemical imbalance and there is little I can do about it'
Attempts to force sleep	Attempts to force sleep include trying to make the mind go blank and trying to get to sleep as fast as possible
Unhelpful thought control strategies[2]	Research suggests that there are a number of strategies that people use to manage unwanted thoughts that occur during the day or the night (Wells and Davies, 1994). Maladaptive strategies include aggressive suppression, and worry: – 'I get angry at myself for having these thoughts' – 'I dwell on other worries'
Looking for signs of not falling asleep[3]	The mind is hypervigilant for signs of falling asleep/staying awake: – 'Am I too hot?' – 'Is my mind busy?' – 'How long is it taking me to fall asleep?' – 'Is there a noise that will disturb me?' The mind is also vigilant for symptoms of fatigue during the day: – 'My eyes are scratchy' – 'I feel unmotivated' – 'My body feels heavy and tired'

Notes: (1) See the Dysfunctional Beliefs about Sleep Scale (DBAS; Morin et al., 2007). (2) See the Thought Control Questionnaire for Insomnia-Revised (Ree et al., 2005). (3) See the Sleep Associated Monitoring Index (SAMI; Semler and Harvey, 2004).

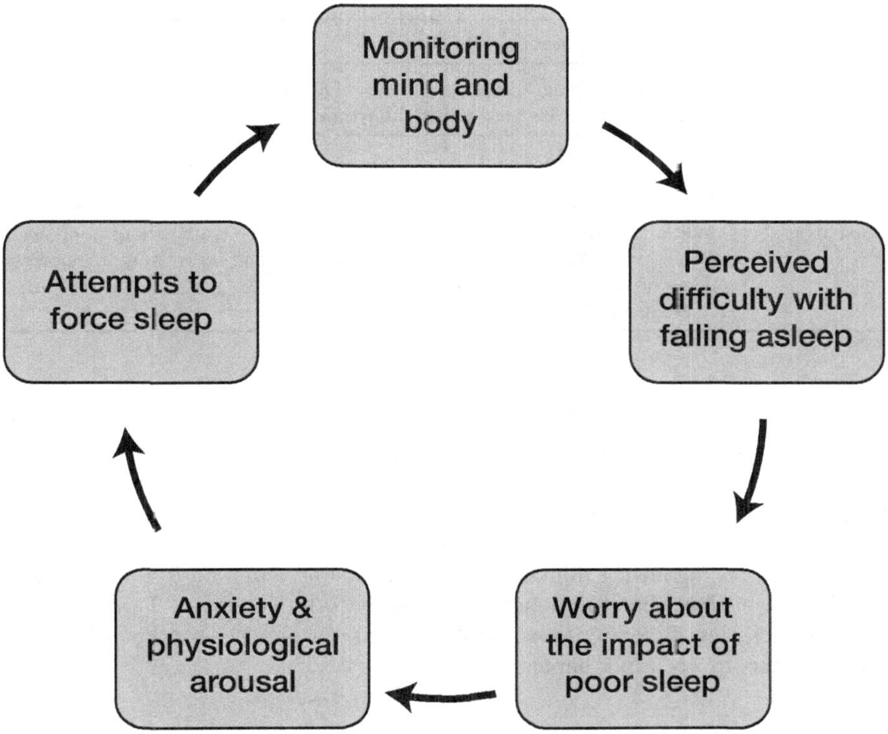

Figure 5.2 Vicious Cycle of Physiological and Psychological Contributors to Insomnia

Conditioned Arousal

For good sleepers, the wind-down period before bed and the bedroom itself are associated with feeling relaxed and sleepy. The bed and bedroom come to trigger a relaxed and sleepy response, as this is the feeling most often experienced in the sleeping environment.

When sleep is disrupted for a period of time, however, there is ample opportunity for the pre-sleep period or the bedroom to become associated with feeling alert and awake. In this case, the period of time before bed and the bedroom itself have become triggers for the mind becoming alert, emotions such as frustration and worry, and physiological arousal.

Going to bed has developed into an automatic trigger for increased alertness and arousal, which interferes with sleep. This is conditioned Insomnia. People experiencing this may describe that they can sense an increasing unease as bedtime approaches. Alternatively, they may report that although they can happily doze on the couch in the evening, they then feel alert when they attempt to sleep in bed.

Tying Things Together: Three Barriers to Restful Sleep

Low sleep drive, body clock disturbance, and elevated arousal are three barriers to restful sleep that operate both day and night. Accordingly, it is important to conceptualise Insomnia

Table 5.4 Three Barriers to Restful Sleep

Barriers	*Typical Behavioural and Cognitive Drivers*
Reduced sleep drive	Sleeping in, napping, dozing in the evening, low mood and motivation, reduced daytime activity levels, and reduced daytime stimulation
Body clock disturbance	Irregular sleep routine, lack of exposure to bright light during the day, exposure to bright light in the evening
Increased arousal	Conditioned arousal, anxiety and worry (this may be worry about poor sleep and/or worry about other topics), stress, lack of wind-down routine before sleep, caffeine or nicotine intake before bed, illicit drug use, and alcohol use (can increase arousal later in the night)

as a 24-hour disorder, not just a disorder of the night. What happens during the day affects sleep at night, and sleep at night affects mood, cognition, and behaviour during the day.

It is helpful to have factors affecting sleep drive, body clock, and arousal in mind when assessing sleep disturbance. Using this framework encourages the clinician to consider specifically how the disruptive factors a client presents with are disrupting healthy sleep regulation. Further, organising thinking about a clinical presentation in this way can assist in the selection of treatment components most likely to be beneficial. Table 5.4 provides examples of each class of barrier to restful sleep. We return to case conceptualisation using the three barriers to sleep in Chapters 7 and 8.

Predisposing, Precipitating, and Perpetuating Factors (the '3-P' Model of Insomnia)

We now move to the consideration of the aetiology of Insomnia, for which the '3-P' model of Insomnia is the most widely cited model (Spielman et al., 1987). In this model, *predisposing* factors combine with *precipitating* factors and *perpetuating* factors to explain the development of Insomnia. A stress of some kind precipitates an acute Insomnia episode in predisposed (vulnerable) individuals. If the Insomnia persists, perpetuating factors likely come into play. These include unhelpful behavioural and cognitive strategies that people employ in response to their poor sleep and tiredness. Perpetuating factors cause the Insomnia to become chronic, and it can continue long after the original stress or disruption has ended.

Table 5.5 provides examples of predisposing factors, precipitating factors, and perpetuating factors in Insomnia, and Figure 5.3 shows how these factors contribute differentially to acute and chronic phases of Insomnia. CBT-I focuses a great deal on the perpetuating factors.

Summary

- Sleep is a state of rest; however, the brain remains active.
- Sleep occurs in 90-minute cycles across the night that consist of four stages corresponding to dozing, light sleep, deep sleep, and dreaming.
- Sleep changes across the lifespan, with reduced total sleep time and deep sleep with advancing age.
- A healthy night of sleep consists of 1 hour or less of deep sleep and between two and five brief wakings.

Table 5.5 Predisposing, Precipitating, and Perpetuating Factors of Insomnia: Definition and Examples

Factors in 3P Model of Insomnia	*Definition*	*Examples*
Predisposing factors	Predisposing factors are individual characteristics that make an individual vulnerable to Insomnia	Family history of Insomnia Biological predisposition to being easily startled and physically tense Advanced age Female gender Altered brain function and sleep architecture
Precipitating factors	Precipitating factors are stressors or circumstances that people can identify as the trigger for the development of Insomnia	Physical illness or injury
	Precipitating factors are the immediate factors or events that have caused the person to present with or experience symptoms now	Onset of depression, anxiety, psychosis
	Without a precipitating factor or event, individuals with a predisposition to Insomnia may never develop the disorder	Adverse life events, grief, relationship conflict A change in situation (occupational, relationship, financial) Financial difficulty A sleep disorder such as OSA
Perpetuating factors	Perpetuating factors are maladaptive strategies that are developed in an attempt to cope with poor sleep (such as anxiety and conditioned arousal) and that keep the problem going	Anxiety about poor sleep (Table 5.3) can become a self-fulfilling prophecy owing to its effect of increasing arousal Spending excessive amounts of time in bed to compensate for poor sleep Increased usage of caffeine and other alerting agents Use of substances (medications, drugs, and alcohol) that help one to fall asleep, but impact on other sleep variables Reduced daytime activity and social contact

- Although the average sleep need is around 7 hours, it is important to recognise that sleep needs vary across individuals.
- Healthy sleep is regulated by an interaction between the sleep drive, the body clock, and arousal, which operate across the 24-hour period.
- It is important to assess for factors affecting the sleep drive, body clock, and arousal when treating Insomnia.
- Insomnia develops in response to a combination of vulnerability and triggering factors.
- Perpetuating factors in Insomnia are a major focus in CBT-I and are important to identify using the three-barriers framework.

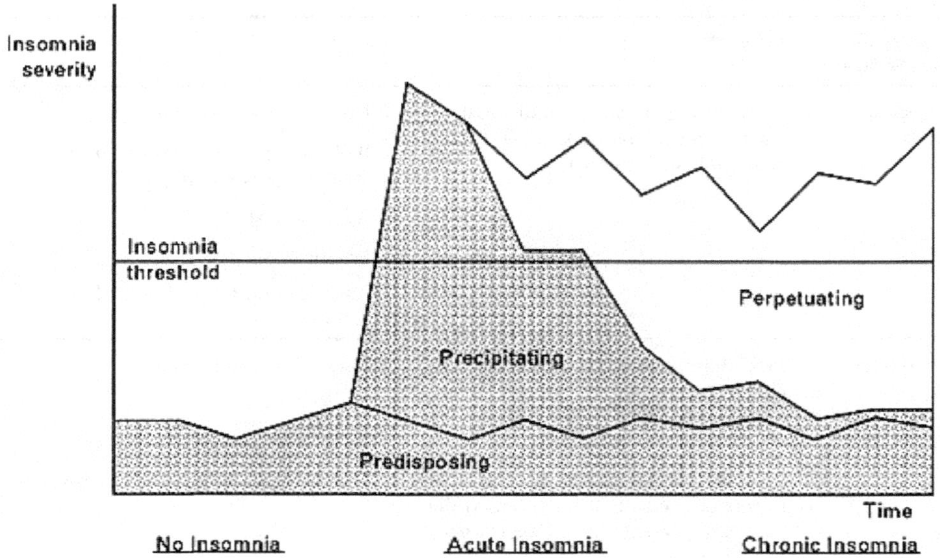

Figure 5.3 Contributions of Predisposing, Precipitating, and Perpetuating Factors in Acute and Chronic Stages of Insomnia

Sources: Spielman et al., 1987; adapted from Pigeon and Cribbet, 2012

References

Bellesi, M., Pfister-Genskow, M., Maret, S., Keles, S., Tononi, G., and Cirelli, C. (2013) "Effects of sleep and wake on oligodendrocytes and their precursors", *Journal of Neuroscience*, 33(36), pp. 14288–14300.

Bonnet, M. H., and Arand, D. L. (1995) "24-hour metabolic rate in insomniacs and matched normal sleepers", *Sleep*, 18(7), pp. 581–588.

Borbély, A. A. (1982) "A two process model of sleep regulation", *Human Neurobiology*, 1(3), pp. 195–204.

Harvey, A. G. (2002) "A cognitive model of insomnia", *Behaviour Research & Therapy*, 40, pp. 869–893.

Hirshkowitz, M., Whiton, K., Albert, S. M., Alessi, C., Bruni, O., DonCarlos, L., Hazen, N., Herman, J., Katz, E. S., Kheirandish-Gozal, L., Neubauer, D. N., O'Donnell, A. E., Ohayon, M., Peever, J., Rawding, R., Sachdeva, R. C., Setters, B., Vitiello, M. V., Ware, J. C., and Adams Hillard, P. J. (2015) "National Sleep Foundation's sleep time duration recommendations: Methodology and results summary", *Sleep Health*, 1(1), pp. 40–43.

Iber, C., Ancoli-Israel, S., Chesson, A., and Quan, S. F. (2007) *The AASM manual for the scoring of sleep and associated events: Rules, terminology and technical specifications* (1st ed.). Westchester, IL: American Academy of Sleep Medicine.

Kripke, D. F., Garfinkel, L., Wingard, D. L., Klauber, M. R., and Marler, M. R. (2002) "Mortality associated with sleep duration and insomnia", *Archives of General Psychiatry*, 59(2), pp. 131–136.

Kunz, D., and Herrmann, W. M. (2000) "Sleep–wake cycle, sleep-related disturbances, and sleep disorders: A chronobiological approach", *Comprehensive Psychiatry*, 41(2, suppl. 1), pp. 104–115.

Lundh, L.-G. (2005) "The role of acceptance and mindfulness in the treatment of Insomnia", *Journal of Cognitive Psychotherapy*, 19(1), pp. 29–39.

Lushington, K., Dawson, D., and Lack, L. (2000) "Core body temperature is elevated during constant wakefulness in elderly poor sleepers", *Sleep*, 23(4), pp. 504–510.

Morin, C. M., and Espie, C. A. (2004) *Insomnia: A clinical guide to assessment and treatment*. Boston, MA: Springer US.

Morin, C. M., Stone, J., Trinkle, D., Mercer, J., and Remsberg, S. (1993) "Dysfunctional beliefs and attitudes about sleep among older adults with and without insomnia complaints", *Psychology & Aging*, 8(3), pp. 463–467.

Morin, C. M., Vallières, A., and Ivers, H. (2007) "Dysfunctional beliefs and attitudes about sleep (DBAS): Validation of a brief version (DBAS-16)", *Sleep*, 30(11), p. 1547.

Ohayon, M. M., Carskadon, M. A., Guilleminault, C., and Vitiello, M. V. (2004) "Meta-analysis of quantitative sleep parameters from childhood to old age in healthy individuals: Developing normative sleep values across the human lifespan", *Sleep*, 27(7), pp. 1255–1273.

Pigeon, W. R., and Cribbet, M. R. (2012) "The pathophysiology of insomnia: From models to molecules (and back)", *Current Opinion in Pulmonary Medicine*, 18(6), pp. 546–553.

Ree, M. J., Harvey, A. G., Blake, R., Tang, N. K. Y., and Shawe-Taylor, M. (2005) "Attempts to control unwanted thoughts in the night: Development of the thought control questionnaire-insomnia revised (TCQI-R)", *Behaviour Research & Therapy*, 43, pp. 985–998.

Scheer, F. A., Cajochen, C., Turek, F. W., and Czeisler, C. A. (2005) "Melatonin in the regulation of sleep and circadian rhythms", in Kryger, M.H., Roth, T., and Dement, W.C. (Eds.) *Principles and practices of sleep medicine*. Philadelphia, PA: Elsevier Saunders, pp. 395–404.

Schulz, H. (2008) "Rethinking sleep analysis: Comment on the AASM Manual for the Scoring of Sleep and Associated Events", *Journal of Clinical Sleep Medicine: Official Publication of the American Academy of Sleep Medicine*, 4(2), pp. 99–103.

Semler, C. N., and Harvey, A. G. (2004) "Monitoring for sleep-related threat: A pilot study of the Sleep Associated Monitoring Index (SAMI)", *Psychosomatic Medicine*, 66(2), pp. 242–250.

Spielman, A. J., Caruso, L. S., and Glovinsky, P. B. (1987) "A behavioral perspective on insomnia treatment", *Psychiatric Clinics of North America*, 10(4), pp. 541–553.

Wells, A., and Davies, M. I. (1994) "The thought control questionnaire: A measure of individual differences in the control of unwanted thoughts", *Behaviour Research & Therapy*, 32(8), pp. 871–878.

Xie, L., Kang, H., Xu, Q., Chen, M. J., Liao, Y., Thiyagarajan, M., O'Donnell, J., Christensen, D. J., Nicholson, C., Iliff, J. J., Takano, T., Deane, R., and Nedergaard, M. (2013) "Sleep drives metabolite clearance from the adult brain", *Science*, 342(6156), pp. 373–377.

6 Understanding Insomnia and Other Sleep Disturbances in Psychotic Disorders

In the previous chapters, we explained how Insomnia and other sleep disturbances develop by way of an interaction between predisposing, precipitating, and perpetuating factors. The same applies to the development and maintenance of sleep disturbance in people with psychotic disorders. This chapter reviews the genetic and other physiological vulnerabilities that act as predisposing factors; the environmental and psychological stressors that may precipitate or trigger difficulties sleeping; and the behavioural and psychological factors that perpetuate Insomnia and prevent individuals from re-establishing normal sleep.

Predisposing Factors

Recall that a predisposing factor (see Chapter 5) is one that increases a person's vulnerability to Insomnia. Multiple neurobiological changes have been identified as predisposing factors to Insomnia in psychotic disorders.

Sleep Architecture

Sleep architecture refers to the way sleep is structured across the night. As discussed in Chapter 5, healthy sleep follows a fairly predictable structure across the night in terms of time spent in each sleep stage and in the ordering of these stages. Irregular cycling, absent sleep stages, and abnormal duration of sleep stages are examples of abnormal sleep architecture. Abnormalities in all stages have been demonstrated in psychotic disorders. These include greater periods of light sleep (stages N1 and N2), which increases the susceptibility to wakings; reduced latency to the first REM period (Monti and Monti, 2005; Benson, 2006; Cohrs, 2008); and decreases in the amount of deep sleep (Keshavan et al., 1990; Hudson et al., 1993).

Sleep spindles, as detected by EEG monitoring, are short bursts of brain activity that occur as NREM sleep becomes deeper. Sleep spindles are not well understood, but they are often seen to be a correlate of cognitive processing and have been linked to memory consolidation, learning, and cortical development. In psychotic disorders, the number of sleep spindles is reduced in comparison with non-psychotic controls (Ferrarelli et al., 2007; Manoach et al., 2010, 2014) and increased in mood disorders (de Maertelaer et al., 1987), together with increases in REM density (Hudson et al., 1993).

Chronobiology and Circadian Rhythms

Chronobiology is a branch of biology that investigates the cyclical nature of biological changes. In humans, chronobiology works towards understanding of how the body clock or circadian rhythm operates. Investigations in schizophrenia and mood disorders have identified dysregulations in the production and timing of hormones such as melatonin and cortisol that are likely causes of body clock dysregulation (Sachar et al., 1973; Van Cauter et al., 1991; Rao et al., 1994; Wulff et al., 2012). Studies suggest that up to 50 per cent of individuals with chronic schizophrenia have abnormally low increases in melatonin during the night, and this is linked to a delay in their sleep–wake timing(Vigano et al., 2001). Therefore, disruptions in circadian rhythms might make it more difficult for people with psychotic disorders to maintain normally timed, regular sleep–wake patterns.

Genetic Vulnerability

Increasing evidence suggests that chronobiological dysregulations may be linked to genetic abnormalities in clock genes. In bipolar disorder, these clock genes have been linked to reduced sleep needs, a preference for evening activity, greater severity of Insomnia, and a higher recurrence of manic episodes (Lamont et al., 2010). Further support for the notion of a genetic contribution to sleep problems in psychotic disorders comes from studies showing that sleep architecture problems are heritable in families in which at least one member has schizophrenia (Sarkar et al., 2010; Manoach et al., 2014) or bipolar disorder (Pagani et al., 2016).

Neurotransmitters

Multiple neurotransmitters are implicated in sleep, and the transition between sleep stages, including high levels of acetylcholine (ACh), low levels of serotonin (5HT), and elevated levels of gamma-aminobutyric acid (GABA). In psychotic disorders, there is also evidence of GABA, dopamine, and serotonin dysregulation (Rao et al., 1994; Dzirasa et al., 2006; Kantrowitz et al., 2009), explaining the close relationship between sleep problems and psychotic disorders. Such neurotransmitter dysfunction would act to disrupt the onset of sleep, increase night-time wakings, and impact on the timing and transition between sleep stages.

Physical Health

Poor physical health, particularly with regards to bodily pain and general health, has been identified as a predisposing factor for Insomnia in the general population (LeBlanc et al., 2009). Similarly, this also applies to people with psychotic disorders, in whom chronic pain and poor physical health are common features. Physical health problems may prompt individuals to perceive a greater need for sleep (where there may or may not be a real need for increased amounts of sleep) and increase concerns about sleep. Lifestyle habits such as insufficient exercise, smoking, and excessive use of alcohol and other substances may predispose individuals to Insomnia through their potential to change sleep drive, increase arousal, affect nocturnal breathing ability, change sleep architecture, and reduce effective coping abilities over time.

Precipitating Factors

Recall that a precipitating factor (Chapter 5) is one that triggers an episode of Insomnia. Sleep disturbances, however, resolve themselves naturally following resolution of the precipitant, unless perpetuating factors develop. Precipitating factors, like vulnerability factors, span the biopsychosocial spectrum.

Stress and Environment

The prevalence of negative life events and trauma, such as physical or sexual abuse, is much higher in people with psychotic disorders than in the general population (Read and Ross, 2003; Galletly et al., 2011). Such stressors serve as a strong precipitator of Insomnia. Common stressful events that precipitate Insomnia in people with psychotic disorders include the death of a loved one, loss of employment, domestic violence, removal of children by child protection services, divorce, and family lawsuit, as well as possible trauma associated with a mental health treatment order. Trauma can have an enduring impact on the ability to fall asleep. It can lead to hyperarousal, fear of sleeping, flashbacks, and chronic nightmares that result in frequent night awakenings and difficulties going back to sleep (Chiu et al., 2016).

Stressful events can also increase arousal by way of worry, irritability, rumination, anxiety, and depressed mood. In addition to night-time arousal, stress can impair motivation to follow a daytime routine. Biologically, stress also impacts on sleep via its effect on the hypothalamic–pituitary–adrenal (HPA) axis, which is our central stress response system. Stress acts to release HPA hormones, which in turn release cortisol. Chronic stress causes HPA hyperactivity and excessive cortisol, which leads to awakenings, shortened sleep time, sleep fragmentation, and night-time awakenings (Buckley and Schatzberg, 2005).

Lifestyle Factors

Owing to their disability, people with psychotic disorders are often sedentary and have lifestyle factors that include daytime napping, smoking, substance abuse and poor diet, and lack of regular daily structure (Galletly, 2012). Such lifestyle issues can act as predisposing, precipitating, and perpetuating factors. Each of these factors has the capacity to trigger Insomnia. A lack of exposure to environmental 'time' cues (zeitgebers), such as fixed activity schedules, exercise and meal times, and daylight exposure, also places people at risk of circadian dysregulation. Many individuals with psychotic disorders are unaware of factors that promote or interfere with sleep (Chiu et al., 2015).

Mental Health Triggers

In people with psychotic disorders, common triggers for Insomnia relate to a deterioration in their mental health. The onset or worsening of psychiatric symptoms is accompanied by a reduced ability to cope with everyday problems, social isolation, and night-time wakings, and can lead to increased time in bed, as an avoidance or compensatory strategy, and the development of other behaviours that are incompatible with good sleep.

As discussed in Chapter 4, an acute psychotic episode is a common precipitant of Insomnia. Heightened arousal occurs in response to delusions, feelings of paranoia, and frightening hallucinations. This is accompanied by a perception of loss of control over one's life, and loss of confidence and self-efficacy. For those with anxiety and panic disorders, nocturnal panic attacks can increase arousal and trigger sleeping difficulties. For clients with trauma, the experience of flashbacks in the middle of the night can cause multiple wakings in a panicked state.

Other Sleep Disorders

There are many sleep disorders that can act as precipitating factors for Insomnia. Respiratory-related sleep disorders such as OSA are a common condition in psychotic disorders. OSA leads to night-time wakings owing to obstruction of the airways causing the sensation of gasping for air. Severe daytime tiredness, which often accompanies OSA, and compensatory behaviours (reduced activity levels, excessive use of stimulants) all get in the way of good sleep habits and, therefore, contribute to precipitating the development of Insomnia.

Parasomnias such as Night-Eating Syndrome are also more common in people with psychotic disorders than in the general population, with a prevalence of 12–25 per cent (Lundgren et al., 2010; Palmese et al., 2013). With large quantities of food being digested overnight, individuals may find that it takes longer to fall asleep, and that they wake frequently during the night. Night-eating has been linked to disruptions to sleep–ake circadian patterns, and it can foster low mood, with feelings of frustration, guilt, and low self-esteem (O'Reardon et al., 2004; Allison et al., 2007; Goel et al., 2009). Other parasomnias, including sleep paralysis and sleep-related hallucinations accompanied by the sensation of a 'felt presence' in the bedroom, also offset healthy sleep–bedroom associations.

Use of and Withdrawal from Substances

A diagnosis of substance abuse is 4.6 times higher among people with psychotic disorders than in the general population. Approximately 47 per cent show some form of substance abuse or dependence (Regier et al., 1990). Although the use of substances (marijuana, amphetamines, etc.) can cause sleep problems in psychotic disorders, so too can the withdrawal of illicit substances (Budney et al., 2004) and long-term use of prescribed medications (Staedt et al., 1996; Chemerinksi et al., 2002). Substance use can be both a precipitating factor and a perpetuating factor.

Medications

Medications can have a direct effect on sleep, either by causing or resolving sleep problems. Some antipsychotic medications are linked to improvements in total sleep duration, the time taken to fall asleep, and overall sleep efficiency (Lieberman et al., 2005; Cohrs, 2008; Winokur and Kamath, 2008), although studies show that difficulties with wakings and daytime tiredness still remain. Changes in sleep architecture (such as increased stage 2 sleep) caused by these medications may contribute to wakings (Ferrarelli and Benca, 2010). Subjective (self-reported) effects on sleep and daytime functions are summarised in Table 6.1.

Perpetuating Factors

Perpetuating factors keep the Insomnia going once it has started, even when precipitating factors are no longer at play. Perpetuating factors include unhelpful behavioural and cognitive strategies that people employ in response to their poor sleep and tiredness.

Behavioural Perpetuating Factors

These are common unhelpful behaviours that develop in an attempt to cope with Insomnia. They include:

- compensating for poor sleep by spending extra time in bed overnight or napping during the day;
- engaging in non-sleep-related activities in bed (e.g. watching TV, eating, smoking, and using computers or social media);

Table 6.1 Effects of Various Medications and Substances on Sleep

Medication or Substance Type	*Self-reported Effects on Sleep and Daytime Functions*
Antipsychotic drugs	– Shorter time to fall asleep – Increased total sleep time – Increased sleep efficiency – Morning tiredness and daytime somnolence – Nightmares – Increased risk of restless leg syndrome, parasomnias, and breathing-related sleep disorders
Antidepressants (tricyclic & monoamine oxidase inhibitors (MAOIs)	– Increased time to fall asleep – Decreased sleep time – Night-time wakings – Daytime somnolence
Antidepressants—selective serotonin-reuptake inhibitors (SSRIs), serotonin-norepinephrine-reuptake inhibitors (SNRIs)	– Increased time to fall asleep – Decreased sleep time – Decreased sleep efficiency – Night-time wakings – Increased frequency and intensity of dreaming – Daytime somnolence
Sedative and hypnotic drugs, including benzodiazepines	– Shorter time to fall asleep – Increased sleep efficiency – Increased total sleep time – Reduced respiratory drive, especially when combined with alcohol – Daytime somnolence and 'hangover' effects
Lithium	– Improved timing of sleep–wake patterns – Increased risk of restless leg syndrome and parasomnias
Melatonin	– Shorter time to fall asleep – Improved timing of sleep–wake patterns
Melatonin-analogues, agomelatine Beta blockers	– Improved sleep efficiency – Improved timing of sleep – Daytime somnolence – Vivid dreams – Nightmares – Increased risk of parasomnias and restless leg syndrome
Antihistamines	– Shorter time to fall asleep – Daytime somnolence
Alcohol	– Shorter time to fall asleep – Decreased sleep efficiency – Night-time wakings – Morning tiredness and daytime somnolence – Delays in circadian sleep phase
Cannabis	– Shorter time to fall asleep – Morning tiredness and daytime somnolence
Nicotine	– Longer time to fall asleep – Reduced total sleep time
Opioid drugs (morphine, heroin, codeine)	– Reduced total sleep time – Morning tiredness and daytime somnolence
Stimulants (caffeine, amphetamine, cocaine)	– Increased time to fall asleep – Decreased total sleep time – Decreased sleep efficiency – Daytime somnolence

- reducing daytime activity levels owing to being tired and having low self-efficacy (e.g. staying inside, social withdrawal, cancelling appointments, lack of engagement in activities);
- use of substances to either stimulate (e.g. nicotine, caffeine, illicit drugs) or sedate (alcohol, hypnotic medication, illicit drug use) to cope with tiredness or facilitate sleep, respectively.

These factors overlap with those listed in the precipitating factors section above. A conceptual rule of thumb is that a perpetuating factor is one that commenced *after* the onset of the sleep disturbance and is employed in response to the poor sleep and tiredness.

Cognitive Perpetuating Factors

People with psychotic disorders have similar types of dysfunctional beliefs and thought control strategies to those that maintain Insomnia in the general community (Harvey et al., 2005; Chiu et al., 2015). In addition to these Insomnia-specific contributors, other psychological factors include intrusive cognitions, worry, racing thoughts, and psychotic symptoms (see Table 6.2).

Other Psychological Perpetuating Factors

A lack of motivation and negative symptoms, such as anhedonia, are major hurdles to improving sleep and engaging in daytime activities. Individuals may comment on the pointlessness of strict sleep routines and resisting the urge to nap, given the limited activities to look forward to (Chiu et al., 2016). CBT-I adaptations for psychosis include motivational interviewing, decisional balance exercises, self-efficacy ratings, the use of carers as support resources, scheduling short sessions later in the day, and simplified material using lay language and visual contents with large print size.

Finally, stigma and shame can perpetuate poor sleep. When a person is in remission, memories of inappropriate activities performed during a psychotic episode can dominate ruminative thoughts. Feelings of guilt, embarrassment, anger, as well as a loss of control and anxieties about the future can perpetuate arousal and negative thoughts at night. The stigma of having a mental illness can also reinforce unhelpful lifestyle behaviours and may be a contributing factor that stops someone seeking help for sleep problems outside mental health settings (Fung et al., 2008).

Summary

- Predisposing factors to Insomnia in psychotic disorders include genetic vulnerabilities and neurobiological changes.
- Precipitating factors might include acute stress, poor mental health, and substance abuse or other sleep disorders.
- Perpetuating factors including poor knowledge about sleep hygiene, compensatory behaviours, unhelpful beliefs about sleep, an external locus of control, and a busy mind, which can be addressed with conventional techniques taught in CBT-I.
- Symptoms of psychotic disorders such as hallucinations, delusions, and low motivation can be addressed with education, a person-oriented approach, and engagement in meaningful and rewarding activities.

Table 6.2 Cognitive Perpetuating Factors in Psychotic Disorders

Cognitive Perpetuating Factors	*Description*
Rumination, and racing thoughts at night	Rumination and racing thoughts are common features of psychotic disorders. They interfere with the initiation of sleep in this clinical group
Maladaptive thought control strategies (e.g., as assessed by the Thought Control Questionnaire Insomnia-Revised; Ree et al., 2005)	People with psychotic disorders report using unhelpful strategies of worry (e.g. 'I dwell on worries') and aggressive suppression (e.g. 'I get angry at myself for having the thought') in order to manage unwanted thoughts. Methods for fostering use of helpful thought control strategies include education about how to process worries and engage the mind away from the unwanted thought
Dysfunctional beliefs and attitudes about sleep (assessed by the DBAS; Morin et al., 2007)	Over-concern about the consequences of poor sleep is common in people with psychotic disorders and may lead to anxiety and behaviours such as 'catch-up' sleep during the day. Therapeutic strategies in CBT-I include relaxation training, cognitive restructuring (forming more helpful beliefs about sleep), and sleep education
External locus of control	Individuals with psychosis tend to attribute the cause of their sleep problems to their psychiatric illness, rather than behavioural and cognitive factors over which they can exert some influence. In other words, they believe that sleep problems are primarily due to (unchangeable) biological factors, rather than a direct influence of (changeable) psychological and behavioural factors. Psychoeducation about sleep and behavioural experiments can be used to improve unhelpful cognitions, behaviours, and gaps in knowledge around how to improve sleep
Hallucinations and delusions	Hallucinations and delusional thoughts often increase in frequency and intensity in the evening, when there is a reduced capacity for distraction and opportunities to engage in other activities. This is associated with increased fear, rumination, and, therefore, arousal and wakefulness. Education and CBT approaches to psychotic symptoms (e.g. Wykes et al., 1999; Casstevens, 2006) may be used as a means of eliciting helpful thought patterns and helpful behavioural strategies

Source: Chiu et al., 2015, 2016

References

Allison, K. C., Grilo, C. M., Masheb, R. M., and Stunkard, A. J. (2007) "High self-reported rates of neglect and emotional abuse, by persons with binge eating disorder and night eating syndrome", *Behaviour Research & Therapy*, 45(12), pp. 2874–2883.

Benson, K. L. (2006) "Sleep in schizophrenia: Impairments, correlates, and treatment", *Psychiatric Clinics of North America*, 29(4), pp. 1033–1045.

Buckley, T. M., and Schatzberg, A. F. (2005) "On the interactions of the hypothalamic–pituitary–adrenal (HPA) axis and sleep: Normal HPA axis activity and circadian rhythm, exemplary sleep disorders", *Journal of Clinical Endocrinology & Metabolism*, 90(5), pp. 3106–3114.

Budney, A. J., Hughes, J. R., Moore, B. A., and Vandrey, R. (2004) "Review of the validity and significance of cannabis withdrawal syndrome", *American Journal of Psychiatry*, 161(11), pp. 1967–1977.

Casstevens, W. J. (2006) Evaluation of a mentored self-help intervention for the management of psychotic symptoms. FIU Electronic Theses and Dissertations.

Chemerinksi, E., Ho, B.-C., Flaum, M., Arndt, S., Fleming, F., and Andreasen, N. C. (2002) "Insomnia as a predictor for symptom worsening following antipsychotic withdrawal in schizophrenia", *Comprehensive Psychiatry*, 43(5), pp. 393–396.

Chiu, V. W., Harvey, R. H., Sloan, N. B., Ree, M., Lin, A., Janca, A., and Waters, F. (2015) "Cognitive and behavioral factors associated with insomnia in inpatients with schizophrenia and related psychoses", *Journal of Nervous & Mental Disease*, 203(10), pp. 798–803.

Chiu, V. W., Ree, M., Janca, A., and Waters, F. (2016) "Sleep in schizophrenia: Exploring subjective experiences of sleep problems, and implications for treatment", *Psychiatric Quarterly*, 87(4), pp. 633–648.

Cohrs, S. (2008) "Sleep disturbances in patients with schizophrenia: Impact and effect of antipsychotics", *CNS Drugs*, 22(11), pp. 939–962.

de Maertelaer, V., Hoffman, G., Lemaire, M., and Mendlewicz, J. (1987) "Sleep spindle activity changes in patients with affective disorders", *Sleep*, 10(5), pp. 443–451.

Dzirasa, K., Ribeiro, S., Costa, R., Santos, L. M., Lin, S.-C., Grosmark, A., Sotnikova, T. D., Gainetdinov, R. R., Caron, M. G., and Nicolelis, M. A. L. (2006) "Dopaminergic control of sleep–wake states", *Journal of Neuroscience*, 26(41), pp. 10577–10589.

Ferrarelli, F., and Benca, R. M. (2010) "Neurophysiology and neuroimaging of human sleep", in Winkelman, J. W., and Plante, D. T. (Eds.) *Foundations of psychiatric sleep medicine*. New York: Cambridge University Press, pp. 36–43.

Ferrarelli, F., Huber, R., Peterson, M. J., Massimini, M., Murphy, M., Riedner, B. A., Watson, A., Bria, P., and Tononi, G. (2007) "Reduced sleep spindle activity in schizophrenia patients", *American Journal of Psychiatry*, 164(3), pp. 483–492.

Fung, K. M. T., Tsang, H. W. H., and Corrigan, P. W. (2008) "Self-stigma of people with schizophrenia as predictor of their adherence to psychosocial treatment", *Psychiatric Rehabilitation Journal*, 32(2), pp. 95–104.

Galletly, C. (2012) "People living with psychosis: The good news and the bad news", *Australian & New Zealand Journal of Psychiatry*, 46(9), pp. 803–807.

Galletly, C., Van Hooff, M., and McFarlane, A. (2011) "Psychotic symptoms in young adults exposed to childhood trauma—A 20 year follow-up study", *Schizophrenia Research*, 127(1–3), pp. 76–82.

Goel, N., Stunkard, A. J., Rogers, N. L., Van Dongen, H. P. A., Allison, K. C., O'Reardon, J. P., Ahima, R. S., Cummings, D. E., Heo, M., and Dinges, D. F. (2009) "Circadian rhythm profiles in women with night eating syndrome", *Journal of Biological Rhythms*, 24(1), pp. 85–94.

Harvey, A. G., Tang, N. K. Y., and Browning, L. (2005) "Cognitive approaches to insomnia", *Clinical Psychology Review*, 25(5), pp. 593–611.

Hudson, J. I., Lipinski, J. F., Keck Jr, P. E., Aizley, H. G., Vuckovic, A., Zierk, K. C., and Pope Jr, H. G. (1993) "Polysomnographic characteristics of schizophrenia in comparison with mania and depression", *Biological Psychiatry*, 34(3), pp. 191–193.

Kantrowitz, J., Citrome, L., and Javitt, D. (2009) "GABAB receptors, schizophrenia and sleep dysfunction", *CNS Drugs*, 23(8), pp. 681–691.

Keshavan, M. S., Reynolds, C. F., and Kupfer, D. J. (1990) "Electroencephalographic sleep in schizophrenia: A critical review", *Comprehensive Psychiatry*, 31(1), pp. 34–47.

Lamont, E. W., Coutu, D. L., Cermakian, N., and Boivin, D. B. (2010) "Circadian rhythms and clock genes in psychotic disorders", *Israel Journal of Psychiatry & Related Sciences*, 47(1), pp. 27–35.

LeBlanc, M., Mérette, C., Savard, J., Ivers, H., Baillargeon, L., and Morin, C. M. (2009) "Incidence and risk factors of insomnia in a population-based sample", *Sleep*, 32(8), pp. 1027–1037.

Lieberman, J. A., Stroup, T. S., McEvoy, J. P., Swartz, M. S., Rosenheck, R. A., Perkins, D. O., Keefe, R. S. E., Davis, S. M., Davis, C. E., Lebowitz, B. D., Severe, J., and Hsiao, J. K. (2005)

"Effectiveness of antipsychotic drugs in patients with chronic schizophrenia", *New England Journal of Medicine*, 353(12), pp. 1209–1223.

Lundgren, J. D., Rempfer, M. V., Brown, C. E., Goetz, J., and Hamera, E. (2010) "The prevalence of night eating syndrome and binge eating disorder among overweight and obese individuals with serious mental illness", *Psychiatry Research*, 175(3), pp. 233–236.

Manoach, D. S., Demanuele, C., Wamsley, E. J., Vangel, M., Montrose, D. M., Miewald, J., Kupfer, D., Buysse, D., Stickgold, R., and Keshavan, M. S. (2014) "Sleep spindle deficits in antipsychotic-naïve early course schizophrenia and in non-psychotic first-degree relatives", *Frontiers in Human Neuroscience*, 8, p. 762.

Manoach, D. S., Thakkar, K. N., Stroynowski, E., Ely, A., McKinley, S. K., Wamsley, E., Djonlagic, I., Vangel, M. G., Goff, D. C., and Stickgold, R. (2010) "Reduced overnight consolidation of procedural learning in chronic medicated schizophrenia is related to specific sleep stages", *Journal of Psychiatric Research*, 44(2), pp. 112–120.

Monti, J. M., and Monti, D. (2005) "Sleep disturbance in schizophrenia", *International Review of Psychiatry*, 17(4), pp. 247–253.

Morin, C. M., Vallières, A., and Ivers, H. (2007) "Dysfunctional beliefs and attitudes about sleep (DBAS): Validation of a brief version (DBAS-16)", *Sleep*, 30(11), p. 1547.

O'Reardon, J. P., Ringel, B. L., Dinges, D. F., Allison, K. C., Rogers, N. L., Martino, N. S., and Stunkard, A. J. (2004) "Circadian eating and sleeping patterns in the night eating syndrome", *Obesity Research*, 12(11), pp. 1789–1796.

Pagani, L., St. Clair, P. A., Teshiba, T. M., Service, S. K., Fears, S. C., Araya, C., Araya, X., Bejarano, J., Ramirez, M., Castrillón, G., Gomez-Makhinson, J., Lopez, M. C., Montoya, G., Montoya, C. P., Aldana, I., Navarro, L., Freimer, D. G., Safaie, B., Keung, L.-W., Greenspan, K., Chou, K., Escobar, J. I., Ospina-Duque, J., Kremeyer, B., Ruiz-Linares, A., Cantor, R. M., Lopez-Jaramillo, C., Macaya, G., Molina, J., Reus, V. I., Sabatti, C., Bearden, C. E., Takahashi, J. S., and Freimer, N. B. (2016) "Genetic contributions to circadian activity rhythm and sleep pattern phenotypes in pedigrees segregating for severe bipolar disorder", *Proceedings of the National Academy of Sciences*, 113(6), pp. E754–E761.

Palmese, L. B., Ratliff, J. C., Reutenauer, E. L., Tonizzo, K. M., Grilo, C. M., and Tek, C. (2013) "Prevalence of night eating in obese individuals with schizophrenia and schizoaffective disorder", *Comprehensive Psychiatry*, 54(3), pp. 276–281.

Rao, M. L., Gross, G., Strebel, B., Halaris, A., Huber, G., Bräunig, P., and Marler, M. (1994) "Circadian rhythm of tryptophan, serotonin, melatonin, and pituitary hormones in schizophrenia", *Biological Psychiatry*, 35(3), pp. 151–163.

Read, J., and Ross, C. A. (2003) "Psychological trauma and psychosis: Another reason why people diagnosed schizophrenic must be offered psychological therapies", *Journal of the American Academy of Psychoanalysis & Dynamic Psychiatry*, 31(1), pp. 247–268.

Ree, M. J., Harvey, A. G., Blake, R., Tang, N. K. Y., and Shawe-Taylor, M. (2005) "Attempts to control unwanted thoughts in the night: Development of the thought control questionnaire-insomnia revised (TCQI-R)", *Behaviour Research & Therapy*, 43, pp. 985–998.

Regier, D. A., Farmer, M. E., Rae, D. S., Locke, B. Z., Keith, S. J., Judd, L. L., and Goodwin, F. K. (1990) "Comorbidity of mental disorders with alcohol and other drug abuse: Results from the epidemiologic catchment area (eca) study", *JAMA*, 264(19), pp. 2511–2518.

Sachar, E. J., Hellman, L., Roffwarg, H. P., Halpern, F. S., Fukushima, D. K., and Gallagher, T. F. (1973) "Disrupted 24-hour patterns of cortisol secretion in psychotic depression", *Archives of General Psychiatry*, 28(1), pp. 19–24.

Sarkar, S., Katshu, M. Z. U. H., Nizamie, S. H., and Praharaj, S. K. (2010) "Slow wave sleep deficits as a trait marker in patients with schizophrenia", *Schizophrenia Research*, 124, pp. 127–133.

Staedt, J., Stoppe, G., Hajak, G., and Rüther, E. (1996) "Rebound insomnia after abrupt clozapine withdrawal", *European Archives of Psychiatry & Clinical Neuroscience*, 246(2), pp. 79–82.

Van Cauter, E., Linkowski, P., Kerkhofs, M., Hubain, P., L'Hermite-Baleriaux, M., Leclercq, R., Brasseur, M., Copinschi, G., and Mendlewicz, J. (1991) "Circadian and sleep-related endocrine rhythms in schizophrenia", *Archives of General Psychiatry*, 48(4), pp. 348–56.

Vigano, D., Lissoni, P., Rovelli, F., Roselli, M. G., Malugani, F., Gavazzeni, C., Conti, A., and Maestroni, G. (2001) "A study of light/dark rhythm of melatonin in relation to cortisol and prolactin secretion in schizophrenia", *Neuroendocrinology Letters*, 22(2), pp. 137–141.

Winokur, A., and Kamath, J. (2008) "The effect of typical and atypical antipsychotic drugs on sleep of schizophrenic patients", in *Serotonin and sleep: Molecular, functional and clinical aspects*, pp. 587–610 [online]. Available at: http://dx.doi.org/10.1007/978-3-7643-8561-3_24 (accessed November 22, 2016).

Wulff, K., Dijk, D. J., Middleton, B., Foster, R. G., and Joyce, E. (2012) "Sleep and circadian rhythm disruption in schizophrenia", *British Journal of Psychiatry*, 200, pp. 308–316.

Wykes, T., Parr, A. M., and Landau, S. (1999) "Group treatment of auditory hallucinations: Exploratory study of effectiveness", *British Journal of Psychiatry*, 175(2), pp. 180–185.

7 Description of Cognitive Behavioural Therapy for Insomnia

This chapter discusses treatment options for Insomnia, focusing primarily on CBT-I. A knowledge of normal sleep and its regulation, as well as the aetiology of Insomnia, is important for understanding the rationale behind CBT-I components. Accordingly, we suggest that you read Chapter 5 on sleep and its regulation before embarking on the current chapter.

This chapter begins by reiterating the importance of treating Insomnia and sleep disturbances in their own right, followed by a brief discussion regarding pharmacological treatment options (including commonly prescribed medications in psychotic populations). Next, we provide a review of CBT-I research outcomes and describe typical CBT-I components. Finally, we outline the main adaptations to CBT-I in the context of psychosis. We apply the three barriers to sleep (arousal, reduced sleep drive, and circadian rhythm disruption) presented in Chapter 5 to sleep disturbance in psychosis. The resulting treatment protocol, the Sleep Well, Feel Well with Psychosis programme, is presented in Parts II and III of this book. Interventions relevant for symptoms of hypersomnia, circadian rhythm disturbance, and nightmare disorder are also mentioned, as these often present in psychotic populations. For brevity, we refer to features of hypersomnia, circadian rhythm disturbances, and nightmare disorders collectively as 'other sleep disturbances'.

The Importance of Independent Treatment of Insomnia and Other Sleep Disturbances

Despite the high prevalence and burden of sleep disturbances in the general population, they often go unidentified and untreated. People often use self-help remedies of limited benefit rather than seek professional help for poor sleep (Morin et al., 2006b). For those Insomnia sufferers that do seek professional help, treatment is usually limited to pharmacotherapy (Charles et al., 2009; Everitt et al., 2014), with as many as 95 per cent of clients receiving hypnotic medication without CBT-I (Charles et al., 2009).

In the context of psychosis, a qualitative study conducted with 14 individuals with schizophrenia-spectrum disorders found that only 50 per cent had sought help from a doctor or other health professional for their sleep difficulties. Of those who sought help, all were given pharmacotherapy, and none was offered CBT-I. Only one was provided with psychoeducation (Chiu, n.d.).

Low rates of referral for psychological interventions such as CBT-I are in part due to a lack of awareness of the techniques it uses and its effectiveness. There is also a perception of it being an expensive treatment option and one that has few properly trained practitioners (see Benca, 2005, for a review). Whether they are treated with CBT-I, pharmacotherapy, or both, we support the view that independent assessment and treatment of Insomnia and other sleep disturbances should become the standard for all clients (Sateia and Nowell, 2004).

Pharmacotherapy as a Treatment Option

Hypnotic medications (commonly referred to as 'sleeping pills') are designed to induce or prolong sleep. These form the most commonly utilised treatment for Insomnia in primary care settings (Charles et al., 2009). Many hypnotics described in this chapter are benzodiazepines (e.g. temazepam, flurazepam, nitrazepam).

There is substantial evidence that benzodiazepines can assist in the initiation and maintenance of sleep; are appropriate for treating transient, short-term Insomnia; and can provide immediate relief. These advantages, however, are moderated by high risk of side effects and long-term dependence. Potential adverse effects of benzodiazepines include dependence, tolerance, altered sleep architecture (increased stages N1 and N2 sleep, and reduced REM and deep sleep), next day 'hangover effects', cognitive performance decrements, falls, and undesired behaviours during sleep (e.g. sleep-walking and sleep-eating). Therefore, they are recommended for short-term use only (Schutte-Rodin et al., 2008; Krystal, 2009).

Another, newer, class of drugs used in Insomnia and circadian rhythm disturbances includes 'non-benzodiazepines', such as *benzodiazepine receptor agonistic modulators* (BzRAs), which are often referred to as '*z-drugs*'. Z-drugs include zolpidem, zaleplon, and zopiclone. Z-drugs show a better side-effect profile and a reduced impact on sleep architecture relative to benzodiazepines (Montplaisir et al., 2003). However, these 'non-benzodiazepines' still have risks and may become habit-forming. Side effects for some people include night-eating, nausea, headache, anterograde amnesia, hallucinations, and nightmares, as well as panic when withdrawal is attempted (Siriwardena et al., 2008; Gunja, 2013). In people predisposed to sleep-walking (somnambulism), they can cause increased sleep-walking behaviours and sleep-driving, particularly when combined with alcohol (Gunja, 2013).

Synthetic *melatonin* (in short-release and sustained-release preparations) and melatonin receptor agonists (melatonin analogues such as ramelteon and agomelatine) are often used to treat poor sleep where there is circadian rhythm disturbance. There is evidence that careful timing of oral melatonin is useful to address circadian rhythm disorders (e.g. Aurora et al., 2010). Sustained-release melatonin is also approved to treat age-related Insomnia in older adults (55 years and older), as melatonin levels tend to decline with age. Studies have shown that low doses of melatonin can improve sleep in older adults and appear to have a lower side-effect profile than hypnotic medications (Zhdanova et al., 2001; Lemoine et al., 2007). For cases of Insomnia that are not age-related and do not feature circadian rhythm disturbance, melatonin has reduced efficacy (Ferracioli-Oda et al., 2013).

Antidepressant and *antiepileptic* drugs are frequently used off-label to treat Insomnia, although their efficacy and safety for the treatment of chronic Insomnia is not well documented (Schutte-Rodin et al., 2008). In the context of psychotic disorders, *antipsychotic medications* are commonly used. First-generation antipsychotics (e.g. thioridazine) and second-generation antipsychotics (e.g. clozapine, olanzapine, and quetiapine) increase total sleep time, sleep efficiency, and sleep latency (Cohrs, 2008; Winokur and Kamath, 2008), although it is noteworthy that Insomnia symptoms and daytime somnolence often remain. Changes in sleep architecture, including increases in stage 2 sleep and reduced deep sleep, may contribute to wakings and daytime sleepiness.

Stimulants, such as methylphenidate or modafinil, or certain antidepressants, may be prescribed to address hypersomnia, excessive daytime sleepiness, and narcolepsy. However, an optimal balance between providing an effective level of daytime stimulation without causing poor sleep at night (leading to increased dose of sedative medication) can be challenging to achieve.

Some drugs are prescribed to help realign sleep–wake cycles to a regular schedule. These include lithium in bipolar disorder, which can act as a synchroniser and stabiliser of circadian rhythms, atypical neuroleptics, and sedatives in the short term (Borodkin and Dagan, 2010).

Finally, non-prescription drugs and naturopathic agents are also frequently used to treat Insomnia. These include antihistamines, analgesics, valerian, hops, and passion flower. Evidence regarding the efficacy and safety of these agents is limited (see Schutte-Rodin et al., 2008).

Cognitive Behavioural Therapy for Insomnia

CBT-I is a multi-component treatment that includes a combination of psychoeducation, including sleep hygiene education, behavioural interventions (stimulus control, sleep restriction therapy, maximising daytime energy, relaxation), and cognitive interventions (managing negative thoughts, managing unhelpful beliefs about sleep, managing a busy mind) to address reduced sleep drive, hyperarousal, and circadian disruption, which are thought to perpetuate the disorder.

CBT is the therapy of thoughts and behaviour:

C = cognition (the 'cogs' of the mind: thoughts, beliefs, worries, attention)
B = behaviour (how people act)
T = therapy

There is overwhelmingly strong evidence that CBT-I is an effective treatment for Insomnia. Research suggests that approximately 80 per cent of clients report clinically significant improvement following CBT-I (Morin et al., 1999). The weight of evidence, along with the minimal adverse side effects, has led to CBT-I being widely recommended as a first-line treatment of Insomnia. Indeed, the American Academy of Sleep Medicine publishes systematic reviews of the evidence supporting its treatment recommendations. Two such reviews (Morin et al., 1999, 2006a) concluded that CBT-I leads to significant improvements in Insomnia, with sustained improvement seen up to 2 years post-treatment. Further, The American Academy of Physicians in 2016 recommends that CBT-I is the first-line treatment for all adults with Insomnia (Qaseem, et al., 2016)

There is also extensive research demonstrating the effectiveness of CBT-I in the context of comorbid conditions (Geiger-Brown et al., 2015). For example, Smith et al. (2005) concluded that treatment effects are generally moderate to large for the use of CBT-I in Insomnia co-occurring with medical and psychiatric illnesses, and are comparable to treatment effects in stand-alone Insomnia. A summary of the emerging evidence base for CBT-I in psychosis is presented in Chapter 9.

A summary of the benefits and features of CBT-I that have resulted in it being the recommended option for the treatment for Insomnia is presented in Table 7.1.

The Interplay between Cognitive and Behavioural Treatment Components

Cognitive and behavioural factors in Insomnia are intrinsically related (Barber et al., 2014). Behavioural changes operate to improve coping and cognitive appraisals (e.g. the behavioural change of establishing an exercise routine can assist in altering the belief that the only way

Table 7.1 Strengths of CBT-I as a Treatment Option for Insomnia

Strength of CBT-I	*Evidence*
1. It is effective	Outcome studies support the use of both individual and group CBT-I interventions (Koffel et al., 2015; Navarro-Bravo et al., 2015). In treatment guidelines, CBT-I is universally accepted as a first-line treatment modality for Insomnia in the long term
2. Benefits are maintained after treatment discontinuation	CBT-I has lasting benefits, with outcomes being sustained during 12–24-month follow-up periods (Morin et al., 2006a) Skills learned during the active phase of treatment in CBT-I can be applied after the treatment phase is complete; this results in longer-term maintenance of gains after treatment discontinuation compared with pharmacologic treatments
3. It is efficacious in comorbid Insomnia	CBT-I is effective when a comorbid disorder is present, and it is often appropriate to treat Insomnia and the comorbid disorder simultaneously (Smith et al., 2005)
4. It can be used concurrently with pharmacotherapy	CBT-I may be used in conjunction with hypnotic medication; Morin et al. (2009) found that clients who used zolpidem for 6 weeks when starting CBT-I did better at 6-month follow-up compared with those who continued to use zolpidem as needed beyond that time, and also those who received CBT-I alone
5. CBT is cost-effective	In depression and Insomnia, CBT-I added to treatment as usual showed improvements in quality of life in a cost-effective manner (Watanabe et al., 2015) CBT has demonstrated cost-effectiveness across a range of disorders, such as panic disorder, social anxiety disorder, health anxiety, depression, chronic fatigue, and psychosis
6. CBT is safe with few side effects and patients often prefer CBT over other therapies	When CBT-I and pharmacotherapy are described to clients, the majority rate CBT-I more favourably (Azad et al., 2003; Waters et al., 2015)

to improve energy is to rest or sleep). Similarly, modifying unhelpful beliefs and thoughts that impact on sleep can promote a better adherence to behavioural routines (e.g. learning to manage overly negative thoughts about the day ahead may assist with adhering to a regular rising time). The clinician will often be employing both cognitive and behavioural strategies within each session.

In order to provide a flavour of CBT-I, we now present a brief overview of its components.

CBT-I Elements

Psychoeducation

Psychoeducation is a crucial element of CBT-I, because it both sets the stage for CBT-I components, but is also a powerful tool for cognitive change in itself. Most people know little about how sleep is regulated (see Chapter 5), and many people hold unhelpful expectations about how much sleep they require, their daytime energy, and the consequences of Insomnia.

Psychoeducation assists in establishing realistic expectations about sleep and daytime tiredness by highlighting: (a) that there is a range of healthy total sleep times (usually 6–9 hours), (b) that most people experience daytime tiredness at least some of the time, and

(c) that there are often effective strategies for improving both sleep and tiredness. In order for psychoeducation to be effectively delivered for Insomnia, it is crucial for CBT-I practitioners to have a good sense of sleep and its regulation.

Elements of psychoeducation typically include:

- the nature and purpose of sleep;
- the cyclical nature of sleep stages, explaining that there are intermittent periods of light sleep during which awakenings are frequent;
- healthy sleep requirements;
- normal expectations for the time taken to fall asleep and nocturnal wakings;
- factors that maintain a consistent sleep–wake cycle;
- the consequences of oversleeping and unhelpful sleep habits;
- an introduction to the causes of daytime tiredness, emphasising that sleep is one of many factors.

Providing psychoeducation about sleep need, sleep regulation, and ways to manage poor sleep is an important tool for encouraging changes in sleep. Psychoeducation is not an expendable treatment component that can be rushed over in order to get to the 'active' treatment components. Indeed, many members of our sample commented that the educational components of the programme were central to the improvements they made.

Sleep Hygiene

An element that should either follow, or run concurrently with, psychoeducation is sleep hygiene education. This refers to the promotion of habits and practices that are conducive to effective sleeping (see Text Box 7.1).

Although the evidence suggests that sleep hygiene as a stand-alone behavioural approach is the least effective CBT-I component in the general population (Morin et al., 2006a), it should not be overlooked in the context of psychosis. Research in this population suggests that there are significant gaps in clients' knowledge regarding sleep hygiene, notably concerning the use of caffeine in the evening, irregular rising times, a lack of pre-sleep wind-down, and extensive napping (Chiu et al., 2015).

In the context of psychosis, establishing a routine that reflects good sleep hygiene can be a complicated process. For example, napping is often associated with medication side effects (for example, naps will often increase dramatically in the 2–3 days after a depot injection). Naps are also often associated with wider psychosocial difficulties experienced by individuals with a psychosis (such as depression, long-term unemployment, reduced community involvement, and social isolation). As a result, a gentler and more flexible approach to napping in those with a psychosis is often required. Plan a schedule for naps in which they are (a) as brief as the client can manage, and (b) as early in the day as possible.

Furthermore, the sleep environment of those with a psychosis is often less conducive to sleep than that of the general population. For example, it is not uncommon for clients in this population group to regularly sleep on a couch, in front of the TV, in a room without curtains, or in an untidy or unclean environment. Working to assist clients in making changes to their sleep environment can be helpful. Additionally, the bedroom may not feel safe for some clients with psychosis. This is particularly so for clients who have a trauma history or who experience nightmares. Strategies to make the bedroom feel safe (e.g. soft light on, favourite soft toy), grounding and relaxation techniques, dream rescripting or journaling, and Imagery Rehearsal Therapy (Krakow and Zadra, 2010) may be helpful in such cases.

Text Box 7.1 Common Sleep Hygiene Recommendations

- **Minimise daytime napping**, as napping can reduce sleep drive. In the general population, napping guidelines suggest that, if required, naps ideally should be before 3 p.m. and last less than 30 minutes.
- **Get up at the same time each day,** even after a poor night of sleep. This helps to regulate the body clock. Further, not sleeping-in helps to increase sleep drive at bedtime.
- **Have a wind-down period before bed.** Choose to do some gentle, nurturing, relaxing activities in the hour or two before bed. Give yourself permission to switch off from the day. Try to avoid emotionally upsetting conversations and activities right before bedtime.
- **Avoid stimulants such as caffeine and nicotine from about 4 p.m.** These substances increase arousal and interfere with sleep.
- **Do not drink alcohol to assist sleep.** Although alcohol is well known to speed the onset of sleep, it disrupts sleep later in the night.
- **Exercise daily.** Vigorous exercise is very beneficial for sleep but should not be within around 3–4 hours of bedtime. Relaxing exercises such as stretching or gentle yoga can be done before bed to help unwind.
- **Ensure adequate exposure to natural light during the day.** Sunlight can help to increase energy and regulate the body clock. A daily minimum of 30 minutes is recommended, but more is better.
- **Use the bed only for sleeping.** It is not a good idea to use your bed to watch TV, listen to the radio, smoke, or eat. Save the bed just for sleeping and sexual activity.
- **Make the sleep environment pleasant and relaxing.** The bed should be comfortable, and the room should not be too hot or cold, or too bright.

Education is only part of the solution when it comes to establishing good sleep hygiene. Often, poor sleep hygiene practices are used because clients do not have the skills to cope in a more helpful way. They might be using poor sleep hygiene practices (e.g. napping or using stimulants) to cope with anxiety, low mood, boredom, tiredness, fears, or psychotic symptoms.

It is important for the clinician and the client to understand what is driving unhelpful behaviours. If an unhelpful behaviour is being used as a way of coping, we refer to it as a '*safety behaviour*'. Safety behaviours are not helpful because they (a) prevent people from experiencing disconfirmation of their unhelpful beliefs, and (b) may make the feared outcome more likely to occur (Salkovskis, 1991). For example, the use of daytime sleep as a safety behaviour may (a) prevent clients learning that they *can* generate energy via methods other than napping, and (b) make poor sleep that night more likely.

Examples of night-time safety behaviours include spending an excessive amount of time in bed (leading to sleep fragmentation) or drinking alcohol (that may promote short-term sleep but is likely to result in poorer quality of sleep). Examples of daytime safety behaviours include cancelling appointments after a night of Insomnia, social withdrawal, napping, and excessive caffeine use. Use of screening questionnaires that assess sleep hygiene knowledge and use of unhelpful behaviours may help with the assessment (e.g. Ree and Harvey, 2004b; see Chapter 8). We return to safety behaviours in more detail in the *Behavioural Experiments* section of the current chapter.

Behavioural Interventions

Behavioural interventions aim to resolve Insomnia and other sleep disorders by changing behaviours. As well as sleep hygiene elements, behavioural interventions include the following techniques:

- stimulus control;
- bedtime restriction;
- maximising daytime energy;
- relaxation.

Stimulus Control

One of the central behavioural techniques in CBT-I is stimulus control, originally developed by Richard Bootzin (Bootzin and Nicassio, 1978). Stimulus control is based on classical conditioning principles and is designed to overcome the unhelpful conditioning that occurs with repeated experiences of going to bed and not sleeping well. As discussed in the *Conditioned Arousal* section (Chapter 5), repeatedly going to bed and not sleeping over a period of time causes associations to develop between the bed/bedroom and not sleeping/ feeling anxious/tense/frustrated. Here, the act of going to bed comes to trigger arousal. (See Figure 7.1)

A common experience for those with Insomnia is that they feel sleepy while watching evening TV on the couch, only to find that they become alert and awake once they turn the light off and attempt to sleep in their own bed. Stimulus control can be effective in reversing this unhelpful association, so that the bedroom becomes associated with sleepiness and relaxation. This is the basis of the 'get out of bed if you can't sleep' (termed 'GOOBICS') instructions that will be discussed in the manual presented in Part II of this this book.

The theory behind stimulus control indicates that it is important for the bedroom to be associated with falling asleep, rather than with being aroused. Stimulus control instructions therefore direct Insomnia sufferers to get out of bed if they are lying awake feeling aroused, distressed, or not sleepy. The individual is instructed to get up, engage in a wind-down activity, and return to bed only when they feel sleepy.

Leaving the bedroom when awake and alert helps to break the association between the bedroom and wakefulness. Additionally, it can help dissipate negative thoughts and arousal.

Insomnia:	*Going to bed* →	*Triggers* →	*Increased arousal, worry, tension, 'sleep anxiety'*
Good Sleep:	*Going to bed* →	*Triggers* →	*Reduced arousal, relaxation, sleepiness*

Figure 7.1 Conditioned Arousal in Insomnia

Many people find that they are better able to calm down when they get up out of bed after a period of tossing and turning, frustration, and worrying. The act of leaving the bedroom can assist with creating a helpful perspective rather than overly negative thinking and also with down-regulating heightened arousal.

Additional elements of stimulus control overlap with elements recommended in the context of sleep hygiene, namely, that: (a) the bedroom is reserved only for sleep (and sexual activity), (b) a wind-down period before bed is beneficial, (c) a regular rising time in the morning should be practised, and (d) that daytime naps should be minimised.

People with psychosis often have particularly high levels of night-time rumination and worry. It is, therefore, important that strategies to address negative and intrusive thoughts are put in place. Muscle relaxation, breathing exercises, nurturing activities (e.g. relaxing shower), jigsaw puzzles, creative writing, craft, and colouring-in before sleep are particularly recommended to reduce night-time cognitive arousal in this group. When clients get out of bed during stimulus control, techniques for addressing worry may also be encouraged (see *Cognitive Interventions*, 69).

Time in Bed Restriction

Often, people with Insomnia experience fragmented, light sleep, with prolonged nocturnal wakings. Time in bed restriction, also called sleep restriction, was first introduced by Spielman et al. in 1987. It aims to consolidate fragmented sleep by restricting time in bed for a designated period of time.

As discussed in Chapter 5, people with Insomnia often cope with poor sleep by increasing time spent in bed. Although this at first appears a sensible way to provide greater opportunity for sleep, it often backfires in the longer term and results in increased sleep fragmentation. In this case, fragmented sleep is the body's way of communicating that it cannot sustain consolidated sleep for the duration that the individual is in bed. Furthermore, time spent awake in bed often means increased likelihood of arousal, thus further prolonging wakeful periods. The rationale behind time in bed restriction is to strengthen the homeostatic sleep drive and increase the propensity for sleep.

Time in bed restriction involves calculating an individual's weekly average total sleep time (ideally from their sleep diary). The client is then asked to shorten their time in bed relative to their average total sleep time plus 30 minutes. For example, a person who spends 12 hours in bed, from 9 p.m. to 9 a.m., but sleeps 8 hours, may be asked to restrict their time in bed to 8.5 hours. In this case, they might go to bed at 11.30 p.m. and rise in the morning at 8 a.m. Detailed plans and problem-solving for how the extra time out of bed will be spent are important.

During time in bed restriction in the general population, clients are also asked to avoid daytime naps. This results in reduced total sleep time and an increasing sleep drive over the initial several days. The increased sleep drive acts to consolidate sleep by reducing the number and frequency of wakings overnight. Once wakings have reduced in number and duration, time in bed is gradually increased (at a rate of about 30 minutes per week), until optimal sleep duration has been achieved. Further information regarding this procedure is presented in Morin and Espie (2004). Time in bed restriction is effective as a stand-alone treatment, but is more typically incorporated in a multi-component CBT-I treatment. Time in bed restriction in the general Insomnia population often brings about very positive results over a 2–3-week period.

It is important to tread cautiously with time in bed restriction in the context of psychosis and bipolar disorder. As severe sleep loss is a common precursor to psychosis onset and relapse, use of time in bed restriction for clients with psychotic disorder is questionable. The literature on sleep restriction is mixed in psychosis, with some studies showing that individuals might be at increased risk of a psychotic relapse with time in bed restriction (Wehr et al., 1987). A recent study, however, failed to replicate these effects in a group of individuals with affective psychosis (Kaplan and Harvey, 2013). In line with the technique of sleep compression outlined by Manber and Carney (2015), a gentler approach in CBT-I for those with a psychosis is recommended, where any time in bed restrictions are minimal and gradual. Often, the process of establishing a regular morning rising time is enough to provide a gentle time in bed restriction. As discussed above, it may not be feasible to eliminate daytime napping, but having a planned schedule around it can be hugely beneficial.

Maximising Daytime Energy

A common belief in Insomnia sufferers is that daytime energy can only be improved with rest or sleep. This renders the person helpless and passive in the face of fatigue and makes unhelpful compensatory behaviours such as sleeping-in, reduced activity levels, excessive caffeine use, and napping more likely. This contributes to the vicious cycle of Insomnia, as the homeostatic sleep drive, arousal levels, and body clock are adversely affected.

Education about fatigue and energy, as well as their sources, is important for helping clients to view sleep as *part* of the equation in determining energy levels. Understanding that energy can be influenced by a multitude of factors is an important treatment goal. When people feel more confident in managing fatigue, they are less likely to overcompensate with sleep, rest, or reduced activity levels. As a result, both sleep and the body clock improve greatly. A list of factors that commonly increase daytime tiredness is presented in Text Box 7.2.

Relaxation

Relaxation is the voluntary 'letting go' of tension. Relaxation training is designed to help reduce problematic arousal. Tension may be physical, such as tension in the muscles, or it may be cognitive or emotional distress.

There are many potential outcomes of relaxation training, which include the following:

- The mind becomes more tranquil.
- Breathing rate decreases as less oxygen is needed.
- The heart rate decreases, and blood pressure drops.
- Muscles relax.
- A feeling of calmness develops.

Research has established that relaxation techniques contribute positively to Insomnia treatments. These techniques exert their therapeutic effects, in part, by facilitating the production of slower brainwave patterns (as demonstrated on EEG recordings). The goal of relaxation practice in Insomnia is to wind down, not to force sleep, trusting that sleep will come if the body is relaxed and in need of sleep. Relaxation training can be useful during the day and/or during the night. It is often best to encourage practice of relaxation techniques during the day, as this can prevent tension building up and allows development of the skill independent of attempts to sleep.

There are several forms of relaxation training, and there is not a single method that is best for everyone. It is appropriate for the clinician to offer clients a range of different

Text Box 7.2 Physical, Behavioural, and Psychological Factors that Contribute to Daytime Fatigue and Reduced Energy

- Pain
- Inactivity
- Physical illness
- Boredom and lack of stimulation
- Low blood sugar
- Caffeine rebound
- Low iron levels
- Overexertion
- Eye strain (reading/screen use)
- Lack of, or too much, social contact
- Dehydration
- Low mood
- Temperature (too hot/cold)
- Over-vigilance (monitoring) of fatigue symptoms
- Hypothyroidism
- Repetitive tasks
- Medication side effects
- Poor diet
- Post-lunch energy dip (circadian rhythm)
- Anxiety and stress
- Circadian disturbances (delayed sleep phase for morning tiredness; advanced sleep phase for early evening tiredness; and irregular circadian rhythms for chronic or unpredictable tiredness)
- Long daytime naps (which can lead to sleep inertia or 'sleep drunkenness')

relaxation exercises and select the form that might be easiest for them to learn. Examples of relaxation techniques will be provided in the Therapist Manual later in this book.

Cognitive Interventions

What a person thinks, how they feel, and how they behave can have a significant impact on sleep and daytime functioning. Overly negative, catastrophic thoughts can lead to strong emotions and unhelpful behaviours that maintain sleep problems. This is regarded as the vicious cycle of Insomnia.

Much research has indicated that cognitions and cognitive processes are important maintaining factors in Insomnia, and that working to reverse these factors is helpful for improving treatment outcomes (for further detail, see Morin et al., 1993; Morin and Espie, 2004; Harvey et al., 2005). Cognitive interventions assist in the management of overly negative thoughts that occur during the day and night, cognitive hyperarousal (busy mind), and unhelpful beliefs and attitudes about sleep.

Thought: 'I can't cope today because I didn't sleep well'

→ ***feelings:*** *low mood and anxiety*
→ ***behaviour:*** *stay in bed until lunchtime*
→ ***consequence:*** *increased daytime lethargy and poor sleep the following night.*

Figure 7.2 Example of the Vicious Cycle of Insomnia

The Role of Overly Negative Thoughts

One of the major assumptions of cognitive therapy (CT) is that a person's thoughts and beliefs influence the emotions experienced and their intensity. CT proposes that events or situations do not directly determine emotional responses. Rather, it is the *interpretation* of these events or situations that determines the emotional response. For example, a person who thinks that a poor result in an exam will mean they will always be a failure is likely to be more distressed and helpless than someone who reasons that the result is disappointing but does not reflect on their success or failure as a human being.

Similarly, a person who reasons that they cannot do anything to improve their poor sleep is likely to feel lower in mood and more helpless than someone who believes they can work to improve their sleep.

It is not the situation that causes emotions: it is thoughts about the situation.

Situation → thoughts → feelings → behaviours

Everyone experiences negative thoughts—these are normal and, when they are accurate, they can be helpful. It is *overly* negative thoughts that CT aims to draw attention to. CT helps people to become more aware of their overly negative thoughts and the impact that these thoughts have on their emotional experience. Clients are taught that it is possible to have a choice in how they respond when overly negative thoughts appear. CT supports clients to make helpful choices about their thoughts (see the cognitive restructuring section below). We emphasise that managing both daytime and night-time overly negative thoughts is important in the context of Insomnia and other sleep disturbances.

Examples of overly negative thoughts common to Insomnia are presented below. Negative thoughts might be about the present moment (*I can't bear this*), the short-term future (*tomorrow will be a disaster*), or the longer-term future (*my Insomnia will make me sick*). Such thoughts place a great deal of pressure on the individual's ability to sleep well. They increase arousal and make sound sleep harder to achieve. Further examples include:

- catastrophising about a poor night of sleep:
  - *What if I die from poor sleep?*
  - *I will have a relapse.*
- jumping to negative conclusions:
  - *I'll never sleep well again.*
  - *I know I won't cope tomorrow.*

- black and white thinking:
  - *There is nothing I can do about this.*
  - *There was nothing good about my day today.*
- overgeneralisation:
  - *I never have any energy.*
  - *I am powerless against my Insomnia.*

For some people, simple awareness of their overly negative thoughts is enough to enable them to actively disengage from them. In this case the client is encouraged to:

- label the thoughts as unhelpful or overly negative;
- repeatedly practise choosing to not engage with the thought: 'I don't have to change/argue with/get rid of this thought' or 'Where would I like my mind to be focused right now?'.

For other people, it is helpful to assist them to change the thought into something more helpful and/or positive. In these cases, cognitive restructuring may be used.

Cognitive Restructuring

Cognitive restructuring can be useful for managing overly negative thinking. This is covered in greater detail in Session 3 of the Therapist Manual. First, clients are educated regarding the impact of their thoughts on their emotions. They are asked to be watchful for any overly negative thinking ('catching' overly negative thoughts). Once these thoughts can be recognised, it becomes possible to make decisions regarding their helpfulness and accuracy ('checking' and 'changing' overly negative thoughts).

Checking and changing thoughts involve the therapist and client examining the evidence for and against thoughts that trigger uncomfortable emotions. For example, the thoughts 'I hate this, I'll never sleep, tomorrow will be a disaster' can be evaluated, and a new, more helpful thought may be developed along the lines of 'If I can wind down, sleep will come if I need it. If I end up not sleeping well tonight, there are things I can do to help myself cope tomorrow'. We employ a simplified '*catch it, check it, change it*' method for assisting clients to identify and manage overly negative thoughts (drawn from Holden and Granholm's 2012 work on CBT for schizophrenia).

Patients with psychosis may have limited ability to evaluate their thoughts and so the simplified technique of developing coping statements with respect to sleep and daytime functioning may be more achievable than cognitive restructuring. Accordingly, different options based on the client's ability are presented in the Therapist Manual in Part II.

The Role of Thought Control Strategies

Research employing the Thought Control Questionnaire for Insomnia-Revised (TCQI-R; Ree et al., 2005) suggests that the strategies of worry to manage unwanted thoughts (e.g. 'I dwell on other worries') and aggressive suppression (e.g. 'I punish myself for having the [unwanted] thought') are unhelpful strategies that are often used in individuals with psychosis (Chiu et al., 2015). Assisting clients to use helpful thought control strategies such as cognitive restructuring, talking to someone about the thought or engaging the mind away from the unwanted thought may be helpful.

Busy Mind

Many people with Insomnia comment that they have a 'busy mind' when they are trying to sleep. This cognitive arousal might be due to negative thinking or it may be just that their mind is overactive. Clients with delayed sleep phase will be particularly prone to the mind remaining busy late at night. Although a busy mind in itself can interfere with sleep, it can also increase the likelihood of overly negative thinking, as frustration and worry about not falling asleep increase with time spent lying awake. In order to assist clients to better manage a busy mind at night, it is important to first understand why the mind is busy. Some common reasons for a busy mind in Insomnia are listed in Text Box 7.3.

Depending on the source of the busy mind, the following strategies may be useful:

- creating a day that is as engaging and positive as possible;
- winding down before bed;
- writing tasks such as journal writing, problem-solving, or making to-do lists can assist in emotional processing and clearing the mind ready for sleep; research has demonstrated that writing about issues, problems, and concerns can be good for psychological well-being and can be beneficial for sleep (Harvey and Farrell, 2003);
- asking clients to experiment with not watching the clock during the night: clock watching tends to lead to calculations regarding how much sleep is likely to be lost/obtained and can thus increase arousal (Tang et al., 2007);
- establishing a regular sleep–wake routine: this may assist the mind to quieten as bedtime approaches owing to increasing melatonin levels.

These approaches are discussed in detail within Session 3 of the Therapist Manual.

Text Box 7.3 Common Reasons for a 'Busy Mind'

- General worries, about work, relationships, finances, the future.
- Rumination about the past.
- Worries about sleep and tiredness.
- Watching the clock overnight (checking how much sleep has been lost).
- Planning (the next day, week, month, year).
- Problem-solving.
- Trivial 'random' thoughts—for example, a song running through your mind.
- Monitoring for signs of sleepiness or alertness (e.g. paying attention to relaxation level, how busy the mind is, physical comfort level, the clock to see what the time is).
- Intrusive, unwanted thoughts (including hallucinations).
- Thought suppression or trying to make the mind go blank, which results in a paradoxical increase in cognitive arousal.
- Fantasies or other positive thoughts/images.
- Thoughts skipping all over the place, from positive to negative and in-between.

Working with Unhelpful Beliefs about Sleep

People with Insomnia often hold rigid and catastrophic beliefs about the consequences of poor sleep and their ability to manage or improve their sleep (Morin et al., 2007). These beliefs often reflect the helplessness that many clients feel about their sleep problems. Research has indicated that people living with psychosis also often have unhelpful beliefs with respect to levels of self-efficacy for being able to improve their sleep ('there is nothing I can do to improve my sleep'; Chiu et al., 2016). Unhelpful beliefs about sleep are thought to trigger overly negative thoughts in the face of poor sleep or daytime fatigue. Assisting clients to modify unhelpful beliefs is considered a longer-term solution that reduces the likelihood of overly negative thoughts occurring. Accordingly, a focus of the current treatment is to bring about change in these beliefs, as a reduction in unhelpful beliefs is associated with improved treatment outcome (Morin et al., 2002).

Examples of unhelpful beliefs include:

- 'I must get eight hours of sleep most nights.'
- 'I should sleep in after a poor night of sleep.'
- 'Insomnia is the result of a chemical imbalance so there is little I can do about the problem.'
- 'I cannot cope after a poor night of sleep.'
- 'I am worried that I may lose control over my abilities to sleep.'
- 'When I feel irritable, depressed, or anxious during the day, it is mostly because I did not sleep well the night before.'

(From the Dysfunctional Beliefs about Sleep scale (DBAS); Morin et al., 2007.)

Emphasis on Experiential Learning in CT: Behavioural Experiments

Behavioural experiments are planned activities undertaken by clients and therapists during, and between, sessions. They can be used to examine and modify unhelpful beliefs, thoughts, and behaviours. Setting up experiences or 'experiments' to help clients evaluate their beliefs can be far more powerful than discussion-based strategies alone. A number of Insomnia treatment studies, including one with bipolar disorder clients (Harvey et al., 2015), have employed behavioural experiments with good effect (Harvey et al., 2007, 2014; Wong et al., 2015). For example, a client may believe that the only way to improve their energy is to rest or sleep. The client could contrast their usual behaviour of retreating to bed when tired with a new behaviour—of going for a gentle 10-minute walk. Contrary to their initial belief, it is likely that the client would find that the walk improves rather than drains their energy levels. This experience helps the client to expand their repertoire of coping strategies beyond retreating to bed and encourages a helpful belief that there are more positive ways to cope with tiredness (see Ree and Harvey, 2004a, for more detail on behavioural experiments in Insomnia).

We encourage clinicians, wherever possible, to use in-session behavioural experiments and make the CBT-I treatment as experiential as possible. Some examples of in-session experiences used on our treatment sample are as follows:

- Instead of discussion about how best to maximise energy, providing an experience of possible strategies is recommended. Have the client rate their energy levels after 5 minutes of sitting and reading compared with 5 minutes of walking with the therapist, telling jokes, or skipping. This can assist them in changing the belief that energy can only be improved by sleep or rest.

- Similarly, with diet as a potential factor in influencing energy levels, the provision of healthy snacks and decaffeinated drinks for clients to try provides an experience of alternatives to junk food and caffeine. This makes the consumption of healthy snacks/drinks at home more likely and provides a first-hand opportunity to observe changes in energy levels.
- When exploring the most suitable relaxation technique, practising the exercises together with the client during the session and asking them to rate level of relaxation and/or enjoyment after each exercise enable them to select a technique that best suits their needs.

Working with Nightmares

Several psychological interventions have been used to treat nightmares (for a review, see Augedal et al., 2013; for practice guidelines, see Aurora et al., 2010). Imagery rehearsal therapy falls under the CBT rubric and is the treatment with the most evidence. Imagery rehearsal therapy asks clients to recall the nightmare, write it down, imagine a change to the nightmare (for example, a client may imagine a more positive outcome), and then rehearse the 'new dream' while awake. There is evidence that clients can displace the unwanted content when the dream recurs after they have practised this technique. The content in the Therapist Manual employs an intervention based on that developed by Krakow (2002) called 'Turning nightmares into dreams' (TNID). For work with nightmares, grounding techniques will often be required, and it is important to do this work in session with the client in order to assess how they respond. More extreme forms of nightmare disorder that are causing a great deal of distress and fear of sleep may require medical treatment by a sleep physician, in addition to the CBT strategies in the protocol.

Managing Daytime Tiredness

Some CBT-I protocols emphasise daytime strategies as much as night-time strategies for managing Insomnia (e.g. Harvey et al., 2004, 2015; Kaplan and Harvey, 2009; Manber and Carney, 2015). In this case, management of daytime tiredness (hypersomnia) is a central component of the approach. Working to make the day as engaging, productive, and pleasurable as possible is important for improving sleep drive, which is known to improve sleep. Making the day more positive also improves mood and reduces worry about sleep, which can lead to improved nocturnal sleep. In our clinical experience, there is a bidirectional relationship in which improved night-time sleep can improve daytime function, and improved daytime function can improve night-time sleep.

Kaplan and Harvey (2009) suggest that motivational interviewing, goal setting, psycho-education, and working to establish regularity in the sleep–wake cycle may be beneficial in management of hypersomnia.

In order to improve daytime energy, principles of behavioural activation (Hubley et al., 2016), in which clients are encouraged to select activities that are engaging and either pleasurable or associated with a sense of mastery, are recommended. Periods of activity are balanced with periods of rest (either sleep or low-key activities such as watching TV, reading, or craft).

If daytime rest periods are to involve sleep, goal setting and planning for the duration and timing of naps are important. A rule of thumb in the general population is that naps should be less than 30 minutes and 8 hours or more before the night-time sleep period.

Although this may be unachievable in many patients with psychosis in the space of a 4-week therapy, scheduling naps in terms of both duration and timing is important.

Medications are a frequent contributor to daytime somnolence (with side effects such as headaches, nightmares, 'hangover' effects, and drug interactions; Chiu et al., 2016). During CBT-I, a review of the timing, type, and dosage of the client's medications is worthwhile in order to arrive at the most effective timing schedule for medication. Of course, it is important that the therapist and/or client discuss with the prescribing doctor before changing medications or their timing.

Stress Management

The vast majority of individuals with psychosis are in life circumstances that are stressful. Many are unemployed, are under financial strain, are socially isolated, have unstable accommodation options, and are managing physical health conditions. Life stress combined with reduced capacity for problem-solving can result in reduced quality of life, increased arousal, and behaviours that impact negatively on sleep and daytime energy levels. As a result, strategies for motivational interviewing (Carey et al., 1999; Compton et al., 1999), structured problem-solving, and goal setting are recommended for individuals with psychosis. Although these are often employed to assist clients with sleep-related problems (e.g. building motivation for establishing a consistent rising time and setting a realistic goal for achieving this, together with problem-solving around expected difficulties in relation to achieving these aims), it is often important to devote some time to the management of stressors that are not directly sleep-related. Clients are encouraged to consider their current life balance and goals for the future. With the client's goals in mind, the clinician and client work to set realistic goals and generate workable plans. The goal of this intervention component is to provide motivation for increased engagement in daytime activity (increase energy and sleep drive); reduce stress (e.g. work towards a life that is overly '*illness centric*') and improve mood (reduce arousal and increase energy); and assist with modification of unhelpful beliefs about sleep (if clients can make positive changes in their life, they are then unshackled from beliefs such as, 'I cannot function without eight hours sleep').

Managing Circadian Rhythm Disruption

Morgenthaler et al. (2007) note that there is evidence for the benefits of planned sleep schedules and timed light exposure in circadian rhythm disorders. Further, Frank et al. (2005) describe positive outcomes for interpersonal social rhythm therapy for managing bipolar disorder and note that establishing regularity in daily, sleep, and social routines can have a protective effect in recurrent bipolar mood disorder.

Treatments emphasising the establishment of a regular sleep–wake routine, planned exposure to sunlight, meals, and periods of activity (including social activity, if applicable) and rest are recommended. These factors assist in the management of Insomnia and daytime energy levels, as well as in the correction of circadian phase delay or advance. More extreme circadian misalignments, or irregular or free-running types, will likely require medical and/or bright light treatment in addition to CBT-I strategies.

Modifications to CBT-I for Use in Psychosis

In view of the multifactorial nature of sleep dysfunction in people with psychosis, as well as the features of many psychotic conditions that impact on learning, there are a number of modifications to standard CBT-I that we adopted:

- simplification of traditional CBT-I with reduced reliance on reading/writing and simplified concepts (for example, client versions of written materials are brief and simply worded; the therapist manual provides more detail);
- modified instructions for time in bed restriction (either gentler instructions or omitted);
- modified approach to daytime napping, emphasising planned napping that is as brief and early in the day as the client can manage; gradual reduction of napping is often useful;
- greater emphasis on sleep hygiene, especially with regards to substance use and creating a sleep environment that is conducive to sleep;
- consideration of the impact of psychotic symptoms (positive and negative) and past trauma when addressing psychological perpetuating factors for Insomnia;
- strategies for hypersomnia;
- strategies for nightmares;
- strategies for intrusive thoughts;
- strategies for circadian rhythm disturbance;
- addressing low motivation;
- addressing low self-efficacy;
- adaptability and being formulation-driven: not every strategy will be relevant for every client; we encourage the use of clinical judgement to identify the strategies that will be most beneficial for each client; for example, nightmare work may be important for one client, whereas work to reduce stimulants near bedtime may require emphasis for another.

Formulation-Driven Approach to Psychosis: Targeting the Three Barriers to Sleep

As discussed in the previous chapter, people with psychosis tend to present with many factors that perpetuate their Insomnia. These may be categorised into three barriers to restful sleep: (a) reduced sleep drive, (b) body clock disturbances, and (c) increased arousal. Consideration of presentations of Insomnia around these three factors can assist with case formulation and selection of appropriate CBT-I interventions. Table 7.2 summarises these factors within the context of psychotic disorders. It is important to understand the rationale behind each CBT-I intervention and to be able to select and/or emphasise the interventions that are most likely to be relevant for each client. Examples of interventions that target each of the three barriers to sleep are provided in Table 7.2.

When CBT-I Should Not Be Administered to People Living with Psychosis: Contraindications

There are some clients with psychosis for whom CBT-I is not appropriate. This is both to ensure client safety and to maximise the likelihood of meaningful gains being made from the intervention. We suggest delaying delivery of CBT-I in the following cases:

- high suicidal ideation: These clients need to have their risk status prioritised and are generally experiencing a very high level of distress that will prevent adequate engagement;
- unresolved anger, low mood, or negative symptoms that reduce motivation and engagement to an unworkable point (e.g. clients who are at the pre-contemplative stage of change);

Table 7.2 The Three Barriers to Sleep in Psychosis and Example Interventions

Barrier	*Perpetuating Factors*	*Example Interventions*
Reduced sleep drive	Lack of exercise Sedentary lifestyle with few interests Excessive and/or late timed napping Oversleeping/excessive time spent in bed Smoking Caffeine and other stimulants Night-eating or diet of high-sugar foods	Psychoeducation about sleep and sleep hygiene Stimulus control (GOOBICS) Reduced or scheduled napping Gentle time in bed restriction Maximising daytime energy/Behavioural activation Work towards appropriate use of stimulants such as caffeine and nicotine
Body clock disturbances	Incorrect timing of medications Stimulating activities at night-time Lack of exposure to morning daylight and other zeitgebers, such as erratic meal times Irregular rising time Irregular bedtime Lack of daytime structure	Establishing regular sleep schedule (emphasising regular rising time) Adequate and appropriately timed light exposure Regular, planned mealtimes Scheduled time outside the home Planned opportunities for social interaction
Increased arousal	Withdrawal from long-term medications or illicit substances Rumination and worrying Dysfunctional beliefs and attitudes about sleep Paranoia Hallucinations Nightmares and flashbacks Elevated levels of depression and anxiety Maladaptive thought control strategies Sleep monitoring behaviours (e.g. watching the clock) Stress (occupational, social, financial, accommodation)	Psychoeducation about sleep and sleep hygiene Interventions for managing overly negative thoughts, intrusive thoughts, hallucinations, and unhelpful beliefs Behavioural interventions of winding down before bed, stimulus control (to correct conditioned arousal), avoid clock watching, and relaxation training Imagery Rehearsal Training for nightmares Stress management

- acute psychotic episode where communication and concentration required for learning are impaired (e.g. distressing voices and paranoid thoughts, high distractibility, formal thought disorder);
- other factors that significantly impair attention and learning;
- acute agitation that manifests as explicit violent behaviour directed at others, or aggression with threats of violence;
- presence of other sleep disorders that are not currently being managed (e.g. OSA, narcolepsy, severe PLMD).

Summary

- CBT-I is the recommended treatment of choice for Insomnia. It includes a combination of psychoeducation, behavioural interventions, and cognitive interventions.
- CBT-I may also be applied to symptoms of hypersomnia, nightmares, and circadian rhythm disruption.

- Psychoeducation is a critical treatment component and can help to shift unhelpful beliefs about sleep and energy.
- CBT-I focuses on the day and night equally to maximise improvements in both sleep and daytime function.
- Special considerations for CBT-I in psychotic disorders include personalised approaches, simplification of content, tackling low motivation, and reshaping beliefs that sleep problems are unchangeable.
- A formulation-driven approach to delivering CBT-I is recommended in which different treatment components are emphasised depending on clinical need.
- Awareness and assessment of the three barriers to good sleep in individuals with psychosis (reduced sleep drive, circadian rhythm disturbance, and increased arousal) can assist with goal setting and selection of CBT-I components.
- There are contraindications for the use of CBT-I in some individuals with psychosis that must be considered.

References

Augedal, A. W., Hansen, K. S., Kronhaug, C. R., Harvey, A. G., and Pallesen, S. (2013) "Randomized controlled trials of psychological and pharmacological treatments for nightmares: A meta-analysis", *Sleep Medicine Reviews*, 17(2), pp. 143–152.

Aurora, R. N., Zak, R. S., Auerbach, S. H., Casey, K. R., Chowdhuri, S., Karippot, A., Maganti, R. K., Ramar, K., Kristo, D. A., Bista, S. R., Lamm, C. I., Morgenthaler, T. I., and Standards of Practice Committee (2010) "Best practice guide for the treatment of nightmare disorder in adults", *Journal of Clinical Sleep Medicine: Official Publication of the American Academy of Sleep Medicine*, 6(4), pp. 389–401.

Azad, N., Byszewski, A., Sarazin, F. F., McLean, W., and Koziarz, P. (2003) "Hospitalized patients' preference in the treatment of insomnia: Pharmacological versus non-pharmacological", *Canadian Journal of Clinical Pharmacology*, 10(2), pp. 89–92.

Barber, L., Rupprecht, E., and Munz, D. (2014) "Sleep habits may undermine well-being through the stressor appraisal process", *Journal of Happiness Studies*, 15(2), pp. 285–299.

Benca, R. M. (2005) "Diagnosis and treatment of chronic Insomnia: A review", *Psychiatric Services*, 56(3), pp. 332–343.

Bootzin, R. R., and Nicassio, P. M. (1978) "Behavioral treatments for insomnia", *Progress in Behavior Modification*, 6, pp. 1–45.

Borodkin, K., and Dagan, Y. (2010) "Circadian rhythm disorders", in Winkelman, J. W., and Plante, D. T. (Eds.) *Foundations of psychiatric sleep medicine*. New York: Cambridge University Press, pp. 186–201.

Carey, K., Purnine, D., Maisto, S., Carey, M., and Barnes, K. (1999) "Decisional balance regarding substance use among persons with schizophrenia", *Community Mental Health Journal*, 35(4), pp. 289–299.

Charles, J., Harrison, C., and Britt, H. (2009) "Insomnia", *Australian Family Physician*, 38, p. 283.

Chiu, V. (n.d.) *Sleep problems in schizophrenia: A qualitative study on help-seeking experiences*. Perth, WA: University of Western Australia.

Chiu, V. W., Harvey, R. H., Sloan, N. B., Ree, M., Lin, A., Janca, A., and Waters, F. (2015) "Cognitive and behavioral factors associated with insomnia in inpatients with schizophrenia and related psychoses", *Journal of Nervous & Mental Disease*, 203(10), pp. 798–803.

Chiu, V. W., Ree, M., Janca, A., and Waters, F. (2016) "Sleep in schizophrenia: Exploring subjective experiences of sleep problems, and implications for treatment", *Psychiatric Quarterly*, 87(4), pp. 633–648.

Cohrs, S. (2008) "Sleep disturbances in patients with schizophrenia: Impact and effect of antipsychotics", *CNS Drugs*, 22(11), pp. 939–962.

Compton, P., Monahan, G., and Simmons-Cody, H. (1999) "Motivational interviewing: An effective brief intervention for alcohol and drug abuse patients", *Nurse Practitioner*, 24(11), pp. 27–8, 31–34, 37–38 passim; quiz 48–49.

Everitt, H., McDermott, L., Leydon, G., Yules, H., Baldwin, D., and Little, P. (2014) "GPs' management strategies for patients with insomnia: A survey and qualitative interview study", *British Journal of General Practice*, 64(619), pp. e112–e119.

Ferracioli-Oda, E., Qawasmi, A., and Bloch, M. H. (2013) "Meta-analysis: Melatonin for the treatment of primary sleep disorders", *PLoS ONE*, 8(5), pp. 1–6.

Frank, E., Kupfer, D. J., Thase, M. E., Mallinger, A. G., Swartz, H. A., Fagiolini, A. M., Grochocinski, V., Houck, P., Scott, J., Thompson, W., and Monk, T. (2005) "Two-year outcomes for interpersonal and social rhythm therapy in individuals with bipolar I disorder", *Archives of General Psychiatry*, 62(9), pp. 996–1004.

Geiger-Brown, J. M., Rogers, V. E., Liu, W., Ludeman, E. M., Downton, K. D., and Diaz-Abad, M. (2015) "Cognitive behavioral therapy in persons with comorbid insomnia: A meta-analysis", *Sleep Medicine Reviews*, 23, pp. 54–67.

Gunja, N. (2013) "In the zzz zone: The effects of z-drugs on human performance and driving", *Journal of Medical Toxicology*, 9(2), pp. 163–171.

Harvey, A. G., Bélanger, L., Talbot, L., Eidelman, P., Beaulieu-Bonneau, S., Fortier-Brochu, É., Ivers, H., Lamy, M., Hein, K., Soehner, A. M., Mérette, C., and Morin, C. M. (2014) "Comparative efficacy of behavior therapy, cognitive therapy, and cognitive behavior therapy for chronic insomnia: A randomized controlled trial", *Journal of Consulting & Clinical Psychology*, 82(4), pp. 670–683.

Harvey, A. G., and Farrell, C. (2003) "The efficacy of a Pennebaker-like writing intervention for poor sleepers", *Behavioral Sleep Medicine*, 1(2), pp. 115–124.

Harvey, A. G., Sharpley, A. L., Ree, M. J., Stinson, K., and Clark, D. M. (2007) "An open trial of cognitive therapy for chronic insomnia", *Behaviour Research & Therapy*, 45(10), pp. 2491–2501.

Harvey, A. G., Soehner, A. M., Kaplan, K. A., Hein, K., Lee, J., Kanady, J., Li, D., Rabe-Hesketh, S., Ketter, T. A., Neylan, T. C., and Buysse, D. J. (2015) "Treating insomnia improves mood state, sleep, and functioning in bipolar disorder: A pilot randomized controlled trial", *Journal of Consulting & Clinical Psychology*, 83(3), pp. 564–577.

Harvey, A. G., Tang, N. K. Y., and Browning, L. (2005) "Cognitive approaches to insomnia", *Clinical Psychology Review*, 25(5), pp. 593–611.

Harvey, A., Watkins, E., Mansell, W., and Shafran, R. (2004) *Cognitive behavioural processes across psychological disorders*. New York: Oxford University Press.

Holden, J., and Granholm, E. (2012) "Group cognitive behavioural social skills training for schizophrenia", in Steel, C. (Ed.) *CBT for schizophrenia: Evidence-based interventions and future directions*. Oxford, UK: John Wiley, pp. 169–190.

Hubley, S., Kaiser, R., and Dimidjian, S. (2016) "Behavioural activation treatment for depression", in Wells, A. (Ed.) *Treating depression: MCT, CBT and third wave therapies*. Chichester, UK: John Wiley, pp. 369–392.

Kaplan, K. A., and Harvey, A. G. (2009) "Hypersomnia across mood disorders: A review and synthesis", *Sleep Medicine Reviews*, 13(4), pp. 275–285.

Kaplan, K. A., and Harvey, A. G. (2013) "Behavioral treatment of insomnia in bipolar disorder", *American Journal of Psychiatry*, 170(7), pp. 716–720.

Koffel, E. A., Koffel, J. B., and Gehrman, P. R. (2015) "A meta-analysis of group cognitive behavioral therapy for insomnia", *Sleep Medicine Reviews*, 19, pp. 6–16.

Krakow, B. (2002) *Turning nightmares into dreams: The authorized audio series and treatment workbook for New Dream Therapy* [CDs]. USA: The New Sleepy Times.

Krakow, B., and Zadra, A. (2010) "Imagery rehearsal therapy: Principles and practice", *Sleep Medicine Clinics*, 5(2), pp. 289–298.

Krystal, A. D. (2009) "A compendium of placebo-controlled trials of the risks/benefits of pharmacological treatments for insomnia: The empirical basis for U.S. clinical practice", *Sleep Medicine Reviews*, 13(4), pp. 265–274.

Lemoine, P., Nir, T., Laudon, M., and Zisapel, N. (2007) "Prolonged-release melatonin improves sleep quality and morning alertness in insomnia patients aged 55 years and older and has no withdrawal effects", *Journal of Sleep Research,* 16(4), pp. 372–380.

Manber, R., and Carney, C. E. (2015) *Treatment plans and interventions for Insomnia: A case formulation approach.* New York: Guilford Press.

Montplaisir, J., Hawa, R., Moller, H., Morin, C., Fortin, M., Matte, J., Reinish, L., and Shapiro, C. M. (2003) "Zopiclone and zaleplon vs benzodiazepines in the treatment of insomnia: Canadian consensus statement", *Human Psychopharmacology: Clinical and Experimental,* 18(1), pp. 29–38.

Morgenthaler, T., Alessi, C., Friedman, L., Owens, J., Kapur, V., Boehlecke, B., Brown, T., Chesson, A., Jr., Coleman, J., Lee-Chiong, T., Pancer, J., and Swick, T. J. (2007) "Practice parameters for the use of actigraphy in the assessment of sleep and sleep disorders: An update for 2007", *Sleep,* 30(4), pp. 519–529.

Morin, C. M., Blais, F., and Savard, J. (2002) "Are changes in beliefs and attitudes about sleep related to sleep improvements in the treatment of insomnia?", *Behaviour Research & Therapy,* 40(7), pp. 741–752.

Morin, C. M., Bootzin, R. R., Buysse, D. J., Edinger, J. D., Espie, C. A., and Lichstein, K. L. (2006a) "Psychological and behavioral treatment of insomnia: Update of the recent evidence (1998–2004)", *Sleep,* 29(11), pp. 1398–1414.

Morin, C. M., and Espie, C. A. (2004) *Insomnia: A clinical guide to assessment and treatment.* Boston, MA: Springer US.

Morin, C. M., Hauri, P. J., Espie, C. A., Spielman, A. J., Buysse, D. J., and Bootzin, R. R. (1999) "Nonpharmacologic treatment of chronic insomnia: An American Academy of Sleep Medicine review", *Sleep,* 22(8), pp. 1134–1156.

Morin, C. M., LeBlanc, M., Daley, M., Gregoire, J. P., and Mérette, C. (2006b) "Epidemiology of insomnia: Prevalence, self-help treatments, consultations, and determinants of help-seeking behaviors", *Sleep Medicine,* 7, pp. 123–130.

Morin, C. M., Stone, J., Trinkle, D., Mercer, J., and Remsberg, S. (1993) "Dysfunctional beliefs and attitudes about sleep among older adults with and without insomnia complaints", *Psychology & Aging,* 8(3), pp. 463–467.

Morin, C. M., Vallières, A., Guay, B., Ivers, H., Savard, J., Mérette, C., Bastien, C., and Baillargeon, L. (2009) "Cognitive behavioral therapy, singly and combined with medication, for persistent insomnia: A randomized controlled trial", *JAMA,* 301(19), pp. 2005–2015.

Morin, C. M., Vallières, A., and Ivers, H. (2007) "Dysfunctional beliefs and attitudes about sleep (DBAS): Validation of a brief version (DBAS-16)", *Sleep,* 30(11), p. 1547.

Navarro-Bravo, B., Párraga-Martínez, I., López-Torres Hidalgo, J., Andrés-Pretel, F., and Rabanales-Sotos, J. (2015) "Group cognitive-behavioral therapy for insomnia: A meta-analysis", *Anales de Psicología,* 31, pp. 8–18.

Qaseem, A., Kansagara, D., Forciea, M. A., Cooke, M., Denberg, T. D., for the Clinical Guidelines Committee of the American College of Physicians. (2016) "Management of Chronic Insomnia Disorder in Adults: A Clinical Practice Guideline From the American College of Physicians", *Annals of Internal Medicine,* 165, pp. 125–133. doi: 10.7326/M15-2175

Ree, M. J., and Harvey, A. G. (2004a) "Behavioral experiments in chronic insomnia", in Bennett-Levy, J., Butler, G., Fennell, M., Hackmann, A., Mueller, M., and Westbrook, D. (Eds.) *Oxford guide to behavioral experiments in cognitive therapy.* Oxford, UK: Oxford University Press, pp. 287–308.

Ree, M. J., and Harvey, A. G. (2004b) "Investigating safety behaviours in insomnia: The development of the Sleep-related Behaviours Questionnaire (SRBQ)", *Behaviour Change,* 21(01), pp. 26–36.

Ree, M. J., Harvey, A. G., Blake, R., Tang, N. K. Y., and Shawe-Taylor, M. (2005) "Attempts to control unwanted thoughts in the night: Development of the thought control questionnaire-insomnia revised (TCQI-R)", *Behaviour Research & Therapy,* 43, pp. 985–998.

Salkovskis, P. M. (1991) "The importance of behaviour in the maintenance of anxiety and panic: A cognitive account", *Behavioural & Cognitive Psychotherapy,* 19(01), pp. 6–19.

Sateia, M. J., and Nowell, P. D. (2004) "Insomnia", *The Lancet,* 364(9449), pp. 1959–1973.

Schutte-Rodin, S., Broch, L., Buysse, D., Dorsey, C., and Sateia, M. (2008) "Clinical guideline for the evaluation and management of chronic insomnia in adults", *Journal of Clinical Sleep Medicine*, 4(5), pp. 487–504.

Siriwardena, A. N., Qureshi, M. Z., Dyas, J. V., Middleton, H., and Orner, R. (2008) "Magic bullets for insomnia? Patients' use and experiences of newer (Z drugs) versus older (benzodiazepine) hypnotics for sleep problems in primary care", *British Journal of General Practice*, 58(551), pp. 417–422.

Smith, M. T., Huang, M. I., and Manber, R. (2005) "Cognitive behavior therapy for chronic insomnia occurring within the context of medical and psychiatric disorders", *Clinical Psychology Review*, 25(5), pp. 559–592.

Spielman, A. J., Caruso, L. S., and Glovinsky, P. B. (1987) "A behavioral perspective on insomnia treatment", *Psychiatric Clinics of North America*, 10(4), pp. 541–553.

Tang, N. K. Y., Anne Schmidt, D., and Harvey, A. G. (2007) "Sleeping with the enemy: Clock monitoring in the maintenance of insomnia", *Journal of Behavior Therapy & Experimental Psychiatry*, 38(1), pp. 40–55.

Watanabe, N., Furukawa, T. A., Shimodera, S., Katsuki, F., Fujita, H., Sasaki, M., Sado, M., and Perlis, M. L. (2015) "Cost-effectiveness of cognitive behavioral therapy for insomnia comorbid with depression: Analysis of a randomized controlled trial", *Psychiatry & Clinical Neurosciences*, 69(6), pp. 335–343.

Waters, F., Chiu, V., Janca, S., Atkinson, A., and Ree, M. (2015) "Preferences for different insomnia treatment options in people with schizophrenia and related psychoses: A qualitative study", *Frontiers in Psychology*, 14(6), p. 990.

Wehr, T. A., Sack, D. A., and Rosenthal, N. E. (1987) "Sleep reduction as a final common pathway in the genesis of mania", *American Journal of Psychiatry*, 144(2), pp 201–204.

Winokur, A., and Kamath, J. (2008) "The effect of typical and atypical antipsychotic drugs on sleep of schizophrenic patients", in *Serotonin and sleep: Molecular, functional and clinical aspects*, pp. 587–610 [online]. Available at: http://dx.doi.org/10.1007/978-3-7643-3561-3_24 (accessed November 22, 2016).

Wong, M. Y., Ree, M. J., and Lee, C. W. (2015) "Enhancing CBT for chronic insomnia: A randomised clinical trial of additive components of mindfulness or cognitive therapy", *Clinical Psychology & Psychotherapy*, 23(5), pp. 377–385.

Zhdanova, I. V., Wurtman, R. J., Regan, M. M., Taylor, J. A., Shi, J. P., and Leclair, O. U. (2001) "Melatonin treatment for age-related insomnia", *Journal of Clinical Endocrinology & Metabolism*, 86(10), pp. 4727–4730.

8 Assessing Sleep

Assessment holds an important place in guiding treatment. The current chapter is designed to help clinicians assess Insomnia and other sleep disorders in the context of psychotic disorders. We outline different types of assessment method and make particular mention of situations when certain assessment procedures are not well tolerated, or may lack validity, in people with psychotic disorders.

Insomnia is assessed on the basis of self-reported symptoms, and so information derived from a thorough clinical interview and questionnaires is important. Sleep diaries are also highly desirable to track sleep–wake patterns, daytime napping, and treatment progress.

Often, clients *underestimate* time spent asleep, and so objective methods such as wrist actigraphy can be useful as an independent measure to demonstrate any discrepancies between subjectively estimated sleep and objectively measured sleep. Wrist actigraphy, although not feasible for everyone, can be a useful method especially if the compliance in completing questionnaires or sleep diaries is low. As a minimum for planning a CBT-I intervention, the use of a clinical interview (Appendix 1) and (simplified) sleep diary (Appendix 2) is recommended.

In addition to gathering important clinical information, the assessment should serve to develop a positive therapeutic relationship between the client and the clinician. It provides an opportunity to build motivation, orient the client to the treatment, and answer any questions the client might have. Enquiry into goals for treatment is also helpful for treatment planning and evaluating motivation to engage in the therapy.

The Clinical Interview

Prior to engagement in the CBT-I intervention, a comprehensive assessment of the sleep complaints, duration, possible causes, and impact should be conducted. Gaining information on the predisposing, precipitating, perpetuating, and protective factors will assist in the planning of therapy.

A semi-structured clinical interview can assist the clinician and is presented in Appendix 1. A description of the clinical interview's components now follows.

Background and Clinical Information

Demographic and clinical characteristics are collected to gain an understanding of the factors contributing to sleep and daytime dysfunction, possible care or referral needs, and levels of psychopathology.

General background information is typically gathered across the following domains:

- **demographic information**, such as age, gender, country of birth, educational attainment, marital status, occupation/trade, employment status, and accommodation type;
- **medical and neurological history**, including physical injuries, chronic pain, diabetes, breathing or respiratory problems, and any neurological conditions;
- **psychiatric history**, such as the diagnosis, length of illness, engagement with mental health services, and previous hospitalisations;
- **mood, anxiety, and other symptom complaints**, and known triggers for an exacerbation of these symptoms;
- **medication** type, dosage, time of day when taken; this includes prescription and 'over the counter' drugs.

Description of Sleep Problems

Information elicited regarding a client's sleep problems should include the following:

Sleep Problems in the Client's Own Words

The client is asked open-ended questions such as 'Tell me about your difficulty with sleep' and 'What is your energy like during the day?'. The clinician is working to discern whether the main concern lies mostly with poor sleep overnight, daytime tiredness, or both.

Questions should then ask for specific details regarding the exact nature of the complaint. For example, does the difficulty lie with getting to sleep at the start of the night, staying asleep, waking too early, and/or sleep being unrefreshing.

The person's perception regarding the link between their mental illness and sleep problems should also be sought, to evaluate whether they believe that their mental illness caused the sleep problems or vice versa.

Sleep Routine

Assessing sleep routine can provide clues about perpetuating factors that reduce sleep drive and the presence of circadian rhythm disruptions (see below). When a person's sleep routine is assessed, the time frame should generally refer to the previous week, unless it was an atypical week, in which case the person should be asked about a 'typical' week. The sleep diary (see below), in addition to the clinical interview, is useful for deriving a good understanding of the person's sleep routine.

Questions about sleep routine should include queries about bedtime, wake time, rising time (which may be later than wake time), time taken to fall asleep ('sleep latency'), number and durations of any wakings during the main sleep period, and the total estimated *sleep* time. This information allows calculation of *sleep efficiency*, which is the proportion of time spent asleep in relation to time spent in bed. Sleep efficiency is calculated by time spent *asleep* being divided by time spent in *bed*. A sleep efficiency of less than 80 per cent is a good indicator of a clinically significant sleep problem. The sleep diary can also be used to calculate sleep efficiency and tends to be more accurate than global estimates gained from interview questions.

A high degree of inter-night variability in sleep routine is common in both Insomnia and psychotic disorders. As they are an important perpetuating factor, sleep–wake routines require careful assessment. Do bedtimes and wake times vary by more than an hour or so from day to day? Questions such as 'What is your earliest bedtime?' and 'What is your latest bedtime?' can assist in the assessment of variability. Is there evidence of sleeping-in late or napping after a night of poor sleep? Does total sleep time also vary? A typical pattern is for a run of poor nights being eventually followed by a longer 'catch-up' sleep.

Assessment of the sleep routine can also provide clues about the presence of circadian rhythm disruption. The Morningness–Eveningness Questionnaire (described below) may also assist the assessment of circadian preference.

As previously discussed circadian rhythm disruptions fall into four major groups:

- Delayed sleep phase: This involves difficulty falling asleep before the early hours of the morning, but then typically sleeping well once asleep. People with a delayed sleep pattern may sleep in until late in the morning or the early afternoon. Delayed sleep phase is more common in adolescents and young adults.
- Advanced sleep phase: This is falling asleep early in the evening, but then waking in the early hours of the morning. Clients may have sufficient duration of sleep, but the timing is timed earlier than they would like or is convenient. Advanced sleep phase is more common in the elderly. In this population, taking sedative medication early in the evening may contribute to a phase advance.
- Irregular sleep–wake disorder: This involves at least three sleep episodes per 24-hour period, with irregular timing from day to day.
- Non-24-hour sleep–wake disorder (or 'free-running type'): There are consecutive delays in falling asleep every day. Generally, the delay is an hour or two, corresponding to a circadian cycle of 25–26 hours. The daily delay in sleep onset causes the patient to gradually 'cycle around the clock', sometimes sleeping during the day and at other times of the month sleeping at night.

Daytime Naps

People with Insomnia often report that they are unable to nap owing to difficulties with down-regulating their arousal levels. People describe being fatigued and tired, but not sleepy. By contrast, individuals with Insomnia comorbid with excessive daytime sleepiness and/or with hypersomnia can, and will, often nap during the day.

Naps can reduce sleep drive at night, particularly if they are longer than 30 minutes and if they occur late in the day (within about 8 hours of bedtime). A further effect of naps is that they can make the day unproductive and unstimulating. Long naps often signal a pattern of disengagement from life and can exacerbate feelings of depression, hopelessness, isolation, and low motivation. If napping behaviours are present, understanding of why they occur is important so that appropriate treatment goals can be established.

Common reasons for daytime napping include:

- excessive daytime sleepiness due to hypersomnia and/or insufficient sleep (screening for sleep disorders other than Insomnia is important in this case);
- sedative effects of medication, alcohol, or illicit drugs such as cannabis;
- to escape from or manage depressed mood, anxiety, hallucinations;
- boredom and lack of stimulation and routine;
- disorganisation and feeling overwhelmed with completing tasks for the day.

Medication and Substance Use

The great majority of people with a psychotic disorder are prescribed medications to address their mental and physical health problems. The therapist should ask whether these medications affect the person's sleep and daytime sleepiness.

Many antipsychotic medications have sedating side effects. Depot injections are particularly sedating, and people may sleep for long periods in the 24–48 hours following the injection. Some people may be prescribed stimulant medication (e.g. modafinil or dexamphetamine) to increase daytime wakings, but, of course, the timing of the ingestion of these medications is crucial for minimising impact on sleep at night.

Around half of all people with psychotic disorders are thought to abuse drugs or alcohol, and unsurprisingly this leads to poor health outcomes. Information on the following should be gathered:

- medications used to assist with sleep or cope during the day, both prescribed and over-the-counter;
- the use of alcohol or illicit drugs to assist sleep at night or coping during the day, and the use of 'uppers' and 'downers'; ask about illicit drug use in a direct, non-judgemental, matter-of-fact manner;
- the use of caffeine to manage fatigue and sleepiness during the day, particularly within 4 hours of bedtime;
- the use of cigarettes and nicotine analogues, especially in the 2 hours before bed.

Sleep Environment

Check that the sleep environment is conducive to relaxation and sleep. Clients with psychotic disorders are more likely than the general population to have a poor sleeping environment, and the degree to which this may be a contributing factor needs to be assessed.

- Ideally, the sleep environment should be dark, quiet, comfortable, safe, not overstimulating, not too hot or cold.
- Does the client sleep in a designed space for sleeping, such as a bed in a bedroom, rather than a couch in a living area?
- Does the person sleep alone, or with a partner in the bed or bedroom? Does the partner cause disturbance? Are there babies/children in the house who might wake at night, or housemates or pets that cause wakings?
- The use of TVs, computers, phones, and other devices with bright screens in bed should also be queried.
- Behaviours such as smoking or eating in bed should be assessed.
- Ask if the client feels unsafe in the bedroom, or perceives a 'sensed presence', which can create feelings of fear and uneasiness.

People with psychotic disorders are often financially disadvantaged and live in supported accommodation, which may be noisy and shared with other residents. Some clients may not be using a proper bed, or have comfortable bedding, or may not have access to heating or cooling elements. The sleep environment may be untidy and/or unclean, with dust and other unhygienic elements contributing to increased arousal or breathing difficulty.

Daytime Sleepiness, Fatigue, and Hypersomnia

As discussed in Chapter 5, there is an important difference between fatigue and sleepiness.

Sleepiness is an individual's capacity to fall asleep, and it can be assessed by the client being asked how likely they would be to fall asleep in various situations (e.g. lying down resting, watching TV, being a passenger in a car, attending an appointment).

In psychotic disorders, excessive daytime sleepiness and/or long sleep duration often co-occurs with Insomnia. Sleepiness may also be a symptom of another sleep disorder, and the therapist should screen for symptoms of OSA, circadian rhythm dysfunction, and narcolepsy, and ask about medication side effects, substance use, and physical ill health (see Chapter 5) in order to better understand any sleepiness.

Excessive daytime sleepiness can be assessed with:

- the number of hours spent asleep (sleep length) or in bed across a 24-hour period;
- the Epworth Sleepiness Scale (Johns, 1991), which assesses a person's chance of dozing in various situations, providing an index of levels of sleepiness;
- the Multiple Sleep Latency Test (MSLT; see p. 94), although it requires the use of a specially equipped laboratory.

By contrast, individuals can experience fatigue without being sleepy. Common to Insomnia is the experience of feeling 'tired but wired'. An assessment of daytime fatigue, its severity, probable causes, and relation to sleep will reveal clues regarding the best ways to manage it. Also, questions about the time of day when clients have more and less energy can provide valuable information in planning treatment.

Common causes of fatigue (in addition to disturbed sleep) to assess include:

- low mood and disengagement from life;
- prolonged periods of stress and anxiety;
- medication side effects;
- poor diet;
- sedentary lifestyle;
- boredom;
- lack of exposure to bright or natural light (vitamin D deficiency, inappropriately timed melatonin production);
- medical problems, such as iron deficiency, thyroid/hormone problems, diabetes.

Nightmares

Nightmares are particularly common in people with a past experience of trauma or adverse events. Nightmares are distinguished from night terrors because they tend to occur in the second half of the night, during REM sleep. The person will usually have a clear memory of the dream's content and will wake from the dream alert.

In contrast, night terrors occur in deep sleep, tending to occur earlier in the sleep period, and the person wakes from them feeling confused and often with a poor memory of the episode.

Questions about nightmares assess the frequency, intensity, and associated distress. People with psychotic disorders may report several bouts of nightmares every night, leading to difficulties going back to sleep and fears about sleep in general.

It is also useful to check for any recurrent themes or dreams, being mindful that themes can include vivid scenes of past trauma or abuse that the client might find difficult or be reluctant to discuss. We have found that any therapeutic work with nightmares relating to past trauma is best done individually, rather than in a group setting.

Other Sleep Disorders

Ask about any previous diagnosis of a sleep disorder, if any treatment was initiated (e.g. CPAP for OSA), and if the client is compliant with treatment (e.g. using the CPAP machine for at least 5 hours a night). In the context of CBT-I, the aim is not to conduct a full diagnostic interview for all sleep disorders, but rather to screen for the presence of sleep disorders and establish whether the client is receiving treatment for that condition.

Questions may enquire about the presence, frequency, and impact of the following:

- snoring at night; waking up gasping for air; waking up with a dry mouth; waking up short of breath (OSA);
- cramps or unusual feelings in the legs in bed, particularly while the client is trying to initiate sleep (RLS);
- leg or arm kicks or jerks during sleep (PLMD).
- 'acting out dreams', which may result in accidental injury such as hitting the wall or their bed partner (REM sleep behaviour disorder);
- sleep-walking, eating, or talking (other parasomnias);
- 'sleep attacks', in which the person has an irresistible urge to sleep during the day, sometimes at inappropriate times (narcolepsy); these may be accompanied by muscle weakness or collapse (cataplexy), hallucinations, and paralysis in the case of narcolepsy;
- strong urges to get up to urinate at night (nocturia); nocturia may be a symptom of OSA;
- incontinence at night (bedwetting), which may be related to medication side effects or a physiological response to a nightmare.

Lifestyle

Questions should assess lifestyle and life balance: for example, 'Tell me about a typical day'. Ask about daily/weekly routines, obligations, hobbies, social support, and satisfaction with current life balance. This assists with the assessment of stress versus understimulation. Furthermore, this line of enquiry provides information for potential motivational hooks. For example, clients who are dissatisfied with their activity level may be able to generate goals based on how they would like to see their situation improve.

Assessment of exposure to bright (sun) light in the morning, during the day, and in the evening is also important. Does the client go outside each day? Question how the client typically spends the 2 hours prior to bedtime (do they have a wind-down routine?), and the first hour or two on waking in the morning (do they have a wind-up routine?).

It is important to take note of whether clients are living a lifestyle that is unconducive to sleep. If not, is the client aware of the ways in which their lifestyle may impact on their sleep? This can prompt the therapist as to whether more work on motivation may be required to enable lifestyle changes. For example, some clients may not enjoy being out in the sun, or they may have social anxieties or paranoia that preclude them from going outdoors often.

Assessment of Self-efficacy and Motivation

Self-efficacy is a person's confidence in their ability to succeed in specific tasks. Low self-efficacy can reduce hope and motivation and can keep people stuck and unlikely to try new strategies. In many cases, people with psychotic disorders report that their sleep symptoms are solely attributable to their psychiatric illness. Consequently, many believe that their sleep problems are a permanent and unmodifiable feature of their condition.

Assessment of self-efficacy involves asking the client if they believe they can work to improve their sleep, or if they believe it to be unchangeable. Low self-efficacy is a barrier to treatment, and an important treatment goal of CBT-I is to demonstrate the factors relating to sleep and tiredness that the client has influence over.

Reduced motivation is common and can be associated with low self-efficacy. It can arise from negative symptoms, medication side effects, comorbid depression or anxiety, and from the impact of other people's stigma about mental illness.

Questions about motivation and self-efficacy may be asked as follows:

- What would be good about learning to improve your sleep?
- What would your life be like 1 year from now if you were sleeping better?
- What is the worst thing about not sleeping well?
- Do you believe you can make changes that will improve your sleep?
- What might be difficult about attending this programme?
- What might be good about attending this programme?
- On a scale of 0–10, how confident are you that you can improve your sleep? (See Figure 8.1.)
- What would it take to make you feel more confident about attending the programme and improving your sleep? (e.g. What might move you from a 5 out of 10 in confidence, to a 6 out of 10?)

Assessment of motivation and readiness for change may also be drawn from Prochaska and DiClemente's (1983) 'Stages of Change' model used in motivational interviewing literature.

They ask the client to identify the stage they feel they are at now, in terms of managing their sleep problem:

- not ready yet (pre-contemplation);
- thinking about it (contemplation);
- preparing to make changes (preparation);
- making changes (action);
- maintaining the changes I have made (maintenance).

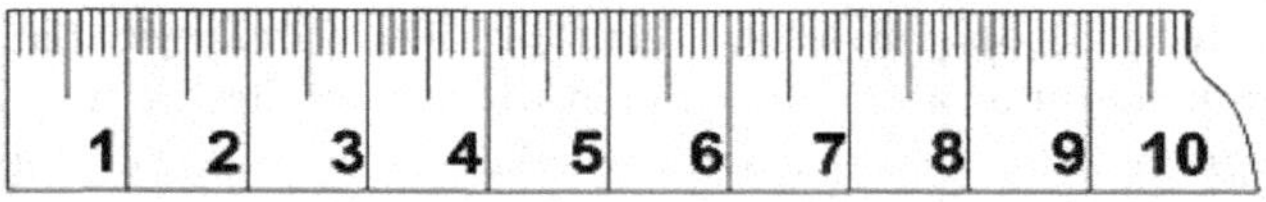

Not Confident at all *Extremely Confident*

Figure 8.1 Confidence Ruler

As treatment progresses, the client is asked to reflect on what stage they are at, aiming for progression from pre-contemplation, to contemplation, to preparation and action, and, finally, to maintenance at the end of the treatment.

Questionnaires

Self-reported questionnaires are measures that are used to quantify the client's self-perceived sleep difficulties and symptoms, and screen for other sleep disorders. They can be an efficient means of gathering standardised information and assessing response to treatment.

Questionnaires to Screen for Sleep Dysfunction

The most commonly used measures to assess Insomnia and other sleep disturbances are as follows:

- *Insomnia Severity Index* (ISI; Bastien et al., 2001): The ISI is a seven-item scale with norms allowing very quick assessment of current Insomnia symptom severity.
- *Pittsburgh Sleep Quality Index* (PSQI; Buysse et al., 1989): The PSQI assesses sleep quality in the previous month and provides information about sleep efficiency, sleep latency, and daytime effects of poor sleep. A global score of 5 or more is used to classify clinically significant sleep difficulties. Responses on the PSQI can help to identify some of the factors contributing to the client's poor sleep quality (e.g. bad dreams, pain).
- *Epworth Sleepiness Scale* (ESS; Johns, 1991): The ESS is the most widely used measure for assessing sleepiness. The patient is asked to rate the likelihood of 'dozing' in eight different circumstances (for example, sitting and reading). A score above 10 indicates clinically significant sleepiness. Patients taking antipsychotic medications will be more likely to have elevated scores on this measure.
- *SLEEP-50* (Spoormaker et al., 2005): The *SLEEP-50* is a 50-item scale designed to screen for nine of the most common sleep disorders and complaints: OSA, Insomnia, narcolepsy, RLS/PLMD, circadian rhythm sleep disorder, sleep-walking, nightmares, factors influencing sleep, and the impact of sleep complaints on daily functioning.
- *The Morningness–Eveningness Questionnaire* (MEQ; Horne and Ostberg, 1976): The MEQ can be used to assess for body clock preferences and is suggestive of advanced or delayed sleep phase.
- *Berlin Questionnaire* (Netzer et al., 1999): The Berlin Questionnaire is a quick ten-item scale that screens for OSA.

If screening indicates the presence of OSA, RLS, PLMD, REM sleep behaviour disorder, or narcolepsy, you should advise the client to obtain further assessment, if possible in the form of an overnight sleep study. This can be done with a referral to a sleep physician.

Questionnaires to Understand Perpetuating Factors to Poor Sleep

- *Dysfunctional Beliefs and Attitudes about Sleep Scale—16-item version* (DBAS-16; Morin et al., 2007): This scale measures 16 common but unhelpful attitudes and beliefs about sleep. Higher scores are associated with Insomnia severity. Larger decreases over the course of treatment are associated with greater levels of improvement.

- *TCQI-R* (Ree et al., 2005): This 35-item measure assesses the different control strategies people employ to manage thoughts that are keeping them awake at night. The thought control strategies of aggressive suppression and worry are unhelpful and appear to worsen Insomnia, anxiety, and mood.
- *Sleep-Related Behaviours Questionnaire* (Ree and Harvey, 2004): This assesses the use of unhelpful behaviours employed to promote sleep and cope with tiredness, with 32 items. Higher scores are associated with Insomnia. This scale can be useful to check for unhelpful strategies that a client may be using during the day or the night to cope with their poor sleep.
- *Sleep Hygiene Knowledge Scale* (SHiK; Chiu et al., 2015): This ten-item measure assesses awareness of and participation in behaviours known to affect sleep in people with psychotic disorders.
- *Sleep Hygiene Index* (Mastin et al., 2006): This 13-item measure asks about the frequency of engagement in behaviours that are bad for sleep hygiene, such as caffeine consumption and exercise before bedtime.

Notes on the Suitability of Questionnaires for Psychosis

Many of the above measures are used widely to screen for sleep problems in people with psychotic disorders. There are, however, some limitations associated with the use of such questionnaires in this population.

A particular note of caution is that most sleep questionnaires fail to assess sleep–wake variability from day to day. This is a particularly important issue in this clinical group, as their most frequent problems are a lack of routine and variability in sleep and wake times. Sleep diaries and actigraphy (see below) are particularly useful for assessing day-to-day variability.

It is important to ensure that clients can read and understand the questions, as many measures require a higher reading ability than many people with psychotic disorders possess. It is also helpful to ask about any learning difficulties that the client may have, to help assess the suitability of reading materials, written work, and cognitive and behavioural strategies used in treatment. Therapists may need to read questions aloud to clients.

Clients who are hypomanic or manic may skew their ratings more positively, whereas others may lack insight into the severity of their sleep problems. Paranoid ideations may lead clients to answer questions more cautiously or skip items.

Finally, scores on sleepiness measures need to be interpreted with caution. Among all the factors that can contribute to daytime sleepiness and hypersomnia, the effects of medication and other substances (drugs and alcohol) may have the greatest influence. It is useful to query the cause of sleepiness if is indicated on a questionnaire. We suggest assessing sleep variables (total sleep time, SOL, wakefulness after sleep onset) distinct from daytime dysfunction. If there is excessive fatigue or sleepiness with normal or high total sleep time, and if no other sleep disorders are suspected, a treatment focus on improving daytime energy and routines is indicated.

Questionnaires to Assess Psychiatric Symptom Severity and Impact

Measures of symptom severity can be useful for understanding where the person sits in terms of established norms and for tracking treatment progress and benefits.

Commonly used scales that are relatively quick and easy to administer include:

- The *Beck Depression Inventory-II* (Beck et al., 1996) and the *Beck Anxiety Inventory* (Beck and Steer, 1993) assess depression and anxiety level, respectively, with 21 items.
- The *Depression Anxiety Stress Scales* (DASS; Lovibond and Lovibond, 1995), which comes with 21 (DASS-21) or 42 questions (DASS-42).
- The *Patient Health Questionnaire for Anxiety and Depression* (PHQ-4; Kroenke et al., 2009) is designed to be an ultra-brief screener of anxiety and depression levels.
- The *Mini International Neuropsychiatric Interview* (MINI; Sheehan et al., 1998) is a short, structured diagnostic instrument for axis 1 psychiatric diagnoses.
- The *Brief Psychiatric Rating Scale* (Overall and Gorham, 1962) is a semi-structured interview that assesses the severity of psychiatric symptoms with 24 items.
- *Psychotic Symptoms Rating Scales* (Haddock et al., 1999) are designed to assess the severity of hallucinations and delusions with 17 items.

Assessment tools are also available for specific symptoms. Detailed scales are available to assess hallucinations in all modalities, delusions, insight, and other psychotic symptoms (see Waters and Stephane, 2015).

Sleep Diaries

Sleep diaries are usually completed over 1 week (7 days) or, more preferably, 2 weeks. Clients are asked to complete the sleep diary every day during this period. The sleep diary gives information about the daily sleep–wake routine. Research suggests that sleep diaries are more accurate than global estimates of variables such as total sleep time. A sleep diary enlarged to A3-size paper may be useful for clients with reading or writing difficulties. Some clients will benefit from daily reminders or prompts to complete the diary. Placement of the diary in a prominent place, such as on the fridge or next to the kettle, can be helpful, as can reminders on the client's phone, or a family member or carer may also assist by reminding them.

The diary collects sleep variables such as the timing of bedtime and wake-up, from which the following information can be drawn:

- variability in bed and sleep time and wake-up time, as well as the frequency and length of daytime naps;
- sleep efficiency, calculated as the percentage of time asleep relative to time in bed; for example a 5-hour total sleep time and 10 hours in bed would mean a sleep efficiency of 50 per cent; sleep efficiency below 80 per cent is usually taken to indicate clinically significant sleep disruption;
- the presence of Insomnia is indicated by a SOL of longer than 30 minutes, night-time wakings with a duration of 30 minutes or longer, or waking more than 30 minutes before a preferred wake time, accompanied by daytime fatigue and/or worry about sleep. In Insomnia, there is also reduced sleep efficiency and, frequently, high inter-night variability;
- hypersomnia, indicated by long sleep duration (shown as time in bed in the diary) over the 24-hour period (9+ hours), daytime naps, and/or persistent daytime tiredness (as shown on questionnaires);
- delayed sleep phase, indicated by prolonged SOL, late lights out time (after midnight), and sleeping in late the next day;

- advanced sleep phase, indicated by a short SOL, early lights out time (before 9 p.m.), and early waking; the person may also doze on the couch in the evening.

Although a sleep log is by no means a diagnostic test, frequent short wakings, together with daytime napping and tiredness, can be indicative of OSA. If accompanied by snoring, gasping, and/or morning headaches, consider referral for an overnight sleep assessment.

Formulation and Case Conceptualisation

After the assessment information has been collected, the next step is to synthesise it into the main factors that contribute to poor sleep and tiredness, paying particular attention to factors that increase arousal, reduce sleep drive, and disrupt the body clock. This information can be used to guide the contents of the CBT-I session.

Factors that Reduce Sleep Drive

These include:

- sleeping in;
- napping;
- reduced daily activity levels;
- reduced daily stimulation;
- low mood/depression;
- use of stimulants.

Factors that Interfere with the Body Clock

These include:

- irregular sleep routine;
- lack of exposure to morning and daytime light;
- exposure to bright light close to bedtime.

Factors that Increase Arousal

These include:

- anxiety about poor sleep/ability to cope;
- general worries;
- external stressors;
- panic symptoms;
- fears;
- trauma-related anxiety;
- rumination;
- nightmares;
- paranoid thoughts, disturbing night-time hallucinations;
- physical stimulation close to bedtime (exercise);
- cognitive stimulation close to bedtime (worrying, ruminating, arguing, social media, planning, problem-solving, stimulating TV shows or computer games);
- stimulants such as caffeine and nicotine.

Objective Assessment Methods

Some issues identified through the screening questionnaires may require further investigation with objective measures of sleep or with independent clinical attention through a referral to a sleep clinic.

A selection of objective methods is as follows:

Wrist Actigraphy

An actiwatch is a device worn on the wrist to record movements from which sleep–wake patterns are inferred. Data from an actigraph can provide information regarding bedtime, sleep time, wake time, and periods of resting or napping during the day. Its output (the 'actigram') can show whether the person has unusual sleep–wake patterns.

Although actigraphy monitoring alone is not valid for the diagnosis of Insomnia, advantages include the fact that it permits 24-hour online recording and may be worn for an extended period of time (up to 30 days on some devices), and it allows assessment of sleep–wake patterns while the individual goes about their normal routine (Sadeh and Acebo, 2002). Seven days of actigraphy recording are sufficient to provide a valuable 'snapshot' of an individual's sleep routine, although longer periods of recording are best.

Data from actigraphy are not always accurate, as a 'sleep period' is assigned by the actigraphy logarithm when the device does not detect movement. Therefore, sedentary periods and time spent reading or watching TV in bed can be interpreted as sleep. To increase the validity of the information it provides, information from concurrent sleep diaries should be used to edit actigraphy data. This is quite time-consuming, however, and may be better suited to research purposes.

Our experience is that people with psychotic disorders tolerate wrist actigraphy very well and, in fact, enjoy wearing the device. They are often appreciative of a printed output showing their sleep–wake patterns. Paranoid thoughts regarding the device's persecutory intent is rare.

Many different devices are available. Philips's brand of Actiwatch is often used in research settings. Increasingly, however, fitness trackers are being used (e.g. Fitbit, Basis Peak, or other brands). Some brands are better than others at assessing sleep timing and efficiency. Although they are more cost-effective than Actiwatches, validation data are still lacking.

Polysomnography

Polysomnography (PSG) is commonly referred to as an 'overnight sleep study'; it involves attaching electrodes to the head and body to permit the recording of overnight brain activity, respiratory functions, and blood oxygen levels (Butkov and Lee-Chiong, 2007). An overnight sleep study may be obtained through a referral to a sleep clinic.

PSG is used to investigate and provide a formal diagnosis of different sleep disorders, including OSA, leg movement disorders, and parasomnias. PSG is not suitable for diagnosing Insomnia Disorder, circadian disorders, or hypersomnia, as it involves the collection of data on only one or two nights of sleep. Longer sleep monitoring periods (also involving daytime monitoring) are needed to assess the clinical features of these other sleep disorders.

Our experience is that the majority of people with a severe mental disorder do not tolerate overnight PSG study in a sleep laboratory, as the laboratory environment appears frightening; the leads and electrodes severely restrict movements, which may cause fear and panic; and the all-night monitoring with video cameras and brain electronics can feed into the person's paranoid ideation. Approximately half of people with psychotic disorders can be persuaded to undergo a home-based PSG. This can also be conducted in the comfort of the person's residence and even hospital ward. Tolerance for the leads, nasal prongs, and finger oximeter can be low, and so a good rapport and some rules should be established before the overnight study is conducted.

Other Procedures and Processes

It is helpful to know that other procedures and processes are available for objective investigation of sleep disturbances. These include the dim light melatonin onset (DLMO) procedure and the MSLT. These are not typically used by therapists administering cognitive and behavioural interventions, but they are mentioned here as they are often sought by sleep physicians to make a formal diagnosis and formulate treatment recommendations.

If circadian rhythm disruptions are suspected, the sleep clinic may initiate a DLMO test procedure to obtain an objective measure of the circadian phase shift by way of the timing of evening melatonin production (Pandi-Perumal et al., 2007). In individuals with a typical sleep–wake schedule, melatonin levels start to rise approximately 2 hours before sleep onset and remain high during habitual sleep hours. DLMO can be used to determine the timing of melatonin secretion through collection of saliva samples under dim light conditions. Saliva samples are then analysed for the assessment of phase delays or advances of rhythms in entrained individuals or of whether the person is in a free-running state (non-24 hours). It can be used also as a tool to aid psychiatric diagnosis in people complaining of sleep and mood disorders (e.g. seasonal affective disorder).

The MSLT can assess how quickly a person falls asleep in a quiet environment during the day, and this objective test of daytime sleepiness is sometimes used for a formal diagnosis of narcolepsy and hypersomnia (Carskadon et al., 1986; Standards of Practice Committee of the American Academy of Sleep Medicine, 2005). The MSLT comprises approximately five scheduled naps during the day, in which the person is asked to go to sleep in a dark, comfortable environment. Sensors measure whether the person is asleep and the stages of sleep. A rapid SOL (less than 8 minutes to fall asleep) indicates excessive daytime sleepiness. A person with hypersomnia may fall asleep quickly, but only a person with narcolepsy will have symptoms of cataplexy and be more likely to experience sleep paralysis or sleep hallucinations that accompany the sudden shift into sleep.

Summary

- Assessment is a critical part of treatment planning, motivation building, and relationship building between clinician and client.
- A clinical interview and sleep diary are the suggested minimum assessment requirements for sleep disturbance prior to CBT-I.
- The clinical interview should ask about the client's description of their sleep problem, sleep parameters, presence of other sleep complaints, coping mechanisms and daytime functioning, sleep environment, as well as levels of motivation and self-efficacy.
- There are several brief questionnaires that can assist with the assessment and provide baseline information regarding sleep disturbance and other symptoms.
- Once assessment data have been gathered, a case formulation is derived that assists in treatment planning. Here, consideration of predisposing, precipitating, and perpetuating factors, as well as the three barriers to sleep, is important.
- Sleep diaries are an important tool for assessing sleep–wake patterns and treatment adherence. Reminders may need to be set up for clients to complete them.

- Wrist actigraphy is an objective measure of sleep that can be useful for assessing sleep–wake patterns.
- Other objective measures of sleep, such as DLMO and MSLT, are not typical in the case of Insomnia but may be useful if other sleep disorders are suspected.

References

Bastien, C. H., Vallières, A., and Morin, C. M. (2001) "Validation of the Insomnia Severity Index as an outcome measure for insomnia research", *Sleep Medicine*, 2(4), pp. 297–307.

Beck, A. T., and Steer, R. A. (1993) *Beck anxiety inventory manual.* San Antonio, TX: Psychological Corporation.

Beck, A. T., Steer, R. A., and Brown, G. K. (1996) *Manual for the BDI-II.* San Antonio, TX: Psychological Corporation.

Butkov, N., and Lee-Chiong, T. L. (Eds.) (2007) *Fundamentals of sleep technology.* Philadelphia, PA: Lippincott Williams & Wilkins.

Buysse, D. J., Reynolds III, C. F., Monk, T. H., Berman, S. R., and Kupfer, D. J. (1989) "The Pittsburgh sleep quality index: A new instrument for psychiatric practice and research", *Psychiatry Research*, 28(2), pp. 193–213.

Carskadon, M. A., Dement, W. C., Mitler, M. M., Roth, T., Westbrook, P. R., and Keenan, S. (1986) "Guidelines for the Multiple Sleep Latency Test (MSLT): A standard measure of sleepiness", *Sleep*, 9(4), pp. 519–524.

Chiu, V. W., Harvey, R. H., Sloan, N. B., Ree, M., Lin, A., Janca, A., and Waters, F. (2015) "Cognitive and behavioral factors associated with insomnia in inpatients with schizophrenia and related psychoses", *Journal of Nervous & Mental Disease*, 203(10), pp. 798–803.

Haddock, G., McCarron, J., Tarrier, N., and Faragher, E. B. (1999) "Scales to measure dimensions of hallucinations and delusions: The psychotic symptom rating scales (PSYRATS)", *Psychological Medicine*, 29(04), pp. 879–889.

Horne, J. A., and Ostberg, O. (1976) "A self-assessment questionnaire to determine morningness–eveningness in human circadian rhythms", *International Journal of Chronobiology*, 4(2), pp. 97–110.

Johns, M. W. (1991) "A new method for measuring daytime sleepiness: The Epworth sleepiness scale", *Sleep*, 14(6), pp. 540–545.

Kroenke, K., Spitzer, R. L., Williams, J. B. W., and Löwe, B. (2009) "An ultra-brief screening scale for anxiety and depression: The PHQ–4", *Psychosomatics*, 50(6), pp. 613–621.

Lovibond, S. H., and Lovibond, P. F. (1995) *Manual for the depression anxiety stress scales* (2nd ed.). Sydney, NSW: Psychology Foundation.

Mastin, D., Bryson, J., and Corwyn, R. (2006) "Assessment of sleep hygiene using the sleep hygiene index", *Journal of Behavioral Medicine*, 29(3), pp. 223–227.

Morin, C. M., Vallières, A., and Ivers, H. (2007) "Dysfunctional beliefs and attitudes about sleep (DBAS): Validation of a brief version (DBAS-16)", *Sleep*, 30(11), p. 1547.

Netzer, N. C., Stoohs, R. A., Netzer, C. M., Clark, K., and Strohl, K. P. (1999) "Using the Berlin questionnaire to identify patients at risk for the sleep apnea syndrome", *Annals of Internal Medicine*, 131(7), pp. 485–491.

Overall, J. E., and Gorham, D. R. (1962) "The brief psychiatric rating scale", *Psychological Reports*, 10(3), pp. 799–812.

Pandi-Perumal, S. R., Smits, M., Spence, W., Srinivasan, V., Cardinali, D. P., Lowe, A. D., and Kayumov, L. (2007) "Dim light melatonin onset (DLMO): A tool for the analysis of circadian phase in human sleep and chronobiological disorders", *Progress in Neuro-Psychopharmacology & Biological Psychiatry*, 31(1), pp. 1–11.

Prochaska, J. O., and DiClemente, C. C. (1983) "Stages and processes of self-change of smoking: Toward an integrative model of change", *Journal of Consulting & Clinical Psychology*, 51(3), pp. 390–395.

Ree, M. J., and Harvey, A. G. (2004) "Investigating safety behaviours in insomnia: The development of the sleep-related behaviours questionnaire (SRBQ)", *Behaviour Change*, 21(01), pp. 26–36.

Ree, M. J., Harvey, A. G., Blake, R., Tang, N. K. Y., and Shawe-Taylor, M. (2005) "Attempts to control unwanted thoughts in the night: Development of the thought control questionnaire-insomnia revised (TCQI-R)", *Behaviour Research & Therapy*, 43, pp. 985–998.

Sadeh, A., and Acebo, C. (2002) "The role of actigraphy in sleep medicine", *Sleep Medicine Reviews*, 6(2), pp. 113–124.

Sheehan, D. V., Lecrubier, Y., Sheehan, K. H., Amorim, P., Janavs, J., Weiller, E., Hergueta, T., Baker, R., and Dunbar, G. C. (1998) "The mini-international neuropsychiatric interview (MINI): The development and validation of a structured diagnostic psychiatric interview for DSM-IV and ICD-10", *Journal of Clinical Psychiatry*, 59(Suppl. 20), pp. 22–33.

Spoormaker, V. I., Verbeek, I., van den Bout, J., and Klip, E. C. (2005) "Initial validation of the SLEEP-50 questionnaire", *Behavioral Sleep Medicine*, 3(4), pp. 227–246.

Standards of Practice Committee of the American Academy of Sleep Medicine (2005) "Practice parameters for clinical use of the Multiple Sleep Latency Test and the maintenance of wakefulness test", *Sleep*, 28(1), pp. 113–121.

Waters, F., and Stephane, M. (Eds.) (2015) *The assessment of psychosis: A reference book and rating scales for research and practice*. New York: Routledge.

9 Evidence for CBT-I in Psychotic Disorders

Therapeutic guidelines for psychosis recommend that non-pharmacological options such as psychological therapies be offered alongside medications (National Collaborating Centre for Mental Health, 2014). Psychological therapies involving cognitive and behavioural components (such as CBT) uphold the principles of recovery-oriented mental health practice by encouraging clients to be actively engaged during treatment, learn self-management skills, and meet their recovery goals. This chapter presents a summary of the empirical evidence to date for CBT-I to treat Insomnia in people with psychotic disorders. Results from our own clinical research are presented. Our research programme—termed the *Sleep Well, Feel Well with Psychosis* programme—forms the context in which our CBT-I Therapist Manual was evaluated.

CBT-I as a Treatment Option

With respect to Insomnia in the general population, as discussed in Chapter 7, CBT-I is the treatment with the most evidence behind it. As such, there is obvious potential for its use in the treatment and management of Insomnia in people with a psychotic disorder. As we discuss in this chapter, there is now emerging evidence that CBT-I can be very effective in psychotic disorders.

Many people with psychotic disorders report a desire to engage in psychological therapies. When given the choice, many view CBT-I as a more acceptable long-term option for the treatment of their sleep disturbances over standard pharmacotherapy (71.5 per cent of respondents versus 22.5 per cent, respectively; Waters et al., 2015).

In the Waters et al. (2015) study, the main benefits of CBT-I cited by participants were as follows:

- long-lasting effectiveness;
- lack of side effects;
- reduced dependence on sleep medications;
- greater sense of autonomy and control;
- empowerment from making their own choices;
- increased human contact, which alleviates loneliness;
- opportunity to learn from others and to offer advice to others when in group settings.

All too often, however, people with psychotic disorders are not given a choice regarding treatment options (González-Torres et al., 2007), with the majority not even offered basic sleep hygiene education (Lyne et al., 2011). This appears to be a significant missed opportunity, as, from an intervention perspective, disturbances in sleep may be considerably simpler to treat than other clinical features of psychosis.

Empirical Evidence for CBT-I

The benefits of psychological interventions to address Insomnia in the general population are well documented (Morin, 2015). Some therapeutic approaches offer behavioural interventions alone (e.g. stimulus control), but most evidence suggests that therapies that address both behavioural and cognitive elements (CBT-I) have most potential for producing reliable and durable change (Spielman et al., 1987; Perlis et al., 2005; Harvey et al., 2014).

In clinical groups comprising individuals with depression, anxiety disorders, and chronic pain, CBT-I has been found to produce longer total sleep time, reduced awakenings, and improved sleep quality (Smith et al., 2005; Edinger et al., 2009; Geiger-Brown et al., 2015). It is also linked to reduced symptoms of psychological distress, such as depression and anxiety, and a tapering-off from sleep medication usage (Dashevsky and Kramer, 1998; Smith et al., 2005).

Evidence for CBT-I in psychotic disorders is slowly building, although much variation exists in the type of sleep therapy, and number of sessions, offered. Although understanding of sleep disorders in psychosis, and how best to treat them, is still developing, there is sufficient evidence to date to justify the use of CBT-I interventions within these populations.

Behavioural Therapies and/or Psychoeducation for Insomnia

Four studies have assessed the benefits of psychoeducation and/or behavioural interventions alone in mixed psychiatric cohorts, with results generally reporting moderate improvements in subjective sleep quality (Holmes et al., 1995; Dashevsky and Kramer, 1998; Haynes et al., 2011; Lyne et al., 2011). Other benefits included increased sleep knowledge (Holmes et al., 1995), decreased worry about sleep difficulties (Dashevsky and Kramer, 1998), and a reduction in the use of sleep medication, a finding that was maintained 6 months later (Dashevsky and Kramer, 1998).

Cognitive Behavioural Therapy for Insomnia (CBT-I)

To date, seven studies have used cognitive and behavioural interventions (CBT-I) to treat Insomnia in psychotic and related disorders. Four studies employed a case-control design:

1. Wagley et al. (2013) provided two individual sessions of abbreviated CBT-I to 20 psychiatric outpatients with mixed diagnoses (and included ten control participants);
2. Freeman et al. (2015) provided four to eight individual sessions of CBT-I to 24 people with schizophrenia-spectrum disorder (26 controls);
3. Harvey et al. (2015) compared eight individual sessions of modified CBT-I delivered to 22 people with bipolar disorder type I (19 controls); and
4. van de Laar et al. (2015) delivered six individual CBT-I sessions to 30 individuals with mixed psychiatric diagnoses (30 controls).

A further three studies provided CBT-I in people with psychotic disorders but did not include a comparison group:

5. Dopke et al. (2004) delivered ten weekly CBT-I group sessions to ten people with mixed diagnoses (predominantly psychosis);
6. Myers et al. (2011) delivered four individual sessions of CBT-I to 15 people with schizophrenia-spectrum disorders; and
7. Sylvia et al. (2014) delivered three individual sessions of abbreviated CBT-I to eight people with bipolar disorder with comorbid anxiety.

Summary of Findings

The findings from the above studies can be summarised as follows:

Sleep Variables

CBT-I provides better sleep outcomes than treatment as usual (TAU) in psychotic and mixed psychiatric disorders. The effect sizes were mixed, and yet findings generally showed moderate to large improvements in sleep variables such as sleep latency, total sleep time, and night-time wakings. Improvements in symptoms of anxiety, depression, and delusions were demonstrated in some studies (e.g. Myers et al., 2011; Wagley et al., 2013; Harvey et al., 2015; van de Laar et al., 2015), but not in others (Sylvia et al., 2014; Freeman et al., 2015).

Number of Sessions

A higher number of sessions was not necessarily indicative of a better outcome, suggesting that session contents should be adapted to the person's need, rather than a fixed number of sessions being provided. In fact, more sessions were linked to a higher drop-out rate (van de Laar et al., 2015), suggesting that 'more is not always better'.

Drop-Out Rates

As with any other medical treatment, treatment drop-out during CBT-I is an important problem, especially in people with psychiatric conditions in whom treatment adherence can be disappointingly low. Available estimates suggest that 14–40 per cent of psychiatric study participants drop out of CBT-I, potentially diminishing the opportunity for improvements in sleep and other related symptoms (Matthews et al., 2013). Enhancing motivation and engagement with treatment may be especially important factors in improving CBT-I adherence for those with a psychotic disorder (see Chapters 4 and 6).

Modifications to Standard CBT-I

To date, few studies have developed modifications to standard CBT-I that address specific features of sleep disturbance in psychotic disorders. The exceptions include: (a) Harvey et al. (2015), who included adaptations for motivation, hypersomnia, and circadian disturbance; (b) Sylvia et al. (2014), who included education on medication and an additional module for hypersomnia; and (c) Freeman et al. (2015), whose study protocol (Freeman et al., 2013) and pilot study (Myers et al., 2011) describe adaptations for psychotic symptoms and comorbid sleep problems (circadian rhythm and fears about sleep). This emerging literature suggests that modifications to standard CBT-I are helpful for addressing the specific challenges and difficulties faced by people with psychosis.

Comorbidities

With an emphasis on controlled methodologies, many of the above studies excluded individuals with comorbidities such as learning disabilities, alcohol/substance dependence, and OSA. Such studies are tremendously important for providing information regarding the benefits of CBT-I approaches without common confounds associated with psychiatric populations. However, the reality is that people with psychotic disorders commonly have comorbid disorders, substance dependence, and learning difficulties, as well as multiple sleep complaints. Thus, the efficacy of treatments must consider the influence of such factors in psychiatric populations.

The Sleep Well, Feel Well with Psychosis Programme

The Sleep Well, Feel Well with Psychosis programme is conducted as part of a broad clinical research programme undertaken by the University of Western Australia and the North Metropolitan Health Service Mental Health, a public mental health service in Perth, Western Australia. The programme seeks to increase accurate detection and management of sleep problems in individuals with severe mental illnesses.

As part of this clinical research programme, a specially adapted CBT-I manual was developed around the needs of people with psychotic disorders. As stated in previous chapters, the intervention has the following characteristics:

- four sessions to ensure low drop-out rates for maximal treatment response;
- the choice of individual or group sessions;
- a personalised approach and a focus on meaningful activity to increase motivation;
- activities to encourage internal locus of control and improved perceptions of self-efficacy;
- strategies to manage hypersomnia, circadian rhythm problems, and frequent nightmares;
- support for managing low mood, anxiety, psychotic symptoms, and intrusive cognitions;
- support for overcoming personal challenges (e.g. stress management and problem-solving);
- lay language to accommodate varying educational levels and reading abilities.

The effectiveness of this CBT-I manual was evaluated against a group of people receiving their usual treatment (TAU).

Participants

Evaluation of the CBT-I manual initially involved a total of 72 individuals with a psychotic disorder. All participants had sleep complaints together with compromised functioning in domains such as work, social engagement, and self-care. Inclusion criteria included: (a) a psychiatric disorder with psychotic features; (b) a stable clinical condition with capacity to provide informed consent, as endorsed by their treating psychiatrist or case worker; (c) self-reported sleep problems resulting in impaired daytime functioning; and (d) a total score of 5 or more on the PSQI, which is indicative of clinically significant sleep problems. People under the age of 18 years were excluded from the study.

Participants consented voluntarily to either the CBT-I programme as an adjunct to their usual medication (n = 50) or a TAU comparison condition (n = 22). The latter group comprised a convenience sample drawn from the same mental health service. The participants in the CBT-I group were only included in the final analyses if they attended at least two of the four treatment sessions. A total of 46 participants (92 per cent) attended at least two sessions, and 32 (64 per cent) attended all four sessions. This reflects substantially lower drop-out rates than other studies and is consistent with reports that attrition rates are improved when clients are able to select which treatment they receive, compared with being randomly allocated (Sidani et al., 2015).

After exclusion of the four participants who failed to attend a minimum of two sessions, statistical analyses were therefore conducted on a total of 68 participants (n = 46 CBT-I; n = 22 TAU).

Both conditions were balanced for gender (50 per cent) and age (CBT-I mean age = 41.7 years, and TAU mean age = 43.3 years). The primary diagnoses for both groups were schizophrenia-spectrum disorders and mood disorders (bipolar disorder or major depression with psychotic features). Psychiatric comorbidities comprising anxiety, borderline personality disorder, and PTSD were present in 80 per cent of participants from both groups. Most participants had low levels of education (86 per cent), and a subset had dyslexia or other learning difficulties. None of the participants worked full time, and all were on a disability pension. A minority worked in part-time supported employment (largely through support from an NGO) in a paid or unpaid capacity.

All participants were taking daily antipsychotic medication (chlorpromazine equivalents mean dose: CBT-I = 418, TAU = 458) and/or a mood stabiliser (sodium valproate, lithium). Other medications included antidepressants and hypnotics, as well as drugs for different medical conditions (e.g. diabetes, high blood pressure, pain). Those suspected of having another untreated sleep disorder, such as OSA, were referred to a sleep clinic for assessment and treatment prior to taking part in this programme.

Treatment Programme and Evaluation

The treatment comprised four weekly or fortnightly group or individual sessions, each lasting 90–120 minutes. Participants were provided with a client resource pack at each session that outlined the skills addressed in that session.

The outcomes for both CBT-I and TAU interventions were assessed at baseline (pre-treatment), post-treatment (approximately 1 week after Session 4), and at follow-up (mean 3 months, range 1–5 months). Only baseline and post-treatment results are presented here. Change across the period of CBT-I treatment was assessed with a sleep change form provided at each session.

Questionnaires included:

- *the PSQI* (Buysse et al., 1989), which provides information about sleep efficiency, sleep latency, the nature of sleep disturbances, and daytime effects of disturbed sleep over the previous month;
- *the MINI psychosis section* (Sheehan et al., 1998), which assesses for the presence of seven psychotic symptoms on a five-point scale; those who reported hallucinations were also asked to rate their distress associated with voices and/or visions;
- *the PHQ-4* (Kroenke et al., 2009), which assesses for psychological distress using four items; scores for anxiety and depression levels can be derived from the measure;
- *the Sleep Hygiene Behaviours Scale* (SHiK-B; Chiu et al., 2015), which assesses for poor sleep hygiene practices in relation to caffeine use, smoking, exercise, substance abuse, sleep schedules, and daylight exposure; the SHiK-B establishes whether respondents engaged in these activities over the previous fortnight;

- *the Sleep Change Scale*, which asked respondents to rate their levels of improvement in the last 7 days from 0 (none at all) to 10 (reflective of a significant amount), in domains of sleep quality, energy and motivation, coping with everyday problems, attention and concentration, and feeling and coping.
- *the Goal Attainment Scale* (Kiresuk and Sherman, 1968), which evaluates post-treatment improvements in sleep quality by asking respondents whether they achieved their treatment goals; scores were rated from 1 to 5, with higher scores indicating greater improvements than expected (1 = much less improvement than expected; 5 = much more than expected).

Results

A detailed evaluation of the results will be published elsewhere (Chiu et al., in preparation). Below, we present an overview of the key findings. First, the effectiveness of the intervention was evaluated with a comparison of measures pre- and post-treatment, using repeated measure analyses. Second, participant progress from session to session was examined with the Sleep Change Scale, and whether treatment goals were attained. Effect sizes were calculated using Dunlap et al.'s (1996) formula for dependent data measurements. Table 9.1 shows the descriptive characteristics of the two groups on PSQI-measured sleep and symptom measures pre- and post-intervention.

PSQI

There were overall significant group differences of moderate effect size (d = 0.6), with significant sleep improvements in the CBT-group, but not in the TAU group (p = 0.12). In the CBT-I group, PSQI global scores (overall sleep quality) improved by an average of 22.7 per cent, with a large effect size (d = 0.88). Daytime dysfunction improved by 25 per cent, with a moderate effect size (d = 0.66), and sleep medication usage decreased by 19.4 per cent.

A closer look at the results showed that the sleep of CBT-I participants improved in several domains. On average:

Table 9.1 Means and Standard Deviations of the Outcome Variables for CBT-I and TAU Groups at Baseline and Post-treatment

Measure	*CBT-I Baseline*	*CBT-I Post-treatment*	*TAU[1] Baseline*	*TAU[1] Post-treatment*
PSQI global score[2]	13.6 (3.0)	10.5 (3.6)***	10.9 (3.45)	9.7 (3.7)
PSQI duration of sleep[3]	1.1 (1.2)	0.7 (1.0)**	1.0 (1.0)	0.5 (0.6)*
PSQI sleep disturbance[3]	2.0 (0.6)	1.5 (0.5)***	1.4 (0.6)	1.4 (0.5)
PSQI sleep latency[3]	2.3 (1.0)	1.6 (0.96)**	2.1 (1.1)	2.0 (0.8)
PSQI daytime dysfunction[3]	2.0 (0.7)	1.5 (0.6)*	1.4 (0.8)	1.2 (0.9)
PSQI sleep efficiency[3]	1.5 (1.0)	1.1 (1.2)	1.3 (1.3)	0.8 (1.0)
PSQI overall sleep quality[3]	2.1 (0.8)	1.3 (0.8)***	1.6 (1.0)	1.4 (0.9)
MINI psychosis total[3]	15.2 (7.2)	13.9 (6.9)*	13.2 (6.7)	12.5 (7.2)
PHQ-4	6.3 (3.1)	4.8 (3.4)**	5.1 (3.1)	4.9 (3.1)

Notes: (1) TAU = treatment as usual; (2) PSQI global score: A global sum of 5 or greater indicates a 'poor' sleeper; (3) PSQI minimum score = 0 (better); maximum score = 3 (worse); * $p < 0.05$; ** $p < 0.01$; *** $p < 0.001$ (repeated measure analyses)

- Total sleep time improved for short sleepers by 1.2 hours (an increase from 5.4 hours to 6.6 hours) and, for long sleepers, by 1.1 hours (a reduction from 10.7 to 9.6 hours).
- SOL reduced from 71.8 minutes to 34 minutes.
- There was a 50 per cent decrease in the number of participants reporting difficulties staying awake during the day.
- There was a 21 per cent decrease in the number of participants reporting bad dreams and nightmares.

The TAU group failed to show any improvements over time on PSQI sleep variables, except for a significant change in total sleep time. A closer examination of the TAU group's data suggests that longer sleepers' sleep duration remained the same, and that the difference was due to a change in three individuals who reported excessively long sleep duration (9.5–12 hours) post-treatment (but not pre-treatment). Therefore, this change in score is not consistent with a normalisation or improvement of sleep, but rather reflects a worsening of sleep in the TAU group.

On the other PSQI variables, the TAU group showed no change on measures of sleep latency, night-time waking, overall sleep quality, bad dreams, problems keeping up enthusiasm, or sleep medication usage.

Symptom Ratings

The CBT-I group also showed:

- significant reductions in total psychological distress (PHQ-4; $d = 0.43$) and in levels of depression and anxiety;
- significant improvements in overall severity of psychotic symptoms (MINI), albeit with a small effect size ($d = 0.18$), which were largely contributed to by significant reductions in paranoia scores ($d = 0.39$).

By contrast, individuals in the TAU group did not show any significant improvements in mood or psychotic symptom ratings.

Sleep Hygiene (SHiK-B)

The CBT-I group also made significant improvements in sleep hygiene (data not shown). After treatment:

- 56 per cent of participants practised more regular bedtime routines;
- 44 per cent sought more natural sunlight during the day;
- 33 per cent reduced their intake of caffeine and nicotine before bedtime;
- 20 per cent stopped napping during the day.

Sleep Change Scale and the Goal Attainment Scale

Subjective improvements in sleep and quality of life were assessed using the Sleep Change Scale and the Goal Attainment Scale (collected at all sessions except the first). Figure 9.1 shows that participants reported steep session-by-session improvements in overall sleep quality, which closely mirrored improvements in 'feelings and coping'. The marked initial improvements in energy, coping, and attention tended to plateau after the third session.

Effectiveness of the intervention was also assessed using the Goal Attainment Scale, which sought participants' ratings of whether they felt they had achieved their treatment goals. Figure 9.2 shows the most commonly cited goals, together with the percentage of participants who improved 'more than expected' (mean of 89 per cent; range 75–100 per cent).

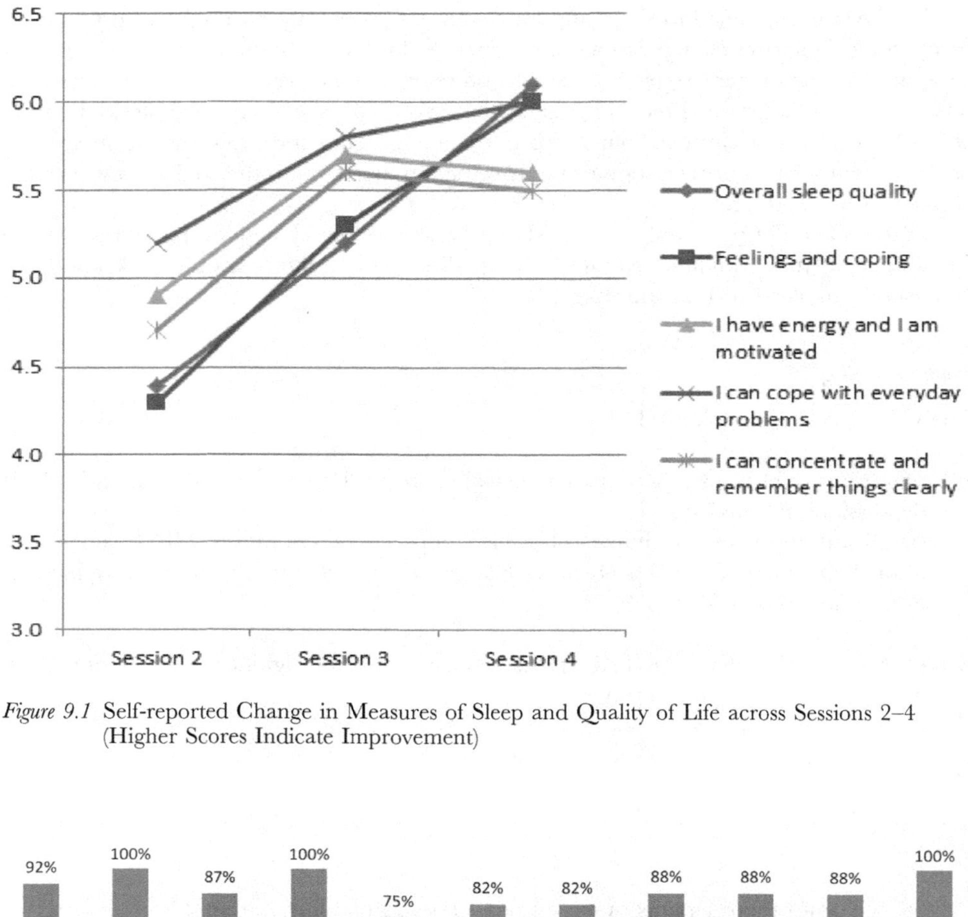

Figure 9.1 Self-reported Change in Measures of Sleep and Quality of Life across Sessions 2–4 (Higher Scores Indicate Improvement)

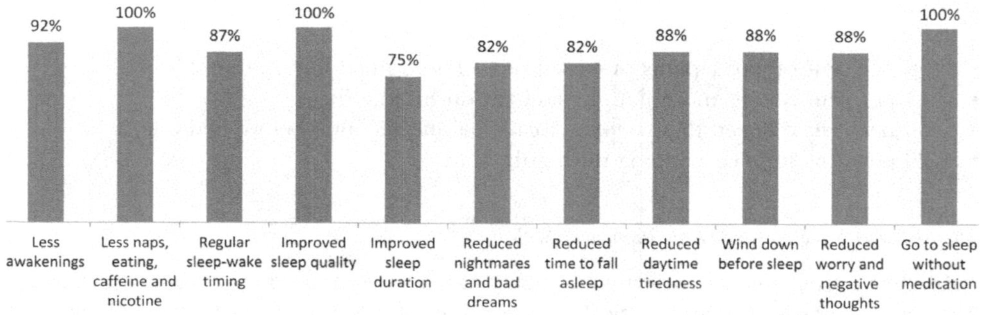

Figure 9.2 Percentage of Participants who Improved 'More than Expected' in Their Treatment Goals

Summary

- Individuals with psychotic disorders can benefit from explicit training in CBT-based sleep and symptom management techniques.
- Our adapted CBT-I intervention showed significant benefits on measures of sleep, daytime functions, and symptoms, and 100 per cent participant satisfaction.
- None of these benefits was shown by the participants who received their usual treatment (the TAU group).
- The low attrition rate found in this study is evidence of strong treatment credibility and positive effects.
- The current intervention looks particularly promising in its effectiveness for treating Insomnia and other sleep problems in people with psychotic disorders.

References

Buysse, D. J., Reynolds, C. F., Monk, T. H., Berman, S. R., and Kupfer, D. J. (1989) "The Pittsburgh Sleep Quality Index: A new instrument for psychiatric practice and research", *Psychiatry Research*, 28(2), pp. 193–213.

Chiu, V. W., Harvey, R. H., Sloan, N. B., Ree, M., Lin, A., Janca, A., and Waters, F. (2015) "Cognitive and behavioral factors associated with insomnia in inpatients with schizophrenia and related psychoses", *Journal of Nervous & Mental Disease*, 203(10), pp. 798–803.

Chiu, V. W., Ree, M., Janca, A., and Waters, F. (in preparation) "Adapted Cognitive-Behaviour and Therapy for Insomnia in psychosis: Who does it work for?".

Dashevsky, B. A., and Kramer, M. (1998) "Behavioral treatment of chronic insomnia in psychiatrically ill patients", *Journal of Clinical Psychiatry*, 59(12), pp. 693–701.

Dopke, C. A., Lehner, R. K., and Wells, A. M. (2004) "Cognitive-behavioral group therapy for insomnia in individuals with serious mental illnesses: A preliminary evaluation", *Psychiatric Rehabilitation Journal*, 27(3), pp. 235–242.

Dunlap, W. P., Cortina, J. M., Vaslow, J. B., and Burke, M. J. (1996) "Meta-analysis of experiments with matched groups or repeated measures designs", *Psychological Methods*, 1(2), pp. 170–177.

Edinger, J. D., Olsen, M. K., Stechuchak, K. M., Means, M. K., Lineberger, M. D., Kirby, A., and Carney, C. E. (2009) "Cognitive behavioral therapy for patients with primary insomnia or insomnia associated predominantly with mixed psychiatric disorders: A randomized clinical trial", *Sleep*, 32(4), pp. 499.

Freeman, D., Startup, H., Myers, E., Harvey, A., Geddes, J., Yu, L.-M., Zaiwalla, Z., Luengo-Fernandez, R., Foster, R., and Lister, R. (2013) "The effects of using cognitive behavioural therapy to improve sleep for patients with delusions and hallucinations (the BEST study): Study protocol for a randomized controlled trial", *Trials*, 14(1), pp. 1–7.

Freeman, D., Waite, F., Startup, H., Myers, E., Lister, R., McInerney, J., Harvey, A. G., Geddes, J., Zaiwalla, Z., Luengo-Fernandez, R., Foster, R., Clifton, L., and Yu, L.-M. (2015) "Efficacy of cognitive behavioural therapy for sleep improvement in patients with persistent delusions and hallucinations (BEST): A prospective, assessor-blind, randomised controlled pilot trial", *The Lancet Psychiatry*, 2(11), pp. 975–983.

Geiger-Brown, J. M., Rogers, V. E., Liu, W., Ludeman, E. M., Downton, K. D., and Diaz-Abad, M. (2015) "Cognitive behavioral therapy in persons with comorbid insomnia: A meta-analysis", *Sleep Medicine Reviews*, 23, pp. 54–67.

González-Torres, M., Oraa, R., Arístegui, M., Fernández-Rivas, A., and Guimon, J. (2007) "Stigma and discrimination towards people with schizophrenia and their family members", *Social Psychiatry & Psychiatric Epidemiology*, 42(1), pp. 14–23.

Harvey, A. G., Bélanger, L., Talbot, L., Eidelman, P., Beaulieu-Bonneau, S., Fortier-Brochu, É., Ivers, H., Lamy, M., Hein, K., Soehner, A. M., Mérette, C., and Morin, C. M. (2014) "Comparative efficacy of behavior therapy, cognitive therapy, and cognitive behavior therapy for chronic insomnia: A randomized controlled trial", *Journal of Consulting & Clinical Psychology*, 82(4), pp. 670–683.

Harvey, A. G., Soehner, A. M., Kaplan, K. A., Hein, K., Lee, J., Kanady, J., Li, D., Rabe-Hesketh, S., Ketter, T. A., Neylan, T. C., and Buysse, D. J. (2015) "Treating insomnia improves mood state, sleep, and functioning in bipolar disorder: A pilot randomized controlled trial", *Journal of Consulting & Clinical Psychology*, 83(3), pp. 564–577.

Haynes, P. L., Parthasarathy, S., Kersh, B., and Bootzin, R. R. (2011) "Examination of insomnia and insomnia treatment in psychiatric inpatients", *International Journal of Mental Health Nursing*, 20(2), pp. 130–136.

Holmes, E. P., Corrigan, P. W., Knight, S., and Flaxman, J. (1995) "Development of a sleep management program for people with severe mental illness", *Psychiatric Rehabilitation Journal*, 19(2), pp. 9–15.

Kiresuk, T. J., and Sherman, R. E. (1968) "Goal attainment scaling: A general method for evaluating comprehensive community mental health programs", *Community Mental Health Journal*, 4(6), pp. 443–453.

Kroenke, K., Spitzer, R. L., Williams, J. B. W., and Löwe, B. (2009) "An ultra-brief screening scale for anxiety and depression: The PHQ–4", *Psychosomatics*, 50(6), pp. 613–621.

Lyne, J., Quinlivan, L., Byrne, C. A., Malone, K., and Walsh, C. (2011) "Sleep hygiene use in a psychiatry outpatient setting", *Irish Medical Journal*, 104(2), pp. 49–50.

Matthews, E. E., Arnedt, J. T., McCarthy, M. S., Cuddihy, L. J., and Aloia, M. S. (2013) "Adherence to cognitive behavioral therapy for insomnia: A systematic review", *Sleep Medicine Reviews*, 17(6), pp. 453–464.

Morin, C. M. (2015) "Cognitive behavioral therapy for chronic insomnia: State of the science versus current clinical practices", *Annals of Internal Medicine*, 163(3), pp. 236–237.

Myers, E., Startup, H., and Freeman, D. (2011) "Cognitive behavioural treatment of insomnia in individuals with persistent persecutory delusions: A pilot trial", *Journal of Behavior Therapy & Experimental Psychiatry*, 42, pp. 330–336.

National Collaborating Centre for Mental Health (2014) *Psychosis and schizophrenia in adults: Treatment and management.* NICE Clinical Guideline 178. London: NICE.

Perlis, M. L., Smith, M. T., and Pigeon, W. R. (2005) "Etiology and pathophysiology of insomnia", in Kryger, M.H., Roth, T., and Dement, W. C. (Eds.) *Principles and practice of sleep medicine* (4th ed.). Philadelphia, PA: Elsevier Saunders, pp. 714–725.

Sheehan, D. V., Lecrubier, Y., Sheehan, K. H., Amorim, P., Janavs, J., Weiller, E., Hergueta, T., Baker, R., and Dunbar, G. C. (1998) "The Mini-International Neuropsychiatric Interview (M.I.N.I.): The development and validation of a structured diagnostic psychiatric interview for DSM-IV and ICD-10", *Journal of Clinical Psychiatry*, 59(Suppl. 20), pp. 22–33.

Sidani, S., Bootzin, R. R., Epstein, D. R., Miranda, J., and Cousins, J. (2015) "Attrition in randomized and preference trials of behavioural treatments for insomnia", *Canadian Journal of Nursing Research*, 47(1), pp. 17–34.

Smith, M. T., Huang, M. I., and Manber, R. (2005) "Cognitive behavior therapy for chronic insomnia occurring within the context of medical and psychiatric disorders", *Clinical Psychology Review*, 25(5), pp. 559–592.

Spielman, A. J., Caruso, L. S., and Glovinsky, P. B. (1987) "A behavioral perspective on insomnia treatment", *Psychiatric Clinics of North America*, 10(4), pp. 541–553.

Sylvia, L. G., Salcedo, S., Bianchi, M. T., Urdahl, A. K., Nierenberg, A. A., and Deckersbach, T. (2014) "A novel home sleep monitoring device and brief sleep intervention for bipolar disorder: Feasibility, tolerability, and preliminary effectiveness", *Cognitive Therapy & Research*, 38(1), pp. 55–61.

van de Laar, M., Pevernagie, D., van Mierlo, P., and Overeem, S. (2015) "Psychiatric comorbidity and aspects of cognitive coping negatively predict outcome in cognitive behavioral treatment of psychophysiological insomnia", *Behavioral Sleep Medicine*, 13(2), pp. 140–156.

Wagley, J. N., Rybarczyk, B., Nay, W. T., Danish, S., and Lund, H. G. (2013) "Effectiveness of abbreviated CBT for insomnia in psychiatric outpatients: Sleep and depression outcomes", *Journal of Clinical Psychology*, 69(10), pp. 1043–1055.

Waters, F., Chiu, V., Janca, S., Atkinson, A., and Ree, M. (2015) "Preferences for different insomnia treatment options in people with schizophrenia and related psychoses: A qualitative study", *Frontiers in Psychology*, 14(6), p. 990.

10 Clinical Cases

This chapter presents two case studies of participants who took part in our CBT-I intervention. The chapter serves to demonstrate the varying presentations that may be encountered with this client group, and to marry together the information that has been imparted in the previous chapters regarding Insomnia Disorder, assessment, sleep and its regulation, sleep dysfunction in psychosis, and evidence for the efficacy of adapted CBT-I in psychotic disorders.

The client details have been altered for confidentiality purposes; however, the outcome data are genuine. We hope that these case studies provide a good sense of how session content may be adapted to suit a client's needs using the fundamental components of CBT-I.

Clinical Case Study 1 (Annie)

Annie is a 44-year-old single mother of three children with a diagnosis of schizophrenia. She completed high school, but she has learning difficulties. She previously worked as a kitchen hand, but was currently unemployed and living on a pension. Her social support network included her mother, who lived overseas but called and texted regularly, and a small circle of friends. She liked to draw, but had not engaged in this hobby for some time.

Two years ago, Annie suffered a deterioration in her mental and physical health after her father passed away; this led to a psychotic episode and difficulty in self-care that resulted in her children being taken away by the Department of Child Protection services. She was only allowed to see them once a week, causing her much anguish.

Annie's psychiatric medications comprised a monthly depot injection (paliperidone, 150 mg) and an antidepressant (mirtazapine, 15 mg nocte), which was prescribed after Annie complained of sleep problems. Her other medications included ventalin, osteo-pandaol, and vitamin D tablets.

Annie had long-term problems with falling asleep, waking 'for hours at night' owing to worrying about her children, and recurrent nightmares that woke her up during the night. The nightmare contents included scenes from a previously abusive relationship and visual images of her children crying and needing her help. During her last psychotic episodes, distress from these nightmares contributed to her poor appetite and extreme weight loss (15 kg). The nightmares improved after she commenced taking paliperidone, but she continued to have bad dreams several times a week.

Annie had chronic hip pain and asthma, which also impacted on her sleep. However, she had recently quit smoking as one of her goals to improve her health and get her children back, and this had helped reduce nocturnal wakings and coughing.

At her first appointment, Annie's appearance was casual but neat. She maintained good eye contact, and rapport was quickly established. Her speech was generally clear, except when she was speaking about child services, when her speech became pressured and loud. Annie's self-reported strengths included drawing and art, and she was very motivated to draw on her creativity when formulating strategies to improve her sleep during the sessions.

Baseline Information: Targets for Therapy

A sleep interview and self-report sleep measures were completed before the intervention. Measures included the PSQI (Buysse et al., 1989) to assess her sleep quality and quantity, the SHiK-B (Chiu et al., 2015), the PHQ-4 (Kroenke et al., 2009), and the MINI Psychotic Disorders module (MINI psychosis; Sheehan et al., 1998). Annie was also asked to keep a weekly sleep diary (Appendix 2) for the duration of the programme to record her sleeping patterns and keep track of her progress. Baseline questionnaire scores and sleep parameter data are shown in Tables 10.1 and 10.2.

Annie's primary complaints were difficulties with sleep onset, sometimes taking up to 2 or 3 hours. She also woke up multiple times at night and started thinking about her children

Table 10.1 Annie's Questionnaire Scores in Selected Domains Pre- and Post-CBT-I

Measure	*Pre-treatment*	*Post-treatment*
PSQI (global)[1]	16	9
PSQI (sleep efficiency)[2]	3	1
PSQI (sleep disturbances)[3]	3	1
SHiK-B (sleep hygiene)[4]	7	3
PHQ-4 (anxiety)[5]	4	1

Notes: (1) PSQI global score: A global sum of 5 or greater indicates a 'poor' sleeper; (2) PSQI sleep efficiency index: Sleep efficiency is calculated and assigned an index score based on a 0–3 scale, where 3 reflects the negative extreme on the Likert Scale; (3) PSQI sleep disturbances index: Scoring of answers is based on a 0–3 scale, where 3 reflects the negative extreme on the Likert Scale; (4) SHiK-B sleep hygiene: Low scores denote better sleep hygiene practices; (5) PHQ-4 anxiety subscale score range is 0–6, with higher scores indicating greater depression severity

Table 10.2 Annie's Sleep Parameters over 7 Days

*Sleep parameters**	*Baseline to Session 1*	*Session 2*	*Session 3*	*Session 4*	*Post-treatment*
Lights out time	21.40	21.09	21.35	21.57	22.55
SOL (minutes)	90	36	45	30	30
Number of night-time awakenings (per night)	4	3	2.5	2	2
Out of bed time	8.30	9.39	9.06	8.35	8.17
Average time in bed (hours)	11.72	12.43	11.41	10.37	9.24
Total sleep time (hours)	5	6.06	7.32	7.38	7.45
Daytime energy and motivation (rating out of 10)**	0	0.4	9.4	9.1	–

Notes: * From PSQI and sleep diary data; ** daytime energy and motivation rating for the week rated on a scale from 0 to 10, with greater score indicating more energy; dash = data missing

and the past, which increased cognitive arousal. Her baseline sleep efficiency was scored at 42.7 per cent.

Annie reported that, although her sleep problems did not impact directly on daytime activities, the potential long-term impact on her health caused her much worry. Annie's nightmares (three times a week) also caused night-time arousal and anxiety. Annie denied any hallucinations or delusions as assessed on the MINI psychosis, although paranoid thoughts were identified during the interview and in her medical notes. She reported no depressive symptoms, but her anxiety levels were high.

Formulation

Formulation of Annie's case is helped by identification of the factors affecting her sleep drive, body clock, and night-time arousal. These were as follows:

Factors Affecting Sleep Drive

These included:

- watching TV in bed;
- sleeping late in the morning to trying and 'catch up' on lost sleep from the night before; average time in bed was nearly 12 hours at Session 1;
- lack of daytime structure and activity

Factors Affecting Body Clock

These were:

- slightly irregular sleep routine: waking up and getting out of bed at different times each day;
- irregular mealtimes (e.g. Annie would go to bed either uncomfortably full or hungry, on an empty stomach).

Factors Increasing Arousal

These included:

- no wind-down period before bed—she went to bed worrying and ruminating about her children; at night, Annie tried to manage negative thoughts by making 'to do' lists;
- drinking coffee and soft drinks close to bedtime;
- alertness and attentiveness to the silence in her house since her children were taken away, increasing her feelings of loneliness and isolation;
- conditioned arousal resulting from remaining in bed for long periods even though not asleep;
- anxiety and fear about the possibility of nightmares and bad dreams;
- pain from a hip injury, making it challenging for her to get into a comfortable position in bed; Annie performs cardio exercises as well as stretching before bed to assist with the pain;
- clock-watching overnight.

Turning Complicating Factors into Positive Sessions

- *Chronic pain*: Regular breaks in CBT-I sessions needed to be provided to assist with pain management and stiffness in Annie's hip. This was taken as an opportunity to experiment with ratings of tiredness before and after stretches, and to discuss the impact of physical activity on tiredness levels.
- *Learning difficulties*: Individual sessions were more suitable than group sessions for Annie, as they provided her with extra time for writing, checking, and spelling. Annie was also supported by the therapist to complete the assessment measures and her resource pack, where key points were highlighted with coloured pens. Drawing on her love of art and drawing, Annie was encouraged to draw and make pictures to help her remember key concepts.
- *Financial limitations*: It was important to devise appropriate strategies for wind-down, daytime energy, and coping strategies within Annie's budget in order to ensure a successful outcome. A most helpful resource was her local community library, where she could borrow books, CDs, movies or TV shows, and puzzles. Comic books and novels aimed at an adolescent audience were particularly appropriate and enjoyable for Annie, as they were easier to read and more visually appealing. She was encouraged to make her own play dough with flour, water, and salt and to sculpt figurines and objects. Knowledge of community networks and social groups (e.g. mental health drop-in centres, churches) that run free art groups, music classes, computer courses, and crochet classes was also beneficial, as these provide free services and activities.
- *Child visitation constraints*: CBT-I appointments needed to be scheduled around visits to her children, which were generally once a week. In case her children or staff from child protection services called her on the phone, Annie requested that her mobile phone be left on during the sessions. This request being allowed enabled Annie to reduce worry and engage better in the session. Disruptions were rare, and phone calls lasted 5 minutes at most. This highlights how it can be helpful to form 'ground rules' before each session.
- *Asthma*: Annie's asthma was well managed, although she understood that a worsening of it could negatively impact on her breathing during sleep. Asthma also influenced the type of daytime activities that she could engage in.

Course of CBT-I

Session 1: Psychoeducation, Sleep Hygiene, Wind-Down, and Stimulus Control

The session began with Annie's goals and motivations for treatment being elicited. Her treatment goals were as follows:

1. wake up in the morning without so much reliance on an alarm;
2. wake up feeling less tired;
3. a reduction in bad dreams.

Annie's motivations to engage in treatment included better physical and mental health, which would improve her chances of getting her children back, as well as better coping and thinking skills, which she hoped would improve the quality of her drawing and art.

In this first session, sleep hygiene was discussed, and psychoeducation was provided about adult sleep needs and the process of falling asleep. Particular attention was given to the importance of a regular wind-down time, to assist her with letting go of worries before bed, and of avoiding staying in bed too long after waking up in the morning, as this would impact on her sleep drive. Stimulus control (GOOBICS) was also introduced.

When discussing factors that get in the way of good sleep, Annie spoke about the silence in the house since her children had been taken away, and said that she had been leaving the TV on overnight for background noise. She was also worried about her daughters and kept her phone near her bed in case they called. Other factors getting in the way of sleep included watching too much TV at night, planning to spend the next day in bed, and going to bed either too hungry or too full.

A behavioural experiment on 'tiredness' was conducted that sought to contrast her levels of tiredness after reading a page in a book compared with after walking around the corridors of the clinic with the therapist. This was used to provide an experience of tiredness levels changing within a short space of time according to choices made, and to show that reading can be a good strategy to help feel sleepy at night, and that light physical exercise would act to wake her up.

Client strategies at the end of Session 1 (homework) were the following:

- *Wind-down time* each night in the hour before bed: Annie chose to read, draw, or colour in a mindfulness book.
- *Reduce night-time arousal*: Annie chose to do gentle stretches for her hip before going into bed and to leave cardio exercises until the morning.
- *Sleep hygiene*: Annie was to avoid caffeinated beverages and soft drinks at night past 5 p.m. and would drink camomile tea or water instead. She would also avoid watching TV in bed.
- *Earlier regular rising time*: Annie's goal for getting up in the morning was 7.00–7.30 a.m. Some clients prefer to work towards their goal gradually over a number of weeks, but Annie preferred to try and get up at 7.30 a.m. from Session 1. The potential benefit of not staying in bed for long after waking up was emphasised. Annie approached this in an experimental manner, contrasting how she felt after lingering in bed for an hour or more after waking versus getting up within 15 minutes.
- *Morning 'wind-up'*: To assist with getting her morning started, Annie decided to have a cup of coffee and perform some hip and cardio exercises.
- *Stimulus control* (GOOBICS): This would be done if she was waking at night and ruminating in bed. Annie decided to try getting out of bed to read, having a warm drink (e.g. milk), or doing some colouring-in, then going back to bed when sleepy.

Session 2: Maximising Daytime Energy, Working with Nightmares

At Session 2, Annie reported encouraging improvements in her sleep, with less time awake at night and shorter SOL. She rated her improvements in sleep as 8.5 (with 0 indicating no improvements at all, and 10 indicating huge improvements). Although sleep onset and wake-up time during the night had improved, nightmares and wake-up time in the morning had not.

Wind-down time had gone well, with Annie describing feeling less 'awake' at bedtime. Annie initially struggled with trying to read a novel and troubleshot this problem herself by borrowing comic books (e.g. Peanuts) from the library. Comic books helped both with her learning difficulties and with managing negative thoughts, through the funny contents.

Between Sessions 1 and 2, a challenge for Annie had been daily worries about her children. Her levels of improvement in feeling and coping were rated as 5.5 out of 10, owing to these worries and ongoing nightmares. The therapist strongly praised Annie for the wonderful steps she had taken with her wind-down routine and emphasised that this change appeared to be helping with her sleep onset. Education about the change process was given, and the notion that managing her worry would require some time and patience was emphasised. Annie was encouraged by the news that there were further skills still to be covered with respect to managing her rumination and nightmares.

Unhelpful beliefs about sleep were evaluated with the DBAS scale (Morin et al., 2007). Annie's low scores suggested that unhelpful beliefs about sleep were not a central feature of her difficulties. However, her beliefs about nightmares—'The nightmares are going to come back', 'Without medications, my nightmares will never end'—were significant. These beliefs reflected low self-efficacy in nightmare management and understandably led to a rather helpless approach in their management.

Socratic questioning was used to encourage Annie to consider whether her bad dreams were part of a conditioned response—for example: *Do you think it is possible that you are having nightmares because you are expecting to? What could be the effect of believing that your nightmares are going to come back? What could be the effect of no longer holding onto this belief?* A strong self-efficacy theme arose from this discussion: 'I'm not helpless in the face of my nightmares; there are things I can do that may help'.

Working to reduce the impact of overly negative thoughts and worry about her children before bed was highlighted as a potential strategy to decrease the frequency of bad dreams about them. Annie decided that she could experiment with allowing herself to fully engage in calming activities (and not worry about her children for this period of time) and observe how she felt. The therapist gave Annie permission to not worry all of the time by encouraging her to entertain the idea that she is a loving Mum, and that she should not worry all of the time. Annie liked the idea of finding a happy medium between thinking about her children at certain times (having a scheduled worry time) and giving herself permission to let go of these worries at other times. For her planned worry time, Annie was given a structure for expressing her worries and problem-solving them. Knowing that she had a time scheduled to think her worries through made it more plausible for her to let go of worries when they intruded close to bedtime.

Additionally, strategies for dealing with nightmares were drawn from a specialised treatment for nightmares (Krakow, 2002). Strategies included stopping (clapping and saying 'Stop!'), grounding (open eyes, focus on the immediate environment), and positive imagery (imagining herself at the beach with her children).

In Session 2, maximising daytime energy was also discussed. By the end of this session, Annie had learned that 'A lot of things can make you feel tired, not just sleep'. This new way of thinking about energy was employed to assist Annie in working towards her goal of rising in the morning without lingering too long in bed. She was aware that once up and out of bed, she had a number of options at her disposal to 'wind up' into the day.

Client strategies at the end of Session 2 (homework) included the following:

- *Push back bedtime if ruminating*: Spend more time winding down if ruminating about the children or after a particularly emotionally draining day.
- *Set aside a 'worry time' during the day*: Dedicate time to expressing worries, planning, and problem-solving.
- *Regular rising time*: This was set at 8.00–8.30 a.m. for the next week.
- *Continue winding down* before bed: Permission was given to Annie to disengage from worrying at this time.
- *Stimulus control—GOOBICS*: Annie was to read comic books and colour in when using this strategy.

- *Energy-generating plan*: Annie was to go for a walk in the morning, have more regular meals (timing and volume and type of food consumed), do some housework, or go for a bicycle ride.
- *Energy-depleting activities to avoid*: Annie was to avoid reading for too long without a break in the day and going to bed during the day.
- *Use grounding and positive imagery techniques*: She was to use these after waking up from a bad dream or nightmare.

Session 3: Managing Overly Negative Thoughts and a Busy Mind before Bed

By Session 3, Annie gladly reported she could get to sleep without worrying so much about her children, and that she had not experienced any nightmares during the week. She was happy with her routine and with the earlier waking time, which was 8.30–9.00 a.m. The week's improvements in sleep and feeling/coping were both rated as 7 out of 10.

Challenges this week had included the summer heat disrupting her sleep (unable to use air conditioning owing to asthma problems) and worries about one of her daughters with special needs. Using a fan and a cold pack in bed and having a cold shower as part of the wind-down routine were suggested. Problem-solving was modelled, and Annie decided that she could ring child protection services about arranging a specialist appointment for her daughter.

Session 3 focused on dealing with overly negative thoughts and a busy mind before bed. This included avoiding watching the time/clock when unable to sleep and brainstorming ways to cope with low mood, anxiety, and intrusive thoughts See Figure 10.1 for Annie's coping strategies.

Reframing overly negative thoughts involved helping Annie to recognise the link between thoughts and feelings, by (a) 'catching' the thought; (b) 'checking' whether the thought was helpful, and how it made her feel; and (c) 'changing' the thought so that it was more accurate and helpful to the situation.

Annie and the therapist worked on a specific recurrent night-time thought ('What am I going to do tomorrow, how am I going to cope?'), as well as an intrusive thought about

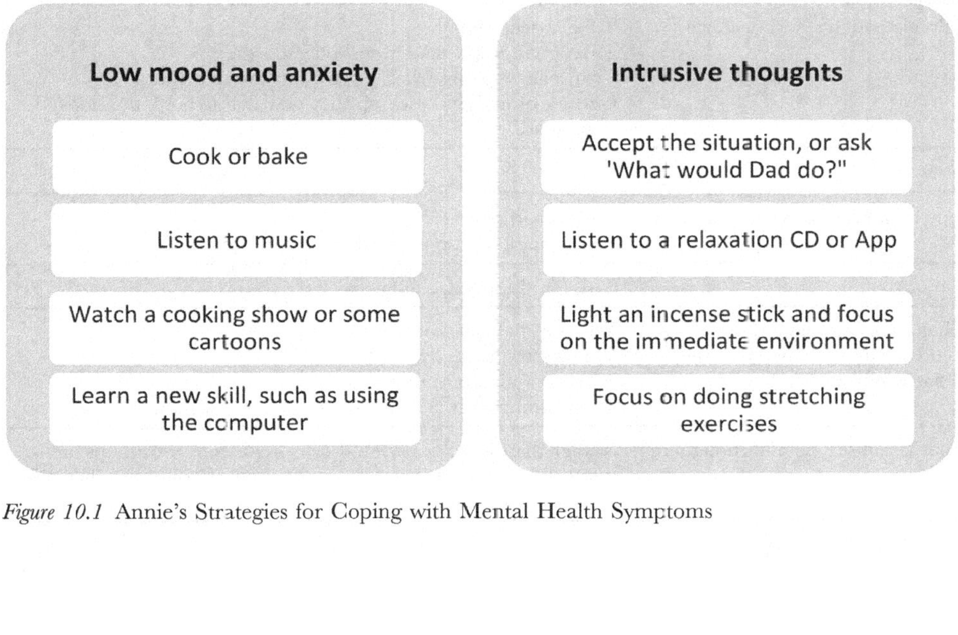

Figure 10.1 Annie's Strategies for Coping with Mental Health Symptoms

her children ('I am a bad parent'; see Table 10.3). Annie and the therapist practised the examining thoughts process together using a worksheet. Annie was also asked to rate her belief in her thought before and after going through the exercise, to demonstrate the positive effects of examining and reframing thoughts.

Client strategies at the end of Session 3 (homework) included the following:

- *Regular rising time*: Get up at 8.00–8.30 a.m.
- *Sleep hygiene*: Have a glass of water with lemon instead of coffee or cordial/red soda in the afternoon.
- *Keep up with winding down*: Use the colouring-in books, draw, and read comics. Also continue doing gentle stretches for the hip before bed.
- *Avoid checking the time* when unable to sleep.
- *Make a to-do list* before wind-down time to help calm thoughts about what needs to be done tomorrow.
- *Watch out for overly negative thoughts and examine them*: Use the thought process worksheets provided in the client resource pack.
- *Continue with worry time during the day.*

Session 4: Review and Maintaining the Gains

At Session 4, Annie felt she was sleeping well and was generally in bed around 10.00 p.m. and up by 8.30 a.m. feeling refreshed. This was a great improvement, both to have reduced

Table 10.3 Reframing Negative and Unhelpful Thoughts with Annie

Sample 1	
Thoughts when unable to sleep:	What am I going to do tomorrow, how am I going to cope?
Feelings:	Drained, tired, frustrated, angry at myself
	Worry that I will have to push back my appointments tomorrow if I can't sleep
Helpful thoughts and strategies:	Take a deep breath Take small steps, take it an hour at a time I can plan my day when I get up in the morning Get out of bed and pick up that new comic book that looked so good
Sample 2	
Unhelpful and distressing thoughts:	I am a bad parent My kids are disappointed that I am not there
Feelings:	Sad, disappointed, ashamed
What advice would a good friend/family member give me? (What would my dad say?)	You are making progress You are trying really hard You can only do the best you can These thoughts don't help me to be a good mum
What is a more helpful thoughts?	Rather than beating myself down, I can concentrate on the things that I can do to be there for them. I could try and make a to-do list for this tomorrow

her time in bed by 90 minutes and to be feeling less tired on waking in the morning. She experienced no prolonged wake-ups at all during the night (and was only waking to go to the toilet). As with the previous week, she reported no bad dreams and felt less stressed at night. This week's levels of improvement with regards to sleep and feeling/coping were rated as 9 out of 10.

Annie found it a challenge 'to close my eyes and feel the stress go', but she had managed to see it as an opportunity to rest her body and mind, rather than worrying. An important observation was that pleasant feelings and thoughts before bed had led to better sleep and fewer bad dreams. Further, the reduced worry enabled Annie to enjoy her day more. A very positive shift had occurred in her compulsion to worry about the children and her parenting before bed.

This last session addressed ways to maintain her sleep improvements over time and planning for a potential setback. A plan was made, summarising Annie's triggers for poor sleep and strategies that she had found most useful (see Table 10.4).

A future goal for Annie was to reduce the dose of her psychiatric medications. The potential short-term increase in nightmares after medication reduction was discussed, and strategies to manage the return of her nightmares were reviewed. This included contacting her mental health support team and seeing a psychologist to help her through the withdrawal effects. If Annie's CBT-I treatment had not been in the context of a trial, the CBT-I clinician would likely be the appropriate person to assist with this goal. Annie also recognised the need for regular meals that will help her to maintain a healthy weight.

Finally, an imagery exercise was used to elicit Annie's perception of her current life balance. She was asked to close her eyes and respond to the statements: 'I spend too much time worrying about . . .', 'I spend too little time doing things such as . . .', and 'What I would like to do differently from today is . . .'. This helped identify that Annie had been spending too much time worrying about her kids and too little time on herself and looking after her health. To address this imbalance, Annie decided to start a hobby (crochet) that she could do without her children but would also be of interest to them and could become a shared activity. Annie also decided to plan ways to improve her physical health, by having a regular weekly swim in the hydrotherapy pool and seeing her GP for a referral to a hip specialist.

Client strategies at the end of Session 4 (homework) were to:

- *address life balance* by working towards small goals in the area of health;.
- *continue to use her sleep wellness plan* and refer back to the client pack at regular intervals.

Post-Treatment Assessment (Week 5)

Post-treatment assessment comprised a structured interview and questionnaires, and data from Annie's sleep diary. Compared with baseline, Annie had reduced her sleep onset time from 90 minutes to 30 minutes and no longer reported difficulties with sleep maintenance or early morning awakenings. She might wake up to go to the toilet, but was able to fall back to sleep rapidly. Her sleep efficiency had increased to 80 per cent, compared with 42.7 per cent at baseline.

Annie was moderately satisfied with her sleep pattern and found her sleep to be more refreshing than before. When rating her achievements in meeting her sleep-treatment goals, she reported they had all been achieved more than she had expected (Table 10.5). A huge accomplishment for Annie was being able to wake up without an alarm clock on 2–4 days of the week, which helped her feel that her sleep pattern was normalising.

Table 10.4 Annie's Individualised Summary Plan

Trigger/Precipitator	
How did the problem first develop?	Stress (death of father, children taken away)
Perpetuators	
What kept it going?	Not coping with children being away Negative thoughts and planning before bed (the mind didn't want to go to sleep because it was problem-solving) Difficulties keeping a routine for waking and sleeping Cigarettes before bed Caffeine and soft drinks before bed Watching the clock at night
Treatment	
What did you learn during the programme about how to overcome the problem?	Do not watch TV in bed Getting up earlier actually helps you feel more tired at night-time and assists with energy during the day (need to have an earlier start) Learning to keep a routine is better, because my mind is more alert Winding down in the evening is important I can deal with stress better when I sleep Avoid building a mountain of stress just before I sleep by managing my thoughts Managing stress means having time where I do other (pleasant) things
What were your most unhelpful habits and thoughts about sleep?	Worrying about the kids Expecting bad dreams to happen
What are the alternatives to these?	Using wind-down time to help me let go before bed (e.g. reading a book/comic, watch a cooking show, or colouring in) Setting worry time during the day Seeing that I am not helpless about my nightmares
How will you build on what you have learned? (What do you think are the most important things to remember to help keep progress going?)	Making an emotional toolbox of different ways to cope (colouring in, comic books, scented candles, relaxation CDs, and a notepad for drawing/making to-do lists, writing down thoughts, talking to my case manager or Mum) Looking after my physical health (diet and exercise) Keeping up routines for the day and the night

Table 10.5 Annie's Self-rated Achievement of CBT-I Treatment Goals

Achievement of Goals	*Perceived Level of Improvement*
1. Wake up with no alarm	Somewhat more than expected
2. Wake up not tired	Somewhat more than expected
3. No bad dreams	Somewhat more than expected

Her scores on selected PSQI, SHiK-B, and PHQ-4 measures also showed significant improvements (see Table 10.1). Other benefits noted by Annie were:

- increased structure in her daily activities;
- a better sense of control, ability to cope, and self-efficacy;
- increased interest in meeting other people and pursuing activities offered in the community.

Follow-up (3 Months Post-Treatment)

Follow-up was conducted with Annie at 3 months post-treatment. Wind-down activities and regular rising time were still practised consistently, and she reported falling asleep more quickly since participating in the programme.

Annie was happy with the progress in her sleep and daytime functions. She also had started attending a parenting course and art classes once a week, where she got to meet new people and felt less isolated. She was also looking for computer lessons to increase communication with her children.

Annie had recently experienced nightmares about her children, which left her feeling sad and frustrated. However, she found that she could fall asleep more quickly following a nightmare by giving herself time to wind down and applying the GOOBICS strategy. She noted that a possible trigger was her children being unable to see each other for 5 weeks because of the carers' conflicting schedules. She agreed that the nightmares might cease after her next visit with her children all together. Grounding strategies learned in Session 2 for dealing with nightmares were revisited and practised. Two weeks later, the therapist conducted a check-up phone call. Annie reported that her nightmares had stopped, her sleep had returned to normal, and that she was in much better spirits.

Treatment Implications of Annie's Case

The implications of Annie's case highlight the importance of adapting treatment strategies to a client's personal situation and stressors. The therapist had to be attentive to and validate Annie's cognitions about her children being taken away and changes to the home environment and daytime structure in their absence.

The delivery of therapy in general needed to be individualised, given Annie's learning difficulties. She needed extra support with written materials, and the therapist needed to be careful to ensure that Annie had understood the material and that she could use it in a helpful way at home.

Managing client expectations was important with Annie. She had actually done terrifically well after Session 1, but she presented as disappointed in her progress, as her nightmares and rumination had persisted. It was important to praise and encourage Annie for the positive and brave steps she had taken and to educate her about the change process being something that takes time and patience.

Financial disadvantage is another element relevant to the majority of this clinical population. Access to information about good community resources can make a huge difference to supporting a client's sleep, coping skills, and life balance goals.

Lastly, the importance of assessment interviews is highlighted by this case. The assessment stage allowed identification of unhelpful cognitions relevant to Annie's nightmares that were not covered in measures such as the DBAS. A thorough initial assessment also assisted in the identification of a range of medical problems that might contribute to the person's Insomnia (e.g. asthma, hip problems).

Clinical Case Study 2 (John)

John is a 25-year-old man with a primary diagnosis of schizoaffective disorder, comorbid with anxiety (agoraphobia) and obsessive–compulsive disorder (OCD).

He completed secondary school but had never worked. He was currently living on a pension. His social support system comprised his parents and his sister, with whom he lived. He had no close friends, but he regularly attended a community drop-in centre and a Hearing Voices Group. Prior to becoming mentally unwell, John described himself as very fit, playing rugby and running regularly. He stopped all sports since his diagnosis at the age of 17. He had since gained 50 kg, which he attributed to medication side effects and a lack of exercise. He now tried to get some exercise by walking the dog after dinner in the evening. John was unhappy and dissatisfied with life, and particularly with not working or studying.

John's psychiatric medications comprised a monthly depot injection (paliperidone, 75 mg), quetiapine (500 mg), sertraline (250 mg), and agomelatine (50 mg).

John complained of sleeping poorly and waking up frequently at night (three to five times during the night). Screening questions did not suggest presence of OSA. He was continuously tired, despite long periods spent in bed. He might sleep for 10 or 11 hours a night, until mid-morning, and then might take a long nap during the day. There was a lot of variation in his rising time across the week. He had difficulties getting up in the morning and would be too tired to get up for work, if he had a job, or if he tried to do any exercise. He felt that his sleep problems were a major hindrance to getting his life back on track.

John also reported nightmares at least twice weekly, which he associated with low and depressed mood the next day. The general theme of his nightmares related to his self-perceived failures and inability to pursue his life goals.

Finally, John reported paranoid thoughts that fed into night-time worry and cognitive arousal. A night-time behaviour associated with his paranoia was to leave a water bottle or piece of scrunched-up paper by the door, so that he could hear if an intruder came into the room. His over-alertness to the sound of paper or the bottle being moved caused him difficulties with falling asleep and frequent awakenings.

Baseline Information: Targets for Therapy

John presented as casually dressed and well groomed, with his hair tied, and rapport was easily established, although he maintained poor eye contact. He would sit comfortably in a relaxed posture most of the time, but occasionally he would fidget with a pen in his hand or an elastic band on his wrist. Speech was well articulated, with a slow rate of speech and occasional long pauses when he was thinking about a question.

A sleep interview and sleep measures were completed before the intervention. Measures completed included the PSQI (Buysse et al., 1989), to assess his sleep quality and quantity, the SHiK-B (Chiu et al., 2015), PHQ-4 (Kroenke et al., 2009), and the MINI Psychotic Disorders module (Sheehan et al., 1998). John was also asked to keep a weekly sleep diary for the duration of the programme, to observe his sleeping patterns and keep track of his progress. John's sleep parameter data at baseline and throughout the course of the intervention are shown in Tables 10.6 and 10.7.

The sleep data confirmed his self-reported symptoms of Insomnia with concurrent hypersomnia. He woke up on average four times a night. His night-time sleep efficiency was 80 per cent (total sleep time at night divided by time in bed), and he spent up to 15 hours per day in bed.

Table 10.6 John's Sleep Parameters over 7 Days

*Sleep parameters**	*Baseline to Session 1*	*Session 2*	*Session 3*	*Session 4*	*Post-Treatment*
Lights out time	22.30	21.45	20.40	21.40	20.45
SOL (minutes)	30	39	18	8	20
Number of night-time awakenings	4	2	–	3	2
Get out of bed time	11.00	7.35	10.30	8.25	7.20
Total sleep time (excluding naps; hours)	10	9.5	11.3	9.4	9.2
Frequency of napping (out of 7 days)	5	5	1	4	3
Time spent napping (hours)	5.5	4.9	4.5	3.9	2.5
Daytime energy and motivation (rating out of 10)**	–	2.32	2.7	3.8	–

Notes: * From PSQI and sleep diary data; ** daytime energy and motivation rating for the week rated on a scale from 0 to 10, with greater score indicating more energy; dash = data missing.

Table 10.7 John's Questionnaire Scores in Selected Domains Pre- and Post-CBT-I

Measure	*Pre-Treatment*	*Post-Treatment*
PSQI (global)[1]	9	5
PSQI (daytime dysfunction)[2]	3	2
SHiK-B (sleep hygiene)[3]	8	3
PHQ-4 (depression)[4]	5	4
MINI (paranoia)[5]	5	4

Notes: (1) PSQI (global): a global sum of 5 or greater indicates a 'poor' sleeper; (2) PSQI (daytime dysfunction): scoring of answers is based on a 0–3 scale, whereby 3 reflects the negative extreme; (3) SHiK-B (sleep hygiene): low scores denote better sleep hygiene practices; (4) PHQ-4 (depression): subscale score range 0–6, with higher scores indicating greater depression severity; (5) MINI (paranoia) = adapted MINI—Psychotic Disorders module, Item 2: scores range from 1 (very untrue) to 7 (very true).

John was uncomplaining about the time it took for him to fall asleep (average of 30 minutes), perhaps because of the beneficial effects of agomelatine (which is an antidepressant that acts on melatonin receptors) and the sedating effects of his other medications. Despite taking agomelatine for 2 years, he still reported irregular sleep time and night-time awakenings. On occasion, his SOL extended up to 165 minutes (3 hours) and this was related to high consumption of sugary foods and/or caffeine, racing thoughts and anxiety, or overstimulation from computer games.

John's scores on validated measures revealed the following profile (Table 10.7):

- global score on the PSQI indicated poor sleep quality;
- very high levels of daytime dysfunction due to sleepiness;
- positive score for depression on the PHQ-4 (score of 5/6);
- elevated rating on items assessing paranoia (score of 5/8);
- poor sleep hygiene.

Formulation

Formulation of John's case is helped by identification of the factors affecting his sleep drive, body clock, and night-time arousal. These were as follows:

Factors Affecting Sleep Drive

These included:

- sleeping late into the day and up to 11 hours a night;
- napping for 3 or more hours on average, and as long as 8 hours after depot injection;
- lack of daily stimulation and routine, with no leisure, work, or study activities;
- depressed mood—a score of 5 out of 6 on the PHQ-4 depression subscale;
- antipsychotic medications that made him feel tired;
- night-time exercise, walking the dog before bed.

Factors Affecting the Body Clock

These included:

- irregular sleep routine, with wake-up any time between 8.20 a.m. and 2.00 p.m.;
- total sleep time ranging from 9 to 14 hours a day;
- lack of exposure to sunlight through staying indoors on the computer during the day and walking the dog in the evening.

Factors Increasing Arousal at Night

These included:

- fears about having nightmares;
- staying in bed while lying awake;
- worrying about not sleeping well;
- delusional (paranoid) beliefs about people entering his room;
- excessive intake of caffeine, soft drinks, and confectionery close to bedtime;
- no wind-down period before bed—going to bed after surfing on the computer or watching TV (simultaneous with the consumption of sugary foods and soft drinks).

Other Factors Contributing to His Sleep Problems

Other factors were:

- belief that feeling tired meant that he had not slept enough;
- long naps as an escape from the boredom and loneliness of the day;
- rumination about past and current perceived failures;
- tiredness that contributed to his reduced self-esteem and self-efficacy, which exacerbated rumination, social avoidance, and further napping.

Enabling and Complicating Factors

When the intervention was started, enablers and barriers to CBT-I were carefully considered. Enablers included good liaison with John's case manager, with whom concerns or questions could be raised. The intervention was offered in the building of John s local mental health clinic, so that John would not need to travel far. John was unemployed, and so he was available to attend sessions any day of the week. Barriers, however, included that the initial sessions needed to be scheduled in the afternoon (2.00 p.m.), owing to his delayed sleeping patterns and low mood and motivation. Furthermore, sessions could not be organised for 2 days after his monthly depot injection, owing to the dangers associated with drowsiness while driving. Extreme sleepiness (somnolence) is a common side effect of the depot injection that may last for a few days (Citrome, 2010), especially when combined with other sedating medications, and clients need to prepare for this. It is unrealistic in many cases for clients to continue to adhere to goals around wake times during this period.

Owing to John's OCD tendencies, the therapist had to be mindful that keeping a sleep diary might feed into his repetitive checking behaviours. John enjoyed keeping a sleep diary and found it helpful for keeping to his routine and recognising patterns in his sleep. It was important to communicate with the client's psychiatrist and case manager to ensure that he was able to withdraw from keeping a sleep diary when his sleep routines improved.

John had been prescribed agomelatine 2 years ago because of his irregular sleep–wake rhythms and prolonged sleep latencies. It had improved his sleep latency, but his sleep hygiene and routines had remained unaddressed, so that the timing of sleep remained very irregular. John's psychiatrist and case manager were contacted to let them know that sleep management with CBT-I could improve these sleep parameters, and that a review of, and adjustments to, his medications might be beneficial following improved sleep. This was especially so in John's case, given some of the side effects of daytime sleepiness associated with his antipsychotics.

Course of CBT-I

Session 1: Goal Setting, Psychoeducation, Sleep Hygiene, Stimulus Control

Session 1 began with John being asked to identify his goals and motivations for engaging in CBT-I.

His treatment goals were as follows:

1. develop a more regular sleep pattern (get up to start the day before 8 a.m.);
2. create a schedule for daytime napping and work to reduce time spent napping during the day;
3. improve daytime energy (starting with working to increase energy from 2/10 to 3/10);
4. increase daytime activity levels and structure (go outside each day).

John was motivated to address his sleep problems as he saw this to be an integral step towards beginning to try to pursue studies or employment. This was discussed at length to enhance motivation for change. The therapist checked with John about his willingness to possibly endure some challenges in the service of working towards his goals, and John indicated that he was 'up for the challenge'.

The session then addressed education about sleep and sleep regulation, including the benefits of sleeping 'efficiently'. Sleeping more efficiently (i.e. within a shorter window of time) helps to consolidate sleep, maximise daytime activities, and reduce time spent awake at night. Consequently, arousal from worrying and rumination in bed are less likely.

The importance of a regular day- and night-time routine was also addressed. Psychoeducation on sleep was provided to start gently challenging unhelpful sleep-related cognitions and worries about the need to nap or sleep longer in response to tiredness. In particular, it was emphasised that the longer the time he spent in bed, the more likely it was that fragmented sleep would occur.

Client strategies at the end of Session 1 (homework) included the following:

- *An earlier rising time*: This would build up a routine, increase sleep drive, and reduce sleep time. The costs and benefits of gradual versus sudden changes to his rising time were discussed, and John opted for quite a dramatic change by setting a rising time of 6.00–6.50 a.m., so that he could help drive his dad to work. Driving his father to work served as a motivator to get up and offered an opportunity for some exposure to sunlight in the morning.
- *Stimulus control* (GOOBICS): This would help reduce conditioned arousal and improve the time taken to fall back asleep.
- *Wind-down activities before bed to ease his anxiety*: John decided to stop playing computer games after dinner. Wind-down activities before bed included reading and watching TV shows for at least an hour before bed.
- *Sleep hygiene*: The aims were to reduce sugar and caffeine intake during the night, and limit their consumption to no later than 5.00 p.m. Suggested alternatives included milk with a little sweetener or honey, decaffeinated teas (e.g. camomile, peppermint), and water. Exercise was also scheduled to take place at an earlier time, with John taking the dog for a late-afternoon walk (3–5 p.m.) rather than at night (7–9 p.m.).

Session 2: Maximising Daytime Energy and Managing Unhelpful Beliefs about Sleep

Since the previous week, John reported major improvements in his sleep (self-reported improvements rated as 7 out of 10), as well as better coping with his mental health symptoms (self-reported improvements of 7 out of 10). He reported success in implementation of the previous week's strategies. He had got into a more regular routine and had started to wake up at a more regular time, within a 2-hour range (6.45–8.25 a.m.). A challenge in the past week had been getting up 'on time', as the cold weather made it particularly hard to resist staying in bed. His original goal of getting up regularly at 6.00 was therefore delayed by 45–60 minutes to help in this matter. John strategised to put on a jumper and drink something warm to help get out of bed in the morning.

John's progress with GOOBICS, winding down before bed, earlier exercise, and reducing intake of sugary drinks was all on track, which represented excellent progress.

The focus of Session 2 was on maximising energy during the day and identifying unhelpful beliefs about sleep that might be driving his poor sleep. John was asked to brainstorm possible reasons for feeling tired during the day, apart from poor sleep. He identified the following factors: being inactive, unhealthy diet (sugary diet, not enough fruit and vegetables), and feeling cold (not wearing enough warm clothes), prompting a need to go back to bed. Potential strategies for addressing these factors were explored, and it was emphasised that these factors were things that John might be able to have an influence over.

An in-session experiment was conducted in which John contrasted how he felt after 5 minutes of quiet reading versus after 5 minutes of brisk walking outside with the therapist. This was quite powerful in demonstrating that his choices could have a large influence over his energy levels. John also mindfully ate (slowly, while paying attention) some healthy snacks that the therapist had brought into the session. He found, with some surprise, that he liked apples and nuts. This was a good opportunity to discuss with John that engaging in activities mindfully (paying attention to them, in detail, in the moment), rather than focusing on negative thoughts or symptoms of tiredness, can make experiences more positive.

John perceived the discussion about mindful engagement in activity to be of significant value, given he might sleep for 12–15 hours at a stretch and feel very sleepy during the day, further disrupting his ability to get into a good sleep–wake routine. Strategies to reduce tiredness were discussed, and John was motivated to implement and refine his 'energy-generating plan' prior to his upcoming depot injection. A balance between realistic expectations about activity levels in the days following his depot injection with hope for some improvement in these days was emphasised.

Unhelpful sleep beliefs were identified by administration of the DBAS scale (Morin et al., 2007) and exploration of how those beliefs could have a negative effect on sleep. The dysfunctional beliefs with which John identified most strongly were:

- When I don't get a proper amount of sleep on a given night, I need to catch up the next day by napping or by sleeping longer the next night.
- The only way to improve my energy is to rest or sleep more.
- I believe Insomnia is essentially the result of a chemical imbalance.

High ratings on these unhelpful beliefs demonstrated that John was feeling quite helpless about his capacity to change his situation with respect to his sleep and poor energy levels. Indeed, John believed that 'having psychosis makes your sleep unchangeable'. Socratic questioning was used to help John explore whether sleep could possibly be improved despite mental health difficulties, with the therapist pointing to the improvements gained since Session 1 as personal evidence and the ideas John had already generated about factors that might contribute to daytime tiredness.

Finally, the impact of nightmares on sleep was discussed. John commented on needing to work on recognising that the nightmares were not real in order to reduce the effect that they had on his mood and motivation the next day. Techniques to help deal with nightmares were practised in session; these included grounding techniques (opening eyes, placing feet on the floor, and focusing on the immediate environment by naming three objects that can be seen in the room), slow breathing, and journaling.

Client strategies at the end of Session 2 (homework) included:

- *a regular rising time* of 6.45–7.30 a.m. (adjusted from the original 6.00–6.50 a.m.);
- *an 'energy-generating' plan*: do journaling in the morning, spend more time on the exercise bike (up to 15 minutes), walk the dog each morning/afternoon, and have a healthy smoothie or eat a piece of fruit, when feeling tired;
- *avoid napping or have shorter naps*, if napping is unavoidable, by using an alarm; time the naps to be no later than 3 p.m;
- *sleep hygiene*: after the success of being able to stay away from sweets and caffeine at night, John decided to aim to reduce his dairy intake for the week, as he believed this would help him feel less sluggish in the day and help with his weight issues;
- *increase wind-down time when fears about nightmares arise*: use grounding techniques, breathing, and journaling.

Session 3: Managing Overly Negative Thoughts and a Busy Mind before Bea

John benefited from experimenting with strategies to improve his tiredness, as described above. He rated his progress in both sleep and coping very highly (7 out of 10). His bedtime was more consistent, he was more active during the day, and he had only napped only once in the previous week. The lack of napping had increased his sleep drive, so that he slept more solidly at night, but that also meant that he woke up later on some days. He was not accustomed to staying awake all day, and it had been a challenging week, but he felt very good about himself. He reported an improvement in his mood and he was experiencing minimal mental health symptoms, if any.

Session 3 focused on dealing with negative thoughts and a busy mind before bed. The increased arousal that can arise from checking the clock overnight was discussed. The contribution of psychotic symptoms, low mood, and anxiety to his sleeping problems was also discussed, and strategies were brainstormed to cope with these situations (see Figure 10.2).

In addition to the strategies that John elicited, relaxation exercises with mindfulness and slow breathing were introduced as a way of calming the mind. Cognitive restructuring was employed by discussion of examples of when his thinking patterns affected his mood. One example linked how thoughts about being unable to sleep can lead to frustration, worry, and depressed mood.

A discussion followed regarding how overly negative thoughts about sleep can be reshaped through the process of identifying ('catch'), evaluating ('check'), and changing the thought, so that it is more accurate and helpful. For example, John expressed the thoughts, 'God is giving me the hard deal' and 'Why do I have a mental illness?', whenever he was unable to sleep and felt powerless about the situation. More helpful thoughts that he developed during the session were: 'It's only one night, I've got plenty more chances to make it better', and, 'I can learn to be more in charge of my sleep'.

Client strategies at the end of Session 3 (homework) included the following:

- *a regular rising time* of 7.00–8.00 a.m.;
- use an alarm clock to put a *limit on naps* (1.5 hour maximum before 3 p.m.);
- *avoid checking the time* when unable to sleep;
- *practise a relaxation or imagery exercise* to help calm the mind: try during the day at first, and then apply at night when sufficiently rehearsed and feeling ready;
- *watch out for negative thoughts and challenge them* using the thought process worksheets provided;

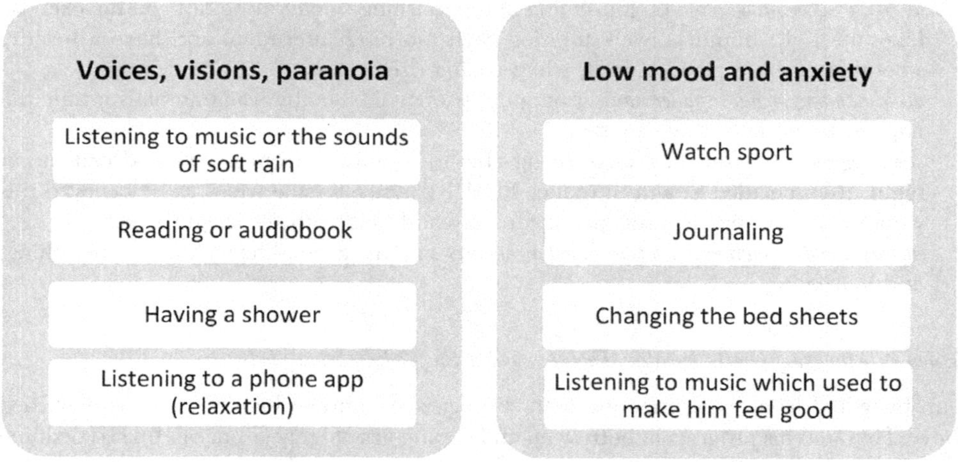

Figure 10.2 John's Strategies for Coping with Mental Health Symptoms

- *coping strategies for his voices, visions and paranoid fears*: listen to an audio book or soft music, have a shower, and journaling.

Session 4: Maintaining the Gains and Stress Management

By Session 4 of the programme, John was reporting a regular bedtime routine and had been able to reduce his time in bed to an average of 9.5 hours per night. He rated his sleep progress since the previous week as 8.5 out of 10, and his improvements in coping and self-efficacy as 7 out of 10.

His attempts to sleep for shorter durations led to him being tired and napping during the day. He also had his depot injection that week, which led to more sleep than in the previous weeks, but less than he had before engaging in this programme. He reported trying to be more active during the day and was going outside nearly every day. He woke up an average of three times per night, but reported he could fall asleep much more quickly since practising GOOBICS.

His demonstration of increased sleep knowledge, coping strategies for tiredness, and better routine showed that the intervention was effective for John, despite the challenge caused by his depot medication.

In Session 4, John discussed with the therapist how best to maintain the improvements made over the intervention, including planning for and management of any setbacks. Setbacks were framed as a normal part of the recovery process, and the therapist highlighted the importance of recognising that the occasional bad night's sleep does not necessarily mean that one is relapsing back into Insomnia. Session 4 also covered the greater need for sleep and the fatigue following the depot injection, but emphasised that this experience is temporary. A plan was made collaboratively with John that included how to deal with next-day effects of the depot injections, get his sleep routine back on track, and increase his confidence about being prepared.

During the session, an individualised summary plan was put together in which the triggers and perpetuators of his sleep problems were re-examined; they were then addressed by recounting of the strategies that John found useful for tackling his sleep-disruptive behaviours and cognitions (see Table 10.8).

In addition, stress management was covered in this session. Through discussion about helpful and unhelpful levels of stress, John acknowledged that he used avoidance as a coping skill for overstress, but consequently found that this led to stagnancy in his life (and then 'rustout' or under-stress). A short imagery exercise that asked John to reflect on his life at present left John with the conclusion that he was spending too much time worrying about the future and not enough time engaging in meaningful activities in the present (learning new skills or taking up hobbies). Based on this information, some small goals were set so that he could achieve a better life balance, which included employment plans and some leisure activities in the next month. It was discussed that engaging in behaviour in the service of valued goals can be very beneficial for maximising energy, sleep, mood, and overall quality of life.

Client strategies at the end of Session 4 (homework) included the following:

- *Address life balance* by initiating small goals towards starting a new hobby (making recordings of his DJ music) and pursuing employment by contacting an employment agency regarding local part-time opportunities.
- *Keep being active* (even in small ways) on the days following depot injections. For example,

take the dog for a short walk in the afternoon and spend a small amount of time with parents instead of being alone in his bedroom all day.

- *Make to-do lists* in the early evening to help manage stress and overthinking at night.
- *Plan tasks and activities to look forward to* for the next day to improve motivation in getting up.

Table 10.8 John's Individualised Summary Plan

Trigger/Precipitator	
How did the problem first develop?	Change in mental health First episode of depression
Perpetuators	
What kept it going?	Continuing episodes of mental health problems (schizophrenia, agoraphobia, OCD) Tiredness from medications Unhealthy food and drink choices Weight gain and lack of exercise Self-critical thoughts
Treatment	
What did you learn during the programme about how to overcome the problem?	Planning tomorrow, today. Having a schedule that helps me spend my time in a more helpful way Strategies to feel refreshed/keep awake (e.g. walking, eating certain foods, and drinking more water, engaging in hobbies) Keeping a sleep diary to recognise patterns in behaviour/ thoughts and sleep Maintain a routine of regular wake-up time and winding-down before bed Having some time outside the house each day—walking the dog and being in the sun.
What were your most unhelpful habits and thoughts?	Eating junk food early in the morning and then going back to bed Thinking that being tired means needing to go back to bed Thinking getting more sleep will reduce mental health problems Believing I am no good, and that there is nothing I can do to improve how I feel
What are the alternatives to these?	Recognising the need to balance daytime activities with sleep Avoiding oversleeping, which can increase tiredness Managing negative thoughts by developing more helpful and positive thoughts: 'There are things I can do to increase my energy', 'Sleeping is not always the best way to respond to tiredness'
What are the most important things to remember to help keep progress going?	Planning for changes in situations (new bedtime and rising time if need to get up early, or start a job) Keeping a routine before bed and in the morning Using energy-generating techniques Keep reviewing sleep facts as opposed to believing sleep myths (e.g. Session 1 information on the process of sleep)

Post-Treatment Assessment (Week 5)

John's post-treatment assessment comprised a questionnaire and data from his sleep diary.

John reported very high satisfaction with the changes in his sleep and daytime function, which included better mental health, and quality of life. He stated that he had been 'the most productive I've been in two years'. He had contacted employment agencies and was currently preparing applications for part-time work.

Table 10.9 shows that John had achieved his specific goals for sleep treatment beyond what was expected.

His sleep data (Tables 10.6 and 10.7) show that John maintained regular bedtime and wake-up times and had reduced total sleep time and time in bed. Other improvements included:

- a decrease in the PSQI global score from 9 to 6;
- increased sleep efficiency (85 per cent), when compared with baseline (80 per cent);
- less-frequent awakenings (two awakenings compared with four at baseline);
- a reduction in sleep latency to 10 minutes;
- he no longer needed to use the sleep medicine;
- a reduction in the number and intensity of bad dreams;
- less-frequent napping and shorter-duration naps;
- reduction in the consumption of sweet beverages and caffeine close to bedtime.

With regards to daytime function, John also demonstrated the following improvements:

- a decrease in PSQI daytime dysfunction;
- improvement in depression (PHQ-4);
- reduction in ratings on paranoid thoughts (MINI psychosis module);
- increased satisfaction with his mental health, relationship with his family, and his life as a whole.

With his sleep continuously improving, a discussion was initiated that he could now concentrate less on his sleep and more on the career and social aspects of his life that felt unbalanced. John was asked to evaluate his progress every 3 weeks and ensure that the sleep strategies remained effective for him when he entered the workforce.

Follow-up (3 Months Post-Treatment)

A session was organised 3 months after the end of John's treatment. With his focus on daytime activities rather than sleep, John was no longer using his sleep diary. Overall, he felt that his sleep was going well, with only a few occasional rough patches. He knew they

Table 10.9 John's Self-rated Achievement of CBT-I Treatment Goals

Achievement of Goals	*Perceived Level of Improvement*
1. Develop a good sleep pattern	Much more than expected
2. Reduce napping in the day	Somewhat more than expected
3. Develop a better routine (going to sleep and waking up at regular times)	Somewhat more than expected

would occur, and so John did not worry excessively about these short episodes. He reported experiencing only one bad dream a week, if any, and that they were less intense and less believable.

John continued to perform wind-down activities before bed most days of the week and noticed deterioration in his sleep whenever he went several days without this strategy. He also maintained a reasonably regular wake-up time in the morning.

As a result of eating a healthier diet and having regular daytime activity (e.g. walking the dog), he had started to lose weight (5 kg), had more energy, and felt much happier in himself. He had completed work experience with an agency and was considering employment opportunities. He felt that the career aspects of his life were being addressed, but that more work needed to be done to address leisure and hobbies.

The ability to wake up earlier improved John's opportunities to access other treatment services (e.g. to attend appointments in the morning, and on time, increased concentration), as well as social and occupational activities. Indeed, the feedback from his mental health team was that John had recently started to attend and engage in many of the group activities, including a group stress management programme.

Treatment Implications of John's Case

As with many other clients living with psychosis, CBT-I was very effective for treating John's sleep problems. Work to increase the sleep drive, regulate the body clock, and reduce arousal was important for John. His case demonstrated the importance of focusing on psychoeducation, motivational issues, and developing daytime energy strategies (Session 2). Emphasising life balance and pursuing goals outside sleep were particularly important for him. John had become so preoccupied with and worried about his poor sleep and tiredness that he had lost sight of important aspects of his life. Of course, this lack of connection with valued activities had a strong negative impact on his self-esteem and self-efficacy, compounding the sleep problem further. Planning ahead, problem-solving, and outlining clear steps to meet goals were very important elements of his recovery journey.

An important note from this case is that, not only should the influence of psychiatric symptoms and medications on sleep be assessed, but also the client's beliefs about the impact they can personally have to bring about improvements. It was important that the therapist worked with John to help him experience that he could influence the resolution of sleep issues, in spite of mental health problems and medication side effects. This important treatment emphasis is drawn from our empirical work that suggests clients feel a 'lack of control' over their sleep, which has implications for their expectations for treatment success and their motivation (Chiu et al., 2016).

References

Buysse, D. J., Reynolds III, C. F., Monk, T. H., Berman, S. R., and Kupfer, D. J. (1989) "The Pittsburgh sleep quality index: A new instrument for psychiatric practice and research", *Psychiatry Research*, 28(2), pp. 193–213.

Chiu, V. W., Harvey, R. H., Sloan, N. B., Ree, M., Lin, A., Janca, A., and Waters, F. (2015) "Cognitive and behavioral factors associated with insomnia in inpatients with schizophrenia and related psychoses", *Journal of Nervous & Mental Disease*, 203(10), pp. 798–803.

Chiu, V. W., Ree, M., Janca, A., and Waters, F. (2016) "Sleep in schizophrenia: Exploring subjective experiences of sleep problems, and implications for treatment", *Psychiatric Quarterly*, 87(4), pp. 633–648.

Citrome, L. (2010) "Paliperidone palmitate—review of the efficacy, safety and cost of a new second-generation depot antipsychotic medication", *International Journal of Clinical Practice*, 64(2), pp. 216–239.

Krakow, B. (2002) *Turning nightmares into dreams: The authorized audio series and treatment workbook for New Dream Therapy* [CDs]. USA: The New Sleepy Times.

Kroenke, K., Spitzer, R. L., Williams, J. B. W., and Löwe, B. (2009) "An ultra-brief screening scale for anxiety and depression: The PHQ–4", *Psychosomatics*, 50(6), pp. 613–621.

Morin, C. M., Vallières, A., and Ivers, H. (2007) "Dysfunctional beliefs and attitudes about sleep (DBAS): Validation of a brief version (DBAS-16)", *Sleep*, 30(11), p. 1547

Sheehan, D. V., Lecrubier, Y., Sheehan, K. H., Amorim, P., Janavs, J., Weiller, E., Hergueta, T., Baker, R., and Dunbar, G. C. (1998) "The Mini-International Neuropsychiatric Interview (M.I.N.I.): The development and validation of a structured diagnostic psychiatric interview for DSM-IV and ICD-10", *Journal of Clinical Psychiatry*, 59(Suppl. 20), pp. 22–33.

Part II
Therapist Manual

11 Tips and Instructions to the Therapist

This manual has been adapted from traditional CBT-I protocols for use in individuals with psychotic disorders. The manual is designed to be useful for psychologists and mental health workers at the 'coalface', who work with individuals who have psychotic symptoms and low psychosocial functioning.

It is recommended that this manual be read in its entirety before the treatment protocol is administered. It is important to be familiar with the contents of each session prior to delivery. This will help you to identify any gaps in your knowledge or skills that may require extra reading or supervision. Furthermore, to deliver CBT-I effectively in the context of psychotic disorders, it is important that you have a good understanding of how sleep is regulated (Chapter 5), the Cognitive Behaviour Therapy model (Chapter 7), how sleep problems manifest in people with psychotic disorders (Chapter 6), and how to assess your client's sleep problems (Chapter 8).

Research has suggested that perceived lack of control within this population is an important factor contributing to their poor sleep. Accordingly, this manual emphasises the development of self-efficacy through clients being helped to have experiences of making choices that improve their sleep and daytime functioning. This is a message that needs repetition and should flow through each session.

Structure and Format

This programme has been designed for use, either in a group format, or one on one with individual clients. There are some points in the manual that are particularly relevant for groups. These can be adapted if you are seeing a client individually.

The manual is structured as a session-by-session treatment programme designed to improve sleep in people with psychotic disorders. This treatment has been designed around 4-weekly (or bi-weekly) sessions that should each last approximately 1.5 hours. All four sessions have a therapist manual and a client resource pack. The client resource pack summarises the main concepts in a simplified way and includes worksheets to be used both during and between sessions. It provides a valuable tool that clients can refer to in the future and, in the case of group CBT-I, should be sent to clients who miss any sessions. The Therapist Manual refers to the relevant activities in the client resource pack.

When a psychological intervention is being delivered, a structured format is most appropriate for clients with significant cognitive impairment and disorganisation (Holden and Granholm, 2012). Sessions may be broken down into shorter, more numerous sessions (e.g. eight 45-minute sessions), if you judge this to be more suitable for your client. The sessions are not intended to be delivered strictly as a script, but example text is provided for maximum clarity.

Depending on individual need, some clients may also benefit from greater time spent on certain sessions, extra support such as between-session check-up calls, and the involvement of additional support networks (e.g. carer, family member, friend, case manager). The involvement of support persons can be particularly useful for this client population.

It is important to adapt the sessions to suit your particular client. For example, sections of low relevance can be skipped over, and optional material can be included if it is particularly pertinent for the client (see Appendices for optional material).

When the programme is delivered in a group format, it is suggested that groups are limited to three to six people. This is consistent with Dopke and colleagues' (2004) suggestions about psychological sleep interventions for people with severe mental illness. In the case of a group format, our experience is that groups of three clients work best for this clinical group. Individual sessions are sometimes preferred for clients with social anxiety, antisocial personality, learning difficulty, or history of trauma impacting on their sleep (which they may not want to share with a group).

Your Role as a Therapist

Ultimately, your role is to help facilitate the client's development of skills to manage their Insomnia and, with time, their independent mastery of these skills. Dopke and colleagues (2004) applied the following strategies in their CBT-I protocol for treating individuals with severe mental illness, which should also be applied here:

- Develop an individualised case formulation together with the client and then select the most important factors that drive their Insomnia (e.g. reduced daytime activity levels, irregular wake time, use of stimulants close to bedtime). Use this to guide the selection of the most pertinent strategies.
- Help group members see links between their behavioural choices and sleep outcomes.
- Assist group members to choose skills most pertinent to them to work on. These skills aim to minimise the impact of their specific sleep problem and also to address the factors perpetuating it.
- Generally, have up to three new key strategies for the client to try each week. Too many strategies can be overwhelming and confusing.
- Provide individualised progress summaries to clients at each session, highlighting the strategies that seemed most helpful, making recommendations, and encouraging continued practice and persistence.

Eliciting Goals and a Formulation

Prior to engagement in the CBT-I programme, conduct an individual sleep interview with each client to assess current symptoms, duration, possible causes, and impact of their sleep difficulties (see Chapter 8). This will assist you in devising appropriate treatment goals and strategies, in addition to gauging the client's motivation to engage in therapy.

Each session should include:

1. identification of personal goals that can meet the client's interest;
2. goal progress discussion;
3. brainstorming ways to overcome barriers to progress, and exercises to encourage discussion;
4. motivation boosts: ask clients to think about how their life would be with improved sleep (e.g. 'What would you do differently if you woke up feeling more refreshed?').

Personalised goals can be elicited using:

- a discussion of recovery goals in the short and longer term;
- other group members' experiences;
- brainstorming;
- breaking down long-term goals into small, manageable steps;
- strategies for overcoming obstacles.

The development of specific, measurable, achievable, relevant, and time-oriented (SMART) goals should be encouraged. For example, a general goal might be to get fit. However, a specific goal would be, 'go for a 15-minute walk each afternoon at 4 p.m.'.

An essential part of CBT-I is working collaboratively with each client to develop a good formulation—or 'blueprint'—for their specific sleep problem. This enables clients to understand their individual cycle of Insomnia/poor sleep and identify particular strategies that may be helpful. This should begin at the outset of the intervention.

The use of weekly sleep diaries and other self-report measures will allow clients to chart their progress throughout the intervention (e.g. length of time taken to fall asleep, number of wake-ups during the night, daytime energy, daytime activity; Appendix 1).

The Contribution of Psychotic Symptoms in CBT-I Treatment

An assessment of how the client's psychiatric symptoms and medications impact on their sleep is essential. Clients' perceptions regarding their psychiatric illness can also provide important information on possible barriers to change. For example, clients may believe that their diagnosis of a psychotic disorder means that they are helpless to improve their sleep or daytime energy. In many cases, clients report that the symptoms of their Insomnia started at the same time as, or just prior to, the onset of their psychiatric illness. Consequently, they feel that their sleep problems are a permanent feature of their condition. Unfortunately, this belief is also often held by mental health professionals (therefore influencing the treatment that is provided to clients). It is important to help clients examine these beliefs with a view to increase their feelings of self-efficacy and control. Even if normal sleep and energy levels are beyond the client's reach owing to the severity of their symptoms or the influence of their medications, moderate improvements can be very meaningful for improving quality of life and keeping the client actively participating in their treatment.

Prominent clinical features of disorders such as schizophrenia include negative symptoms that can lead to amotivation and a pattern of disengagement. As a therapist, you need to stay supportive, assertive, persistent, and encouraging. In addition to disengagement, other possible barriers to treatment are summarised in Table 11.1.

Consultation with Others

Working Collaboratively with the Case Manager or Treating Clinician

Where possible, your client's progress and goals should be discussed in a multidisciplinary team context, so that the client's case manager or treating clinician can reinforce the use of strategies and support their client in achieving their goals.

Most clients will start CBT-I with concurrent pharmacological medications. There may be cases where your client is able to work towards a reduction in sedative medication.

Table 11.1 Barriers to Treatment and Suggested Approach

Barriers to Treatment	*Suggested Approach*
Beliefs that the psychiatric diagnosis means poor sleep is not treatable	Emphasise the contribution of environmental, behavioural, and cognitive factors in the maintenance of Insomnia Encourage the client to discover that they are not helpless. This can be done by providing experiences that demonstrate the influence of their behavioural choices
Styles of coping that include anxious avoidance or dissociation	Be aware of the frequency of, and triggers for, dissociation or avoidance Be watchful in the session for signs of increased anxiety/distress Develop a strategy with the client for how to handle increased anxiety/distress (e.g. grounding techniques)
History of traumatic experiences with mental health treatment	Emphasise the collaborative nature of the process, that the client makes choices together with the therapist Validate past negative treatment experiences in a supportive therapeutic manner Express a genuine desire to explore solutions that work for each individual client—in other words, not expecting that the same strategies work for everyone
Limited reading and writing ability	Simplified written materials Audiotape the session goals and homework (on a CD, phone, or tablet) Use reminders such as follow-up phone calls to act as a prompt or reminder between sessions; use reminders on the client's phone (e.g. alarm set at 3 p.m. to go for a 15-minute walk)

Thus, it is important to raise this possibility with the client's prescribing doctor. Discussions about the optimal timing of medications with sedative properties (such as antipsychotic drugs) can also be of benefit to minimise daytime sedation. Although beyond the scope of this manual, information exists regarding tapering of hypnotic medications (e.g. Kirmil-Gray et al., 1985; Morin et al., 2004). Some information on this issue is presented in Appendices 15 and 16.

With the Sleep Physician

Sometimes, symptoms of Insomnia will be comorbid with another sleep disorder. If screening suggests the presence of other sleep disorders, such as OSA, referral to a sleep physician for an overnight sleep study is indicated. The use of CBT-I is often still helpful for clients with OSA, as the knowledge gained about good sleep habits and self-efficacy can be used as they adapt to CPAP or other treatment strategies for OSA. If another sleep disorder fully accounts for the presenting sleep complaint, CBT-I is not required.

Manual Structure

Aspects of Sleep and Functioning Addressed in this Programme

Eight topics are addressed in the four sessions as follows (See Figure 11.1):

- Session 1: Learning about Sleep and Good Sleep Habits;
- Session 2: Maximising Energy and Working with Unhelpful Beliefs about Sleep;
- Session 3: Managing Worries and a Busy Mind and Introducing Relaxation;
- Session 4: Maintaining Wellness and Working with Triggers for Poor Sleep.

Session Structure

After the previous week's tasks and goals have been reviewed, each subsequent session then introduces sleep facts and the rationale for each new strategy, before moving to the application of skills ('sleep skills training'). This is achieved by making a specific plan of how and when strategies will be practised during the week. Sessions conclude with a motivation boost, summary, and plan for the week ahead.

The Therapist Manual contains information and activities to illustrate particularly important issues. Throughout, 'Therapist notes' provide additional suggestions and information regarding treatment administration.

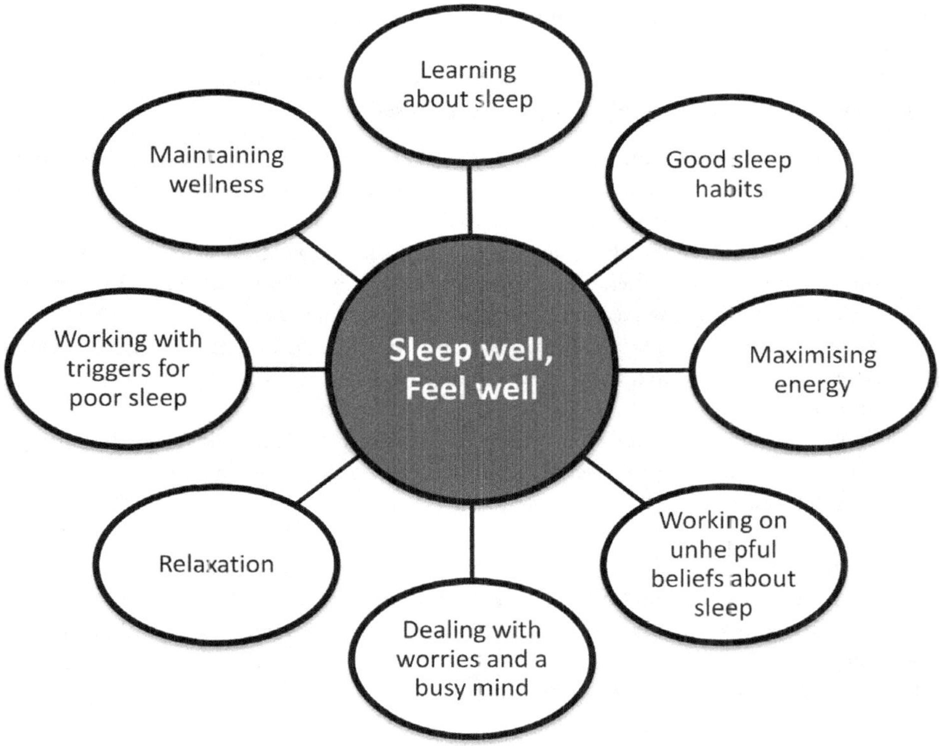

Figure 11.1 Topics Addressed in the *Sleep Well, Feel Well with Psychosis* Programme

The following icons refer to therapeutic activities that encourage clients to try a new strategy or think through a particular issue. Ideas can be discussed verbally or written down in the client resource packs, on a whiteboard or on a large sheet of paper.

Worksheet Activities in the Client Resource Packs

These activities require clients to make notes relevant to their particular sleep issues in their client resource pack.

Group Discussion

An activity involving a verbal discussion of the client's personal experiences (no worksheets provided).

Activities and group discussions can also include the following activity types:

- ***Brainstorm***: This is an activity in which clients generate alternative responses to or ideas for a question or scenario. If clients appear very tired, we suggest having them get up and write their answers on a whiteboard or piece of butcher's paper to help increase levels of alertness.
- ***Barriers to change***: This is an activity that requires clients to problem-solve and plan ahead for how best to implement sleep strategies. The therapist should be active in gently suggesting barriers that the client may not have thought of. The client's emerging insight into their sleep difficulties will assist them in completing an effective relapse plan in the last session.
- ***Motivation boost***: The motivation boost is a suggested component in each session that aims to identify and address low perceived self-efficacy:
  - Session 1 comprises an imagery exercise for clients to consider what they look forward to, what they think will be hardest about the treatment programme, and what will help motivate them to stick with treatment.
  - Session 2 requires clients to explore their beliefs regarding whether living with mental illness makes their sleep unchangeable. The client and therapist consider how this belief might feed into the cycle of Insomnia.
  - Session 3 involves a motivational statement to remind clients that, even when sleep is not going well, there is still much they can do to improve their daytime functioning.
  - Session 4 comprises suggestions to assist clients in dealing with future setbacks in their sleep and reflecting on their improvement since participating in the sleep programme.

Colour versions of the Therapist Manual and client resource packs, which include images and space in the manual for the therapist to make notes, are available upon request. If you would like access to this version of the manual, please contact the authors for an electronic copy.

All the best with delivering the programme!

References

Dopke, C. A., Lehner, R. K., and Wells, A. M. (2004) "Cognitive-behavioral group therapy for insomnia in individuals with serious mental illnesses: A preliminary evaluation", *Psychiatric Rehabilitation Journal*, 27(3), pp. 235–242.

Holden, J., and Granholm, E. (2012) "Group cognitive behavioural social skills training for schizophrenia", in Steel, C. (Ed.) *CBT for schizophrenia: Evidence-based interventions and future directions.* Oxford, UK: John Wiley, pp. 169–190.

Kirmil-Gray, K., Eagleston, J. R., Thoresen, C. E., and Zarcone, V. P. (1985) "Brief consultation and stress management treatments for drug-dependent insomnia: Effects on sleep quality, self-efficacy, and daytime stress", *Journal of Behavioral Medicine*, 8(1), pp. 79–99.

Morin, C. M., Bastien, C., Guay, B., Radouco-Thomas, M., Leblanc, J., and Vallières, A. (2004) "Randomized clinical trial of supervised tapering and cognitive behavior therapy to facilitate benzodiazepine discontinuation in older adults with chronic insomnia", *American Journal of Psychiatry*, 161(2), pp. 332–342.

12 Therapist Manual Session 1

Learning about Sleep and Good Sleep Habits

General Instructions to the Therapist

Establishing a strong case for the effectiveness of CBT-I from the outset of the session is important, as this assists in increasing a client's motivation to actively participate in treatment. Although the evidence for potential benefits for sleep and daytime functioning should be highlighted, it is equally important to establish realistic expectations for the client. In addition to discussing the evidence base for CBT-I, encourage clients to think about their personal motivations to improve their sleep and daytime functioning. Emphasise that the programme will ask clients to be active participants, and that you, as the therapist, will work with them to discover ways to improve their sleep and daytime well-being.

Difficulties with motivation and self-efficacy can be a significant obstacle towards engagement in therapy for clients with a psychotic disorder. Consequently, it is important to gauge each client's confidence regarding their ability to initiate change, and take time to identify their goals and motivation for improving their sleep.

Session 1 Structure

The structure for Session 1 is as follows:

- A general introduction: If in a group setting, clients introduce themselves, stating their name and why they are interested in attending the programme.
- What is CBT-I?
- What is Insomnia?
- What the benefits of engaging in the programme are.
- How to get the most out of the programme and to create effective change in their sleep
- Myths and facts about sleep.
- Sleep skills: sleep hygiene, wind-down before bed, GOOBICS, working towards a regular rising time.
- Motivation boost.
- Summary and weekly plan.

Material Needed

- Client Resource Pack (Session 1)

Supplementary (Optional) Handouts

- *Sleep diary* (Appendix 2): This can be used to identify patterns in clients' sleep–wake routines, and to help track the progress in the timing and quality of their sleep.
- *Sleep hygiene diary* (Appendix 3): This worksheet is a helpful way for clients to monitor their use of good sleep habits during the pre-sleep period on a daily basis.
- *Some interesting facts about dreaming* (Appendix 4): The information from this sheet can be used to help answer queries that clients might have about dreaming.
- *Decision balance sheet* (Appendix 5): This worksheet can be used with clients who are ambivalent about changing an unhelpful behaviour. It takes the client through the process of thinking about the pros and cons of their behaviour, and whether it is worth giving change a try.

Session Content: Introduction

What Is Insomnia?

Insomnia is not just a poor night's sleep that everyone gets now and then. It is a long-term problem with falling asleep, staying asleep, or having unrefreshing sleep, despite enough opportunity to sleep. It can cause a lot of distress and affect many areas of your day. It can influence your mood, thinking skills (such as your concentration and your memory), and energy to go out to see friends or family. Mental health symptoms can cause sleep problems, but Insomnia and other sleep problems can also influence mental health problems, with sleep difficulties making mental health symptoms worse. People often think that their mental health diagnosis means they will be stuck with poor sleep for good. However, as we will discuss today, poor sleep can be improved if you understand it, and know how to manage it, even if you experience mental health difficulties. An important message today is that you can do a lot to improve your sleep and your daytime energy. We will show you how over the next four sessions.

What Is Cognitive Behaviour Therapy?

Cognitive Behaviour Therapy (CBT) is a type of treatment that helps people to develop helpful thinking habits and behaviours. This programme uses CBT to assist you in developing helpful 'sleep skills' for managing sleep problems, such as Insomnia. We will cover things such as: (a) how to make your bed and bedroom more sleep-friendly, (b) how to make a healthy sleep routine, (c) how to deal with unpleasant thoughts, (d) how to set up a structure for the daytime, and (e) how to reduce worry. CBT is not a quick fix for a sleep problem. Instead, it requires steady practice over time. You may get frustrated if you expect results straight away. We will take care to support you through the programme as you learn to manage your sleep and improve your energy.

Benefits of Engaging in the Programme

Sleep is a natural process that will automatically adjust itself with a little bit of knowledge and a structured approach. Cognitive and behavioural therapy can improve different aspects of your sleep, such as the time it takes you to fall asleep, waking during the night, nightmares, and the regularity of your sleep routine. It can also benefit how you feel during the day, such as your level of tiredness, alertness, motivation, and mood. When people sleep well, they tend to have better mental functioning (such as their memory and concentration), as well as better motivation for the day. In addition, the body also gets a well-deserved rest after working so hard during the waking hours. During sleep, the brain and heart clean up toxins in the body, as well as consolidating mental processes that occurred during the day.

Let's have a brief think about what the benefits of attending this programme might be for you.

Identifying Goals and Motivations

Activity 1: Identifying Benefits, Goals and Motivation for Attending the Programme

This worksheet contains space to write down the following:

- Your GOALS for the programme: Let's try and identify three or four realistic goals.
- Your MOTIVATION for treating your Insomnia: Why is it important to you to meet your goals? How might sleeping better and having more energy improve things for you?

The worksheet also includes an '*importance ruler*'. Please rate, on this scale from 0 to 10, how important is it for you to treat your Insomnia.

Therapist notes*: Use the information gathered in the sleep interview assessment (see Chapter 8) to help each client identify specific goals and to complete the Client Resource Pack Activity 1 ('Identifying goals and motivations', Client Resource Pack Session 1). Endeavour to assist each client to establish a strong incentive for completing the programme.*

The following motivational interviewing prompts may assist the client in this activity:

- *What brought you to this programme for treatment?*
- *How you are coping with your sleep difficulties right now?*
- *What is going well for you right now with regards to your sleep? Are there things that aren't going quite so well? Are there any areas you think could be improved?*
- *It sounds as though you would like things to change. Do you have ideas about what you might be able to do differently?*
- *What changes are you thinking about making?*
- *How would you like things to turn out with your sleep?*
- *What difference would it make for you to sleep better?*
- *What difference would it make for you to have more energy during the day?*
- *What do you think it would be like if you kept sleeping how you are now?*

At the end of Session 1, the 'Motivation boost: Cost and benefits' exercise is also intended to assist with motivation.

Some goals commonly expressed by people with psychotic disorders include:

- *'fall asleep faster' (encourage development of a specific goal, e.g. 'reduce time to fall asleep to less than 2 hours');*
- *'wake up less during the night' (e.g. 'from a baseline of 3 hours awake');*
- *'worry less about sleep' (rate on a scale of 1–10, pre- and post-CBT-I);*
- *'take fewer sleeping pills at night' (e.g. reduce dose from 20 mg);*

- *'get into a more normal sleep pattern (sleep at night and wake up in the morning, e.g. 'get out of bed by 10 a.m. six days a week, and be in bed with the lights out by midnight')';*
- *'learn to relax enough to go to sleep' (measured by rating of relaxation at bedtime and time taken to fall asleep);*
- *'reduce my 'nanny naps' and be less tired in the daytime' (measured by time spent napping each week and ratings of daytime energy).*

For the above goals, note down the current starting point, so that progress can be measured (e.g. average 3 hours of wake time overnight; average level of anxiety before bed (out of 10); average 4 hours in bed during the day).

How to Get the Most out of this Programme

***Therapist notes**: It can be useful to cover this as a brainstorming activity. You can utilise guidelines, such as those below, written on a whiteboard or piece of paper. Clients may come up with additional points that would help them to feel safe and motivated to engage in sessions.*

1. **Attend all the sessions**: The programme is here to help you achieve your goals. It is normal to have times when you don't feel like coming; however, you will find that you often feel worse rather than better for not attending.
2. **Contribute**: Be willing to talk openly and honestly. Put your own issues forward.
3. **Ask**: Ask questions if you don't understand or disagree with something that was said. Never go home being confused about instructions on tasks for the week. We understand that we are presenting new information to you and we are happy to explain things until they are clear to you.
4. **Listen**: Some topics discussed may not seem so relevant to you now, but may become useful later. The information that other people share in the sessions may also be helpful to you.
5. **Don't compare yourself with other group members**: Remember that no two people are exactly the same. Even if they have the same goals, what works for you might not work for them, and vice versa. It is important that you develop strategies that work for you.
6. **Maintain confidentiality in group sessions**: People must feel relaxed that what they say will remain private.
7. **Take responsibility**: Remember that, in therapy, 'What you put in = what you get out'. Being non-active in the programme tends to create little or no positive change.
8. **Use the sleep resources**: It is helpful to read over the material learned at home each week.
9. Other: ____

Let's get started!

Aspects of Sleep and Daytime Functioning Addressed in this Session

This session addresses myths and facts about sleep and teaches skills that will encourage better sleep. Sleep skills for today include healthy sleep habits, winding down before bed, and what you should do if you can't sleep and feel agitated.

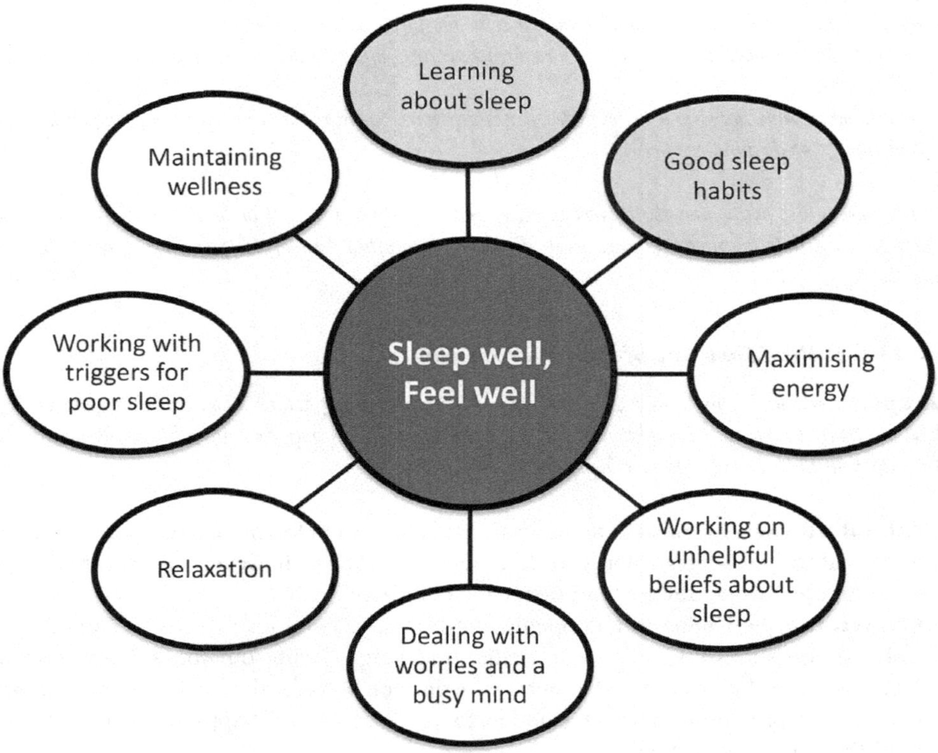

Figure 12.1 Topics Addressed this Week (Session 1)

Myths and Facts about Sleep

What Happens in Normal Sleep?

Activity 2: What Happens in Normal Sleep, and Common Sleep Complaints

***Therapist notes**: The psychoeducation component of CBT-I is important and should not be skimmed over. Learning about the processes of sleep and waking can help the client build realistic expectations about sleep and reduce anxieties around what constitutes normal sleep. Refer the client to the graph shown in the Client Resource Pack for Activity 2.*

Sleep is like sailing along the ocean. When it is going well, it feels relaxing as we sail smoothly across the waves. However, when sleep is not going so well, it often feels like sailing through a storm, where the waves are rocky and unpredictable. Look at the graph in your client resource pack for Activity 2 ('What happens in normal sleep, and common sleep complaints') as we go through some myths and facts about sleep. The little boat's speech bubbles reflect some common worries that people have about their sleep.

There are different stages of sleep, referred to as: (a) light sleep, (b) deep sleep, and (c) dreaming. As we go from one stage of sleep to the next, it is like sailing up and down a wave. Just like sailing on the ocean waves, the transition between stages is not abrupt, but gradual. Falling asleep is a gradual change from wakefulness to a state of relaxation and sleep. When we wake, the body gradually 'comes to', and it takes a while to become fully alert. When the body falls asleep, the brain undergoes changes and it cycles through the sleep stages (i.e. light sleep, deep sleep, and dreaming). Each type of sleep—not just deep sleep—is important.

Therapist notes: *The analogy of a 'wave' is helpful to demonstrate that:*

- *It takes time to fall asleep, and falling asleep is a gradual process, requiring progressive relaxation and changes across a whole host of hormones and other physiological processes.*
- *Just as it takes some time to wind up into the day to become fully alert after a night of sleep, so too does it take time for the mind and body to 'wind down' from wakefulness into sleep.*
- *Brief periods of awareness are a natural part of sleep. It is normal for brief awakenings to occur throughout the night. If the wakings are brief, we often don't remember them in the morning, which is why many good sleepers think that they haven't woken up at all (when really they have).*

Let's talk in more detail about each of these processes.

Falling Asleep

Our bodies naturally do many things to help us fall asleep. For example, body temperature drops, our heart rate slows down, cortisol levels go down, and our bodies release certain hormones, such as melatonin. It is normal to take up to 30 minutes to fall asleep. However, it can take much longer when you are dealing with mental health problems, because you may have many things on your mind, and you might find it hard to switch off. It may also be that you have napped during the day, meaning you are less sleepy at bedtime.

Group Discussion: What Makes it Harder for You to Fall Asleep?

We often hear from people suffering a psychosis that difficulties falling asleep are due to medications, lack of activity in the day, cigarettes in the evening, being on a computer until bedtime, stressful events, or problems with racing thoughts, fears, voices, and visions.

Some people may simply take longer to fall asleep and not know why. It is helpful to identify factors that make it harder to fall asleep, so that we can put helpful strategies into place. This programme aims to reduce the time it takes to fall asleep, or at least make the time pleasanter.

Staying Asleep

Did you know that it is normal to briefly wake up (for less than 5 minutes) when we move from one stage of sleep to the next?

Most of our deep sleep happens in the first half of the night, whereas light sleep and dreaming happen more in the second half of the night. This means that waking up from sleep is more likely to happen during the second phase of the night. Many people simply do not notice or remember that they have had these brief periods of waking during the night, and they fall right back asleep.

Therefore, expecting to fall asleep instantly and not wake from sleep during the night is unrealistic.

We can, however, usually work to improve aspects of sleep for those who take a long time to fall asleep, or who have long wakings during the night.

When you notice that you are not falling asleep quickly or that you have woken up, sleeplessness can be frustrating and stressful. It can cause you to spend a lot of time in bed worrying or feeling tense. Anxiety and frustration overnight often play a big part in how tired we feel the next day.

If we can experience our times awake at night as *relaxing*, this will help reduce how fatigued we feel the next day, even if the amount of time sleeping has not increased.

Waking Up

Have you ever wondered, 'Why do I feel so tired when I wake up, even when I've had about seven hours of sleep?'

Nearly every morning, most of us feel dazed and groggy for up to 45 minutes after waking. This is part of the process of moving from sleep to wakefulness, and we call it sleep inertia. Luckily, this process is only temporary and does not necessarily mean that you have had a bad night's sleep.

Waking up can be a slow process. The brain and the organs of the body all need to 'wake up', and this can take some time. If you go from light sleep to awake, it generally doesn't take as long to feel alert as if you go from deep sleep to awake. If you wake up from a deep stage of sleep, it is quite natural to feel tired when waking and find yourself sailing the 'groggy' wave for longer. It can also take longer to feel awake in the morning if you are taking sleep medication, as it may still be in your system, making you feel groggy.

Some tiredness on waking is normal, and it often lifts after 45 minutes or so. There are things that can help with managing morning drowsiness.

Group Discussion: What Are Strategies for 'Winding Up' in the Morning?

- Do some stretching exercises (even before you get out of bed).
- Take three deep breaths.
- Get dressed. This sends a clear message that you are intending to start the day. Try laying your clothes out by the bed the night before.
- Take a quick walk outside.
- Have a morning coffee or an ice-cold drink.
- A shower can be very effective for helping you to feel more awake.
- Don't skip breakfast and have some healthy breakfast options ready.
- Get some bright light (sunlight is perfect).
- Do work that requires moderate effort, such as tidying up or cleaning.
- Put on some uplifting noise, such as a radio programme or music.
- Importantly, get up at the same time each morning (more on this later).

Sleep Needs

The average amount of sleep healthy adults need is between 6 and 9 hours a night. Some people function fine on as little as 5 or 6 hours of sleep, and there are people who need 10 or more hours. It is a myth that everyone needs 8 hours. In addition, medications often make you sleep longer, and so it is normal to expect that you have longer sleep time if you are on certain medications.

The key is to find the right amount of sleep for you. One way to work this out is by: (a) setting up a healthy daytime routine (not too much activity, but not too little—more on this next session), (b) managing any health problems as best you can, and (c) and observing how well you function on the sleep you are getting.

Oversleeping

Some people benefit from *more* sleep to recover from a mental health relapse (that is, when symptoms increase a lot), medical problems, or stressful times. There are also people who would benefit from *less* sleep. Sometimes, people oversleep because they enjoy sleeping and it feels good, or it can be an escape from boredom, low mood, anxiety, or stress. However, this can make them feel even more tired and low in mood during the day.

Group Discussion: Do You Ever Oversleep? Why Does This Happen?

Sleeping in the day lessens your need for sleep at night. By reducing the time you spend oversleeping in the morning, you make your body more ready for sleep that night.

***Therapist notes**: We find that roughly 20 per cent of clients have long sleep duration (sleeping 10–14 hours over the 24-hour period). This is generally encountered as one block of sleep, but there are also clients who regularly take extended naps (of 3–4 hours) on top of their usual sleep during the night-time.*

Common reasons reported for oversleeping have included: feeling tired after eating a large meal, boredom, being overweight, sedation from medications (particularly after a depot injection or having taken extra PRN medication the night before), avoidance of stressful problems or not wanting to face the day, depression, headaches or migraines limiting daytime functioning, pain, having nothing to look forward to, drug or alcohol abuse, or untreated sleep apnoea. It is important to assess whether oversleeping may be the result of an undiagnosed sleep disorder (e.g. sleep apnoea) or medical condition (e.g. vitamin D deficiency, cancer, hormone problems) that the client may not be aware of.

Sleep Skills: Sleep Smarter to Sleep Better

There are many factors that impact on sleep. Identifying things that help or hinder good sleep can provide you with greater control towards achieving better sleep. Although it is not always possible to solve all the problems that impact on sleep, you may be able to control some factors, or put strategies in place to reduce their impact.

***Therapist notes**: The following short exercise can provide a quick indication of the degree of influence of low self-efficacy. This could also be asked during the pre-treatment assessment period and used to monitor change across the sessions. For clients who are rated as having low self-efficacy (a score of less than 4 out of 10 on the scale below), it is useful to revisit this at the end of the session to check for any improvements in their rating. A central goal is for clients to leave the session with at least one factor that they are confident they can influence.*

Group Discussion: How Much Control Do You Have over your Sleep Problem?

On a scale of 1–10 (1 = little control; 10 = a lot of control), how much influence or control do you believe you have over your sleep problem? Why do you think that is?

***Therapist notes**: Clients with low perceived control over their sleep problems may make comments such as, 'I've tried all the sleep hygiene rules and none of them have worked', 'I've been a bad sleeper since I was a child', 'Without sleeping tablets, I don't get any sleep at all', 'Until my noisy neighbour goes away, my sleep will never get better', and 'My sleepiness over the day feels overpowering—I constantly feel like taking a nap', 'it is just the way I am'.*

Perceived Control over Sleep

Although having a mental illness may make you more prone to sleep problems, this doesn't mean that you can't ever have good sleep. It is similar to fair-skinned people being more prone to sunburn. Rather than avoiding the sun forever, they can learn to manage their fair skin, for example by making sure they wear sunscreen and a hat and not staying in the sun for too long. Similarly, CBT-I teaches you how to manage poor sleep, even though your mental illness may make poor sleep more likely. Hopefully, during this programme you will be able to try out a few different strategies that help you to see how much influence you can have.

Although we cannot force sleep to happen, we can look at the things that get in the way of good sleep and work on reducing them.

***Therapist notes**: The aim of the following activities is to emphasise that there are many factors that clients have at least some control over. Aims here are to give hope, build motivation, and educate clients about factors that influence sleep.*

Treat the next activity (Activity 3) as a behavioural experiment: Have the client read a short passage from a book or their client resource pack for 5 minutes and then rate their fatigue level. Then take them for a short walk around the room/building/grounds, tell them some jokes, or do some stretches or gentle jogging on the spot. Alternatively, a short break may be taken as part of the exercise, for the client to recharge. Ask the client to rate their fatigue after the activation exercise. We usually find that fatigue levels improve as activity increases. If the client experiences that reading makes them more tired, this may be suggested as a potential wind-down strategy in Activity 6 ('Winding Down before Bed').

Activity 3: How Our Choices Affect Tiredness

- How tired or sleepy (or lacking in energy) are you feeling *now*, on a scale of 0–10?
- How do you rate your tiredness after doing a bit of *reading*?
- How do you rate your tiredness after *a short walk*?
- What conclusions can you draw from this?

As we can see from this activity, sleepiness can be affected by the choices we make.

Factors that Impact on Sleep: Sleep Hygiene

***Therapist notes**: Individuals with psychosis and Insomnia are often reasonably knowledgeable about sleep hygiene 'rules', although they may show some important knowledge gaps (see Chapter 6). Often, they have done their own research into the cause of their sleep problems. This may lead to claims that 'they already know' about sleep hygiene, although further questioning might reveal that their knowledge is incomplete and incorrect, or that it has not been applied consistently. It is, therefore, important to carefully assess for knowledge gaps when working through this component of Session 1, to ensure that the client understands the importance of good sleep hygiene and a behavioural routine.*

Our behaviour and environment have a big impact on how well we sleep and how we feel during the day. The trick is to work out what is helpful or unhelpful for you.

***Therapist notes**: There are two activities within this section. The client may need to be prompted if they have difficulty generating relevant factors on their own. In this situation, information gathered from the initial assessment may assist in identifying issues specific to the client.*

Activity 4: What Factors May Be Impacting on Your Sleep?

Let's brainstorm a range of factors that might be impacting on your sleep for better or for worse. Specifically, can you remember a night or a period of time when you slept well?

- Can you think why this good sleep happened?
- What happened during the day and evening, and how were you feeling?

On the other hand, let's take an example of a night or period of time when you slept poorly.

- What do you think led to this?

Further, can you think of a day when you had more energy?

- What were you doing, and what was happening?

Finally, tell me about days when you had very low energy.

- What are you doing, and what was happening on those days?

Once this is finished, let's asterisk (*) the factors over which you have some control.

Therapist notes: *In this activity, clients tend to have difficulty generating answers at first, as they have not thought about these factors before. Some good prompts for clients are: (a) whether they like noise in the environment (e.g. the sound of the rain; many leave a fan or TV on overnight, as they find it hard to sleep in complete silence); (b) whether they sleep better in complete darkness or with a dim light on; (c) what helps them relax before bed (e.g. reading, TV, praying); (d) whether factors that make them worry or sad (such as watching the news, having an early appointment the next day) affects their sleep; and (e) whether they have nightmares.*

Clients tend to report that they sleep better if they have had a busy and fulfilling day. It is useful for the therapist to draw connections between how behaviours and scheduled activities—that the client has some control over—can directly influence how well they sleep at night. This presents us with an opportunity to encourage the client to observe and experiment with different behaviours before bed, and to monitor what effect this has on their sleep using the sleep diary.

Activity 5: Sleep Hygiene Checklist

This worksheet follows from the previous activity and contains a list of factors that can make sleep better and those that can make sleep worse. Tick the factors that apply to you. This will help identify behaviours that are already 'helpful' and areas that may be useful to work on.

Now that we have identified some factors that contribute to poor sleep, it is time to discuss them. For each factor that is problematic, let's identify alternative options and generate strategies that might be helpful and feasible in your situation.

Behaviours that often need to be addressed include:

- napping during the day;
- sleeping in late;
- watching TV in bed;
- using a device with a bright screen in the 2 hours before bedtime;
- consuming drinks that contain caffeine in the late afternoon or evening;
- drinking alcohol;
- eating a heavy meal within 3 hours before bedtime;
- staying in bed despite lying awake for long periods of time;
- staying inside all day;
- smoking before bed.

***Therapist notes**: A gentle, but thorough, discussion should follow that aims to assist the client to explore alternative behaviours. It may be useful to select one behaviour at a time to work on gradually. This way, the client does not become confused or overwhelmed when completing the activity at home. It is crucial that you're confident that the client will be able to consistently make the changes that you agree on in session within their daily life.*

For example, for a client who spends several hours of the day in bed, it may be unrealistic to ask them to reduce their time in bed during the day to less than 30 minutes. In this case, a structured plan for reducing time in bed during the day and for exploring alternative activities may be appropriate.

Coming back to information gleaned in the assessment is also important. For example, why is this client spending hours in bed each day? Is it owing to medication side effects? Low mood? Avoidance? Anxiety? Lack of activities to engage in? Understanding what is driving the behaviour is important for helping to generate effective strategies for change.

Winding Down before Bed

It is often unrealistic to expect that you can quickly shift your mind and body from daytime mode to sleep straight away. Just as it takes some time to wind up in the morning (as we discussed earlier), it takes time to wind down before bed and get the mind and body ready for sleep. Even if you are going to bed later than usual (e.g. if you have been out late or been busy later than usual), it is still helpful to have some wind-down time before you turn the lights out to sleep. Staying up an extra 30 minutes to wind down may mean that you take far less time to fall asleep.

Try scheduling some wind-down time where you do something that makes you feel happy and relaxed for 30–60 minutes before you go to bed. Your wind-down time may need to be longer if your day has been physically, mentally, or emotionally busy.

Group Discussion: What Activities Could Help You Wind Down before Bed?

What might get in the way of wind-down time (see below)?

Activity 6: Winding Down before Bed

Using the Winding Down before Bed worksheet, write down your planned wind-down activities for the week and possible solutions to any barriers that might get in the way.

These should include:

- a winding-down activity to do 1 hour before bed, as well as at bedtime (refer to the table for 'Making a Bedtime Routine' in Activity 6);
- addressing what might get in the way of these wind-down activities (refer to the table for 'Barriers to Bedtime Routine' in Activity 6).

***Therapist notes**: Some common barriers to winding-down and suggested alternatives include:*

- ***Distraction by social media**: Have 10–15 minutes of social media time, put phone on silent/switch off computer, and then start wind-down time in another room.*
- ***Calls from a friend/family member**: Consider putting the phone on silent when wind-down time is starting (can you make sure any phone calls are made prior to your wind-down time?).*
- ***Good show on TV**: Still have wind-down time after the show, even if it is only for 20–30 minutes before bed, or record the show to watch the next day in the morning/afternoon.*

- ***Partner/family member obstructing wind-down time***: *Explain the importance of incorporating wind-down time into your night for better sleep, go into a different room when winding down, or choose a wind-down activity that can be done together (e.g. puzzles, colouring-in, scrapbooking, doing stretches, listening to a meditation).*
- ***Particularly stressful/distressing day***: *Try to do some journaling, call a helpline/friend to help de-stress, or do an extra relaxation exercise.*
- ***Reading difficulties***: *Try reading a comic book, magazine, or children's book with larger print instead.*

GOOBICS

Therapist notes: *GOOBICS is otherwise known as stimulus control therapy in CBT-I. As this strategy asks clients to set a regular rising time each morning, this may restrict their time in bed and thus serve as a gentle 'time in bed restriction' intervention. Refer back to Chapter 7 for a description of the theory behind these strategies.*

The aim behind 'Getting Out Of Bed If You Can't Sleep' (GOOBICS) is that we want the bed and bedroom to be associated with feeling relaxed and sleepy, and *not* with feeling awake and upset.

People with Insomnia often spend a lot of time awake in bed while they are trying to sleep. In this case, after multiple instances of being awake in bed, the mind and body 'learn' to be awake in bed rather than asleep. Making matters worse, people may also do things in bed other than sleeping, such as watching TV, smoking, eating, playing computer games, tossing and turning, or worrying. When the bed and bedroom are paired with not sleeping (and feeling anxious or frustrated), the bed and bedroom become a cue for being awake. Now, the bedroom can become something of a 'chamber of horrors', because going to bed has become a trigger for unpleasant emotions and wakefulness. This, of course, makes it harder to sleep.

The GOOBICS strategy is very useful for relearning to associate the bed and bedroom with feeling relaxed and sleepy rather than awake and tense. It can be particularly useful for those who have trouble falling asleep. It teaches the mind to make the bed and bedroom a trigger for sleep, so that you can expect to fall asleep easily when you go to bed or wake up during the night.

To learn this skill, follow these five steps:

Step 1: Only use the bedroom for sleep. Do not use your bedroom for activities such as eating, watching TV, smoking, talking on the phone, working, or arguing.

Step 2: Only go to bed when sleepy. Only go to bed when you feel sleepy, not because of a standard routine. You take much longer to get to sleep if you go to bed before being sleepy or drowsy.

Step 3: Get out of bed when you can't sleep. If you lie in bed awake for a long time, you are accidentally training yourself to be awake in bed. If you do not fall asleep within a short period of time, say 30 minutes after going to bed and turning off the lights, *and* you are feeling restless, frustrated, or anxious: *Get out of bed, go to another room, and do something relaxing.* However, if you are feeling really dozy and close to sleep, it is OK to stay there, as you are possibly sleeping lightly or about to fall asleep.

(***Note***: *Don't check the clock to determine how long you have been lying in bed awake—just guess!*)

If you do get out of bed, when you feel sleepy again, go back to bed and give yourself another chance to fall asleep. If you do not fall asleep quickly, repeat this step again. You should not try hard to fall asleep, as that would make you feel more alert instead.

What should I do while I'm out of bed? (This could be similar to your wind-down activities.)

Step 4: Get out of bed at the same time each day. This includes weekends, even when you stay up later than usual. If you set your alarm for a regular wake-up time, you will be more likely to get sleepy at about the right time each night to allow yourself to get the sleep you need. Choose a rising time that suits your usual situation.

Getting up every day at the same time is also a great way to reduce excessive time spent in bed. Having a window of 1 hour for 'rising time' is OK. It is really important to work towards getting up at the same time and going to bed only when you feel really sleepy. Remember to be realistic when setting goals and, if setting a regular rising time is a big change for you, work towards it over the next few weeks.

What is your chosen getting-up time? Between _____ and _____.

***Therapist notes**: Do not ask clients to make adjustments of more than 1 hour a day to their rising time (and, for many clients, daily increments may be just 30 minutes). For example, if the goal rising time is 7 a.m., and the current average rising time is 10 a.m., suggest that the client gets up first at 9 a.m., then at 8 a.m., and then at 7 a.m. on the third day.*

When planning a regular rising time, suggest that clients, (a) use more than one alarm, (b) ask friends and family to help, and (c) have a wind-up plan for what to do once out of bed (for example, have a shower or a coffee, get outside for some morning light).

*Clients may ask about what time they should go to bed. We advise clients to go to bed when sleepy (not just tired), rather than setting a specific time. That said, do be mindful with clients who may be retiring to bed **very** early. Spending too long in bed overnight often leads to taking a long time to fall asleep and also to restless sleep overnight. If a client is regularly taking hours to fall asleep at the beginning of the night and they are going to bed early, it is advisable to set a guideline for bedtime. Suggest that bedtime each night is calculated based on the goal get-up time and hours of sleep that the client thinks they need. For example, if a client is aiming to get up at 7 a.m., and they need 8 hours of sleep, they should not go to bed much before 10.30 p.m. The bedtime window can be a little longer than the getting-up window—up to 2 hours. In the current example, bedtime might be when the client feels sleepy between 9.30 p.m. and 11.30 p.m. Once the regular wake-up time has been established, the bedtime becomes more regular.*

For those clients who are not sleepy until very late (after 1 a.m.) and would like to get into an earlier pattern, suggest that they (a) establish a wind-down routine in the evening, and (b) set a goal for rising earlier in the morning. The gradual advancing of the morning rising time will result in a corresponding advancement of onset of sleepiness in the evening, and (c) this effect can be enhanced with 30 minutes' exposure to bright light in the morning (sunlight or via a light box).

Step 5: Avoid or reduce napping. Sleeping during the day weakens your need for sleep at night. If possible, do not nap during the day—even after a night of little sleep. If you really must nap, ideally it should be 30 minutes or less, and before 2 p.m. Set an alarm to help you avoid oversleeping.

***Therapist notes**: We found it was unrealistic for many clients to eliminate naps. Sedation and symptoms were often too strong. It was, however, still important and helpful to work with clients to reduce naps as much as they could. Often, a lot of discussion was required to assist clients in planning engaging alternative activities.*

Activity 7: GOOBICS

These five steps are presented on the worksheet. Please think about activities you might engage in when you have trouble falling asleep, and also activities that will help you at your chosen regular rising time.

Motivational Boost: Cost and Benefits

Activity 8: Which Stage Do You Think You're at Right Now in Terms of Treating Your Insomnia?

Look at the figure in your client resource pack for Activity 8. Right now, *which stage do you think you are at in terms of treating your Insomnia?*

- ❐ thinking about it (not quite ready);
- ❐ preparing to make it happen;
- ❐ making it happen;
- ❐ maintaining a good thing for life.

Making changes to improve your sleep might be hard, but we will be here to help you through this.

Let's finish off with this exercise on willingness (*Optional*). It is about exploring your motivations for improving sleep and any apprehension you may feel about pursuing the strategies applied in treatment. There are no right or wrong answers.

An Exercise in Willingness

Imagine you're climbing a mountain and you're halfway up. Suddenly, the clouds roll in, it starts to rain, and it gets windy.

You have a choice: You can either head back down or you can carry on.

If you carry on, it is not because you like the feeling of being cold and wet. It is because you value the idea of reaching the top. So, in other words, you are *willing* to go through some difficulties to achieve what's important to you.

In this example, there is no right or wrong answer, in that what is right for one person may not be right for the next. One person may choose to go back down the mountain, and this may be right for them if they weren't that motivated to reach the top. On the other hand, if climbing this mountain had been a lifelong dream for the person, the right decision for them may be to push through the discomfort of the weather (as long as it's safe!) and keep going.

Therapist notes: *In this exercise it is important to emphasise that there will likely be challenges associated with the treatment. However, these need to be balanced against the important and valuable personal benefits that improved sleep and energy may bring the client.*

It is common for clients to ask for answers or quick fixes. In CBT-I, it is important that the therapist encourages clients to explore and discover the solutions themselves, as this strengthens both the learning and the sense of ownership over the change process. A simple phrase reminding the client of their autonomy is useful:

> *You are the expert on you, so I'm not sure I am the best person to judge what will work for you. I can give you an idea of what the evidence shows us and what other people have done in your situation, and we can then work out a plan together for you to test out some new strategies.*

Let's assume that this treatment will be tough at times. Think about some *costs and benefits* of working on your sleep issues:

- What can you look forward to when your sleep/tiredness improves?
- What do you think will be the hardest part about sticking to your treatment plan?
- What will help to keep you motivated to stick with treatment, even when you're finding it tough or don't feel that things are improving?

Summary

Summary of Key Points

Activity 9: The Main Things I Learned Today

Let's write down the key points about today's session that apply to you.
Take-home messages are as follows:

- Motivation for change—what might you gain from treatment?
- It is normal to feel tired during the day. There are things you can do to help manage this.
- It is common to take 30 or more minutes to fall asleep or to wake up during the night.
- There are things you can do to help improve your sleep—wind down, GOOBICS, regular rising time, reducing naps, sleep hygiene.
- Achieving goals—let's be proactive about this.

Action Plan for the Week

Activity 10: My Action Plan for the Week

This worksheet should contain your planned sleep strategies for the week, including:

- what I will do for wind-down before bed;
- some changes to my sleep hygiene or environment that I may start making;
- what to do when I get up because I can't fall asleep/get back to sleep quickly;
- my regular wake-up time for *each* morning;
- plan for reducing napping:
  - my goal for napping this week is to nap for _____ (hours/minutes), no later than _____ (time of day);
  - activities I can engage in instead of napping.

Confidence ruler: On a scale of 0–10, how confident are you about trying out your action plan for the week?

Therapist notes: *Remember that you might select just two or three of the above elements of the action plan for use with some clients. Asking them to work on every element at once may be overwhelming. It is important that the client is confident that they can achieve the goals set out in their plan. We often ask for a confidence rating out of 10. If the client rates less than 7 in their confidence that they can achieve the goal, it requires discussion and/or modification.*

Make sure you have a written copy of the client's tasks from each session so that you can ask them specifically about their progress at the start of the next session.

Further Reading

Miller, W. R., and Rollnick, S. (2013) *Motivational interviewing: Helping people change* (3rd ed.). New York: Guilford Press.

Retimertechnologies (2012) *Prof. Leon Lack Public Lecture on Sleep Psychology* [video]. Available at: www.youtube.com/watch?v=4Eiwap0jZV0 (accessed November 29, 2016).

13 Therapist Manual Session 2

Maximising Energy and Working with Unhelpful Beliefs about Sleep

Instructions to the Therapist

The primary objectives of this session are to discuss strategies to improve daytime tiredness, address unhelpful beliefs and attitudes about sleep, and, if appropriate, discuss strategies for unpleasant dreams and nightmares. A continuing theme is building a sense of hope and self-efficacy.

Continuing Work on Sleep Hygiene

Improving sleep hygiene will usually require continued attention. This may be troubleshooting changes planned in Session 1 and/or identifying one or two more unhelpful behaviours that the client engages in (e.g. drinking caffeine or smoking at night), together with work on motivating clients to change these behaviours. Lay a lot of groundwork to ensure that the change is important to them. Decision balance sheets may be useful. Discuss downsides and positives to changing the unhelpful behaviour (see worksheet in Appendix 5), in addition to pros and cons of staying the same. Focus on the pros and cons that resonate with the client, for example, 'How would it improve your life if you weren't spending so much money on coffee?'.

Healthy Snacks for Daytime Energy (Optional Activity)

During this session, we weave an introduction to healthy snacks into the discussion of daytime energy. We bring snacks such as bananas, apples, carrots, nuts, dried fruit, yoghurt, hummus, avocado, and so on, for clients to try during the break. This is a great way to facilitate their experiential learning about how healthy foods can taste great, be easy to prepare, and help generate energy. It also helps in identifying potential barriers to healthy eating (e.g. can't find healthy snacks they like eating, difficulty chewing hard foods). A homework activity can be for clients to purchase one new healthy snack during the week.

Working on Dysfunctional Beliefs and Attitudes about Sleep

Some beliefs about sleep increase worry about sleep and lead to behaviours that can perpetuate poor sleep. Session 2 assesses the specific beliefs that may be playing an unhelpful role in the client's Insomnia, using an abbreviated version of the Dysfunctional Beliefs and Attitudes about Sleep scale. Some items have been removed for the sake of simplicity for this client group. See Morin et al. (2007) for the full scale.

Here, we use seven items from the original scale, which are:

- When I don't get a proper amount of sleep on a given night, I need to catch up on the next day by napping or by sleeping longer the next night.
- I am worried that if I go for one or two nights without sleep, I may have a nervous breakdown.
- I have little ability to manage the negative consequences of disturbed sleep.
- When I feel tired, have no energy, or just seem not to function well during the day, it is generally because I did not sleep well the night before.
- Medication is probably the only solution to sleeplessness.
- The only way to improve my energy is to rest or sleep more.
- I believe Insomnia is essentially the result of a chemical imbalance.

Your role as therapist is to identify relevant beliefs and illustrate the connection to Insomnia in simplistic terms. If a particular client does not have any strongly held dysfunctional beliefs, or does not have the cognitive capacity to benefit from this work, don't spend too much time on this section. Have a brief, simple discussion about the effect of beliefs and refer clients to the 'Strategies for Unhelpful Beliefs about Sleep' section. For clients for whom this information is important, see the example provided in the 'Challenging Unhelpful Beliefs about Sleep' section of this therapist manual for more detail. We have also included additional information on other commonly held unhelpful beliefs about sleep, which may be discussed with clients as an optional component.

Cognitive Capacity

Standard CBT-I programmes work on changing maladaptive beliefs and attitudes about sleep as a central component of the therapy. However, many clients may have cognitive impairments that limit their ability to fully engage, explicitly (e.g. with written worksheets), in this aspect of therapy. Accordingly, this programme places a stronger emphasis on the identification of unhelpful behaviours and on building motivation and commitment to produce helpful changes.

Within this framework, overtly and directly challenging 'beliefs and attitudes' may, in some cases, be a secondary component of the session. The behavioural and educational components are, however, intended to help clients change the thoughts and beliefs that perpetuate their poor sleep. In these sections, your role is to design and provide experiences that facilitate belief change. Because of the heavy cognitive and reflective components necessary for these sections, content needs to be adapted according to the cognitive capabilities of each client.

Time in Bed Restriction as an Optional Strategy

Time in bed restriction (also known as sleep restriction) is a common, evidence-based technique used in CBT-I to help clients deepen and consolidate fragmented sleep by limiting the amount of time a person spends in bed (see CBT-I description in Chapter 7). Its use in psychosis, however, is uncertain, and the therapist needs to tread carefully in recommending it.

Sleep loss is a common precursor to psychosis onset and relapse, and clinical studies using time in bed restriction have reported mixed findings. For example, some research in bipolar disorder reported symptoms of mania and psychosis after a sleep restriction procedure (Wehr et al., 1987). A more recent study, however, failed to replicate these effects in a group of individuals with affective psychosis (Kaplan and Harvey, 2013).

For many clients, a mild version of sleep restriction will already have been implemented in Session 1, with the instruction to make morning rising time regular, and not to go to bed too early. For many clients, this may well be enough. The protocol for time in bed restriction is, therefore, presented as an optional component in the appendix (see Appendix 7). If using time in bed restriction with a client, monitor carefully and apply Kaplan and Harvey's (2013) guidelines:

- Do not allow more than 3 hours' worth of sleep deprivation from the original total sleep time when instructing individuals on their 'time in bed window'.
- Do not allow sleep restriction resulting in less than 6 hours in bed.

Clinical Safety

As a precautionary measure, a 'Symptom Safety Plan' is included towards the end of the session to encourage clients to let the therapist know if they experience a deterioration in their clinical symptoms as a result of the sleep strategies being practised.

Establishing a good rapport is, of course, also needed for the clients to inform you in the event of deteriorating mental health.

Our experience of clients developing worse symptoms in relation to sleep skills practice was rare. It occurred mildly in an instance where the client had placed much pressure on themselves to succeed in the programme. This increased their attentiveness to their progress and increased arousal and anxiety. The situation was quickly resolved, with the therapist reminding the client that recovering from Insomnia is a gradual process over time and reassuring them that they were making good progress and that there was no need to rush in their recovery. It is also helpful to conceptualise the programme as a way to help clients experience sleep as an enjoyable and relaxing process again, rather than a chore. Establishing a good rapport and advising clients to inform you of deteriorating mental health are important, so that concerns can be promptly addressed.

It is also important to be aware of the client's medical comorbidities. For example:

- *With diabetes*: Ensure you don't suggest substitutes for caffeine or energy-generating snacks that are too high in sugars/glucose.
- *With severe obesity, heart, or respiratory problems*: Suggest activities that will not be too strenuous for the client and plan for exercise to be increased in small increments if this is a very new change for them. Consult with the client's medical team if in any doubt.
- *With drug-induced photosensitivity*: For clients who are on medications that increase skin photosensitivity, ensure that they follow sun protection measures (sunscreen, hat, etc.) when pursuing daytime strategies that increase their time outdoors.

Session 2 Structure

The structure for Session 2 is as follows:

- weekly review;
- daytime tiredness;
- unhelpful beliefs about sleep;
- managing nightmares;
- motivation boost;
- summary and weekly plan.

Material Needed

- Client Resource Pack (Session 2).
- Healthy snacks (apple, banana, nuts, etc.).
- In-session feedback (Appendix 6—to be administered at the beginning of each session).

Supplementary (Optional) Handouts

- Sleep Diary (Appendix 2).
- Decision balance sheet (Appendix 5).
- Time in bed restriction instructions (Appendix 7): Time in bed restriction is a form of controlled sleep restriction used as a technique to help the client consolidate their sleep, particularly if they experience numerous awakenings throughout the night (possibly owing to oversleeping). Waking up at the same time each day is also a form of sleep restriction.
- Snacks that provide energy throughout the day (Appendix 8).
- My Personal Cycle of Insomnia Worksheet (Appendix 10).

Session Content: Weekly Review

Aspects of Sleep and Functioning Addressed in this Session

Activity 11: A Review of the Skills We Have Been Learning

In the last session we learned about:

- facts about sleep;
- sleep hygiene: habits and strategies that can help us sleep well on a regular basis;
- winding down before bed—making a bedtime routine;
- getting out of bed if you can't sleep (GOOBICS);
- regular wake-up time and morning wind-up;
- reducing napping—don't oversleep!

We also spoke about trying to avoid spending too much time in bed overnight.

Did you manage to put any of these sleep skills to the test, and how did you find it?

- What went well?
- What was challenging?
- How did you find getting out of bed if you couldn't sleep (GOOBICS)? How did you fill your times awake during the night?
- How did you find waking up around the same time every day? What time(s) did you get out of bed in the mornings?
- Let's brainstorm some ways to get around these challenges.

Therapist notes: *Make sure you have a written copy of the client's tasks from Session 1 so that you can ask each client specifically about their progress on each goal.*

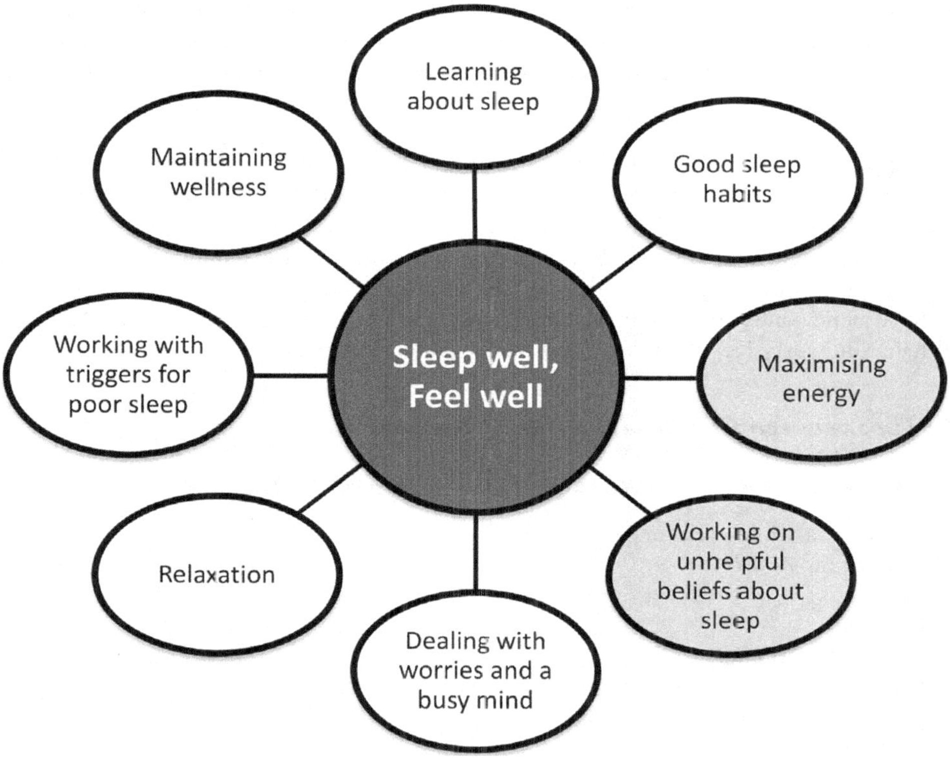

Figure 13.1 Topics Addressed this Week (Session 2)

Tiredness

The Link between Tiredness and Sleep

***Therapist notes**: Tiredness and daytime fatigue are common complaints in people with psychosis. There can be multiple causes of tiredness, of which poor sleep may be one. The following exercises are designed to explore the many causes of tiredness and to arrive at a position that reflects that there are likely several factors clients can have influence over that they can use to remediate low energy levels. See Ree and Harvey (2004) for further details and ideas regarding behavioural experiments and generating energy in Insomnia.*

Group Discussion: Is Tiredness Entirely Related to Sleep?

Many people believe that, if they have a poor night of sleep, they will definitely feel tired and lethargic for the whole of the next day, and that if they have a good night's sleep, they will feel energetic the next day. This way of thinking would mean that lack of energy during the day is almost completely because of bad sleep. Let's explore this idea.

- Can you think of a time when you had a poor night's sleep and you functioned better than expected the next day?
- Can you also think of a time when you slept quite well but felt tired and couldn't get going the next day?

Most people answer 'Yes' to these questions, and this suggests that tiredness and sleep may not be so closely linked after all. What might have been happening in the above examples that would help us to understand that sleep didn't match the energy level the next day?

- Is it possible that there are other factors that add to feeling tired and lethargic in the day?
- Is it also possible that energy can come from sources other than sleep?

There's actually a lot you can do to help lessen the impact of Insomnia. We can almost always improve our energy in the day without improving sleep. It is important to feel that you have some control over your daytime energy, even if you had a bad night's sleep. This will help you worry less about sleep and get you more motivated.

The Link between Our Behaviour and Tiredness

Group Discussion: What Are Some Reasons for Feeling Tired during the Day?

(Complete on a whiteboard or large sheet of paper.)

Some examples are:

- boredom;
- too much napping;
- lack of activity/exercise (being in 'couch potato' mode);
- poor diet (overeating, not eating enough);
- medications;
- low mood;
- post-lunch dip (i.e. our natural body clock rhythm);
- heavy workload or stress;
- drinking camomile tea;
- being hung-over;
- being stressed;
- lack of vitamin D or iron;
- thyroid problems;
- symptoms of sleep apnoea.

So, here, we can see that, although poor sleep can impact on tiredness the next day, believing that poor sleep is the only influence on daytime tiredness is not very accurate. It's probably more accurate and helpful to know that many factors affect our energy levels in the day.

If you're able to find the factors other than sleep that increase and decrease your energy, then you are in a good place to have more influence over how you feel during the day and reduce your worry about sleep.

Activity 12: Sources of Daytime Tiredness

With the answers to the brainstorming exercise in mind, complete the pie chart in your booklet by writing in the different factors that may be contributing to tiredness and low energy levels for you. (See Figure 13.2 for example.)

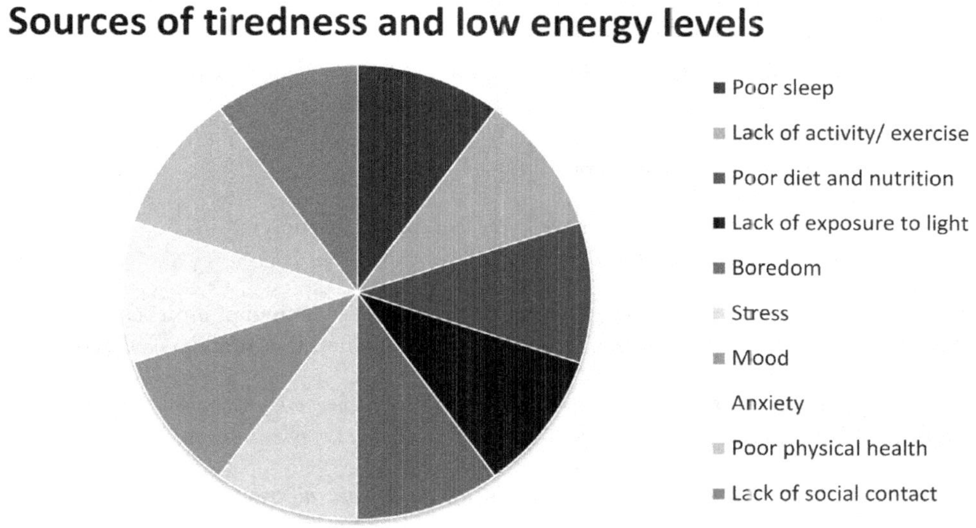

Figure 13.2 Example of Pie Chart Activity

Managing Tiredness during the Day

Blaming poor sleep for daytime tiredness can leave you rather stuck:

- First, you don't have much control over how tired you feel, and all you can do is hope for a good night's sleep the next night.
- Second, worry and concern about your sleep develop. These don't lead to any real improvement, and may actually make the problem worse.
- Third, you may find yourself trying to conserve energy during the day by sleeping in, having a nap, cancelling appointments, avoiding exercise, or avoiding social contact. These strategies can actually lead to *lower* energy levels.

It is often more helpful to engage in activities that will generate energy—such as exercise or doing something that is mentally stimulating or challenging.

What we do *during the day*, not just what we *do at night*, influences how tired we feel and how well we sleep!

Group Discussion: If You Had More Energy in the Daytime, how Might this Help with Your Insomnia?

What do you feel you are missing out on now because of tiredness?

Activity 13: How Behaviour and Activity Affect Energy Levels

Therapist notes: *This is a replication of an in-session experiment conducted during Session 1. We suggest that you experiment with different activities from that used in Session 1. We found it useful to repeat this experiment to give clients more experience with the notion that energy levels can be influenced by the client.*

Now, let's test how our choices can affect energy levels.

- First, how energised are you feeling *now*, on a scale of 0–10?
- Second, let's try a couple of activities:
  - go for a short walk around the building or do some star jumps;
  - have a small, healthy snack (e.g. eat a piece of fruit);
  - tell some jokes;
  - stretch your neck, arm, legs;
  - have a cold drink;
  - listen to some music that makes you feel happy or energised;
  - watch a video that makes you laugh.

Now, how do you rate your energy levels after trying these activities, on a scale of 0–10? Was one activity more effective than another? We should find that tiredness levels decrease as activity increases.

***Therapist notes**: The activity above is to be used as a behavioural exercise for clients to have an experience of how even small changes, such as a healthy snack, can improve tiredness.*

- *When using this exercise, be sure to check that the client is not allergic to the healthy snacks (e.g. nuts) that you bring in for them to try. Also check if the client is diabetic, as it may not be advisable for them to try eating certain fruits that are high in sugar.*
- *Give clients the handout in Appendix 8 ('Snacks that Give You Energy throughout the Day') after they have tried this exercise. It may be used to help the client pick a healthy snack as part of their ideas for the following activity on trying energy-generating strategies.*

Generating Energy during the Day

Let's talk about some things you can do to help you feel better during the day (and sleep better at night). Resting and napping for long periods can make you feel more tired and can interfere with sleep the next night. Instead of conserving energy, it is often better to work towards 'generating' energy during the day instead.

Activity 14: How Can We Generate Energy during the Day?

List some activities and strategies to try out to make you feel more energised. You can also list some 'energy depleting' activities that we should avoid doing, as they generally make us feel more tired.

Look back to your sleep hygiene checklist (Activity 5) to see if there are any habits that might be unhelpful for your daytime energy.

Use of 'Bright Light' during the Day

There are many benefits of getting some bright light each day. These include:

- aligning your body clock with the time of the day;
- improved mood;
- improved alertness and concentration.

For good natural sleep, it is important to have both a healthy sleep routine and a body clock that works at the right time. Morning exposure to bright light (i.e. 30 minutes of natural sunlight) helps to reduce drowsiness and increase alertness for the day by reducing the level of hormones that usually make our bodies feel sleepy at night (e.g. melatonin).

To help your body clock, make sure you are exposed to some bright light (sunlight or a light box) each day. You may even find that getting more sunlight during the day improves your mood.

If you feel very tired most mornings, try getting some sunlight after waking up to help start your day (e.g. take a walk or have breakfast outside in the sun).

Getting more light during the day and avoiding bright light at night will make you feel more alert during the day and sleepier at night.

Activity 15: Use of Bright Light during the Day

Let's make a list of:

- things you can do to get more light during the day;
- things you can do to reduce bright lights at night.

Activity 16: Beliefs about Sleep

Studies show that some beliefs about sleep can fuel worries and anxiety and play a part in keeping Insomnia going.

The statements in the resource pack reflect some beliefs and attitudes that people may have about sleep. Show how much you agree or disagree with these statements by placing a mark (/) along the line to reflect your answer for each.

1. When I don't get a proper amount of sleep on a given night, I need to catch up on the next day by napping or by sleeping longer the next night.
2. I am worried that, if I go for one or two nights without sleep, I may have a nervous breakdown.
3. I have little ability to manage the negative consequences of disturbed sleep.
4. When I feel tired, have no energy, or just seem not to function well during the day, it is generally because I did not sleep well the night before.
5. Medication is probably the only solution to sleeplessness.
6. The only way to improve my energy is to rest or sleep more.
7. I believe Insomnia is essentially the result of a chemical imbalance.

After completing this activity, can you look back and see how these beliefs may be unhelpful for a good night's sleep?

Let's take the top two statements you most strongly agree with and discuss how they could be influencing your sleep and tiredness in unhelpful ways.

***Therapist notes**: In our experience, the unhelpful beliefs that most commonly resonated with clients were: (1) 'When I don't get a proper amount of sleep on a given night, I need to catch up on the next day by napping or by sleeping longer the next night'; (2) 'I am worried that if I go for one or two nights without sleep, I may have a nervous breakdown' (particularly as they may have experienced a manic or psychotic episode after days of sleep deprivation before); and (3) 'When I feel tired, have no energy, or just seem not to function well during the day, it is generally because I did not sleep well the night before'.*

After having completed Activities 12 and 13 in this session, we tend to find that clients report less agreement with Statement 6 ('The only way to improve my energy is to rest or sleep more'). If not, ensure that you reiterate the points from these previous activities to the client.

When clients disagree with beliefs on the measure items, enquire as to why as a way to test their learning and understanding of sleep. Typically, we find that the psychoeducation from Session 1, as well as the activities done so far in Session 2, has started to shape these clients' beliefs and expectations about sleep in a more positive direction. You may even like to ask, 'How much did you agree with these statements before having started attending this sleep programme?', to help identify the unhelpful beliefs that were relevant to the client's case conceptualisation.

How Beliefs and Attitudes about Sleep May Be Driving Insomnia

If a person has unhelpful beliefs about sleep, it is likely that they will worry more about their sleep during the night and day. This can make their sleep worse and reduce mood and energy during the day.

Beliefs → Thoughts/worries → Feelings → Behaviour

When we worry about sleep, it is more likely that we won't sleep very well and we'll end up feeling worse during the day.

Challenging Unhelpful Beliefs about Sleep (Optional: Appendix 9 Handout)

Here is an example of how an unhelpful belief about sleep can affect us, and how we can go about addressing it. (See Figure 13.3)

Belief:
I feel my insomnia is the result of a chemical imbalance (and unless this is corrected by medication, there is nothing i can do to improve my sleep).

Thoughts/ worries/ behaviours/ outcomes that this belief leads to:
- Over-reliance on medications.
- Not feeling motivated to find non-medical solutions to the sleep problem.
- Feeling helpless and powerless.

Evidence for this belief:
- My doctor has told me that certain chemical processes in the brain can make it harder to sleep.
- I only seem to sleep well when I take a sleeping pill.

Evidence against this belief:
- I can see that my worry about sleep makes it harder to sleep.
- I can understand that sleep routines could be helpful in correcting poor sleep.
- Research suggested that CBT for insomnia has more effective treatment outcomes than medication.

What are the benefits of this belief?
- I don't put pressure on myself to change my habits or behaviour.

What are the costs of this belief?
- Reduces the likelihood that a long term solution will be found.

Is there a more helpful or realistic belief?
- It is not helpful to focus solely on external causes for my sleep problem as they are not in my control.
- Regardless of the initial cause of my insomnia, there are likely to be things that I could change about my thinking and daily habits to improve my sleep and daytime energy.

Figure 13.3 Challenging Unhelpful Beliefs about Sleep

Establishing Helpful Beliefs about Sleep

Let's see what strategies or thoughts we can use to challenge the unhelpful beliefs about sleep. (See Table 13.1)

Table 13.1 Strategies for Unhelpful Beliefs about Sleep

Unhelpful Belief	*Helpful Thoughts and Strategies to Try Instead*
When I don't get a proper amount of sleep on a given night, I need to catch up on the next day by napping or by sleeping longer the next night	If we always try to catch up on lost sleep by napping or sleeping longer the next night, this may actually make it harder for us to get into a good sleep pattern. A good sleep pattern is important for helping to relieve Insomnia Try generating energy by going for a walk or eating something healthy instead If you do need to nap, keep it short (less than 30 minutes ideally) and more than 8 hours before you go to bed that night
I am worried that if I go for one or two nights without sleep, I may have a nervous breakdown	Worrying about not having enough sleep can make it even harder to get to sleep at night Winding down each night will help you start feeling more relaxed again and sleep better Although short-term lack of sleep can make mood and anxiety worse, it generally won't lead to a nervous breakdown. Remember that, if you can stay relaxed, poor sleep on one night will make it more likely you will sleep better the next night (as your body wants to catch up) There are things you can do during the day to help prevent worse mood and anxiety, for example, talking to someone about worries, getting some light exercise, or trying relaxation strategies
I have little ability to manage the negative consequences of disturbed sleep	We can't force sleep to happen, but there are many things we can do to set up good conditions for sleep and lessen the impact of poor sleep on health Research shows that people with Insomnia can successfully learn to manage their sleep using various skills and coping strategies. This programme aims to teach you these skills. Can you tell me a couple of ideas?
When I feel tired, have no energy, or just seem not to function well during the day, it is generally because I did not sleep well the night before	Poor sleep can lead to feeling more tired and less energetic during the day, but is not always the main culprit Think about what other factors could also be making you feel tired and less energetic, such as: exercise levels, diet, hormones, medications, boredom, etc.

continued . . .

Table 13.1 Continued

Unhelpful Belief	*Helpful Thoughts and Strategies to Try Instead*
Medication is probably the only solution to sleeplessness	Medications are not the only solution to sleeplessness. Making some healthy changes to our thinking and lifestyle is often just as useful. Remind yourself that sometimes other good solutions just take a bit more time and practice
The only way to improve my energy is to rest or sleep more	There are actually lots of ways to improve your energy, aside from sleep, like doing some exercise or eating a healthy snack (e.g. apple, banana, celery, carrots, oats, nuts, and dried fruit)
I believe Insomnia is essentially the result of a chemical imbalance (This belief was dealt with with above in Figure 13.3, Appendix 9)	It is not helpful to focus solely on external causes for my sleep problem, as they are not in my control Regardless of the initial cause of my Insomnia, there are likely to be things that I could change about my thinking and daily habits to improve my sleep and daytime energy

Additional Commonly Held Beliefs about Sleep, and more Helpful Thoughts (Optional)

'The myth of 8 hours of sleep'

Most people think that we need at least 8 hours of sleep to stay healthy. However, to recap from the first session:

- The amount of sleep that we need to feel alert during the day varies from person to person.
- Sleeping too much can be just as much of a problem as sleeping too little.
- Remember that some daytime tiredness is normal.

'I wake up in the middle of the night or early morning feeling wide awake. This means I will not be able to fall back to sleep.'

- It is normal to initially feel alert if you awaken at the beginning or end of a dream. Drowsiness will soon follow if you don't get yourself overly worked up.
- If you awaken after about 5.5 hours of sleep, you have obtained your core sleep. If you do not fall back to sleep, you will be OK.

'I will not be able to function tomorrow.'

- In most cases, the worst thing that may happen is that you may not be in the best mood during the day.

- Sleep loss does not *always* have a huge impact on daytime functioning.
- You can learn to reduce the effects of sleep loss.
- Worrying this way is not helping you and, in fact, makes it harder to sleep.

'I slept very little or not at all last night.'

- You are probably getting more sleep than you think you are.
- Sleep is very difficult to estimate. Poor sleepers tend to think they've slept significantly less than they actually have.

'It's going to be a miserable day because I didn't sleep well.'

- It's not just how much sleep you lose that affects your daytime functioning, but also your worry about your sleep loss.
- If you can reduce negative thoughts about your sleep loss, you will reduce the effects of Insomnia on your mood and functioning.
- There are choices you can make today to help yourself feel better, even though you didn't sleep well.

Realistic expectations about sleep are important, as they will help to reduce worry about sleep.

Managing Unpleasant Dreams and Nightmares

Occasional nightmares are normal. Sometimes, they may be related to past trauma, stressful events, or something scary seen on TV or online. Other times, nightmares may be completely unrelated to life experience or the day's events. Addressing problematic nightmares that occur often (more than once a week) can assist in improving sleep.

Group Discussion: Are Nightmares Adding to Your Sleep Problems?

- Do you get nightmares?
- How often do they occur (e.g. nightly, weekly, or monthly)?
- Is it the same or a similar dream each time?
- How long have you suffered from nightmares? When did the nightmares start happening regularly?
- How do your nightmares affect you the next day?
- Do you ever feel afraid to fall asleep?

It is common to feel anxious or scared in bed after waking up from a nightmare. When this happens a lot, an association between the bed and these negative feelings may develop. This can make sleeping difficult, as it can make you feel anxious about being in bed or falling asleep.

Therapist notes: *This can be related back to last week's session on classical conditioning and the reasoning behind the GOOBICS strategy.*

If you regularly have nightmares, some questions to ask yourself are:

- Do your nightmares feel uncontrollable?
- Could you be having nightmares because you're expecting to?

Turning Nightmares into Dreams

'Turning nightmares into dreams' (TNID) is a sleep therapy for nightmares designed by Dr. Barry Krakow, who is a sleep disorders specialist. In TNID treatment, Dr. Krakow recommends seven strategies to help manage unpleasant images and nightmares.

Activity 17: Seven Strategies to Manage Unpleasant Images and Nightmares

If you have trouble with nightmares, try these seven strategies and see if they make a positive difference to your sleep (Krakow, 2002).

Let's practise these together first.

1. *Stop*: Clap hands while saying 'Stop!'.
2. *Breathe*: Breathe in deeply, and exhale the image away.
3. *Ground yourself*: Open your eyes, put your feet on the floor, and focus on your immediate environment. Perhaps turn on a dim light. What can you see, feel, hear, and smell?
4. *Talk it out*: Talk to a friend or family member about the images or nightmares.
5. *Write it down*: Write down images or nightmares in a diary.
6. *Acknowledge and move on*: Without accepting or denying, *acknowledge* the unpleasant image and then *return to pleasant ones*.
7. *Choose*: Consciously *choose* to return to pleasant images without feeling that it is a struggle to do so. What are some pleasant images that you can think of?

Therapist notes*: For clients without a friend or family member they could talk to about the nightmare/images, you could suggest that they speak with a helpline, their mental health team, peer support worker, or the therapist (you) via a phone call or scheduled appointment.*

Ensure that you help clients develop a pleasant image or 'safe place' in their mind following a nightmare, as part of the strategies. They can go to this place in their mind following a nightmare, as part of the steps outlined below.

There is evidence that muscle relaxation techniques may be useful for those with whom nightmare imagery work is too challenging (Aurora et al., 2010). Other strategies that our clients have found helpful are GOOBICS (stimulus control; e.g. get a glass of water, read a funny comic, or watch a short video clip of something heart-warming such as baby animals), or using a phone app with relaxing music to enable them to fall back to sleep after a nightmare.

Nightmares have been considered a non-dangerous place for the mind to simulate, rehearse, and problem-solve threatening situations. We found that this information can be used to educate clients, normalise nightmares, and increase motivation to engage in rescripting therapy. This way of thinking about nightmares helped clients to learn that nightmares are not necessarily a 'premonition' of the future.

The Motivation Boost: Sleep and Mental Health

Therapist notes*: A theme in this programme is recognising that many people believe that their sleep problem cannot get better because of their mental health condition. This belief can leave people feeling powerless and reduces motivation to be more active in searching for solutions to tackle the sleep problem. We revisit this theme now, at the end of Session 2.*

Activity 18: Sleep and Mental Health

Many people believe that their sleep problem cannot get better because of their mental health problems. This belief can leave people feeling powerless and reduce motivation to be active in searching for solutions to tackle the sleep problem.

- On a scale of 0–10, how much do you believe that having a mental illness makes your sleep unchangeable? _____
- If you scored 6 or above, think about the impact of this belief, and whether it forms part of your cycle of Insomnia.

Mental health problems are often linked to difficulties with sleep. However, this does not mean that your Insomnia will not get better. It is important to know that your sleep can be improved—you just need a little time and the right tools to help you with it!

Symptom Safety Plan

What do you do if you notice your symptoms (voices, visions, etc.) getting worse as a result of the sleep skills you're trying?

1. Let the group facilitator know as soon as you can.
2. Talk to a family member, friend, or case manager about it.
3. Write about it in the comments section of your sleep diary for the week.

Summary

Summary of Key Points

Activity 19: The Main Things I Learned Today

Let's write down today's key points on your worksheet.

Take home messages:

- Blaming poor sleep for all low mood, poor performance, and low energy can be unhelpful. It tends to result in people giving up and feeling helpless.
- There are lots of factors that can make people feel tired during the day.
- It is often better to try different ways of *generating* energy during the day, as this can help poor sleepers cope better with sleep loss.
- Even if you have a mental health problem, there are things you can do to help improve your sleep.

Action Plan for the Week

Activity 20: My Action Plan for the Week

Write down your planned sleep strategies for the week, including:

1. continue winding down before bed;
2. continue with GOOBICS;

3. my regular rising time for *each* morning is: _____;
4. changes to my sleep hygiene that I will work towards;
5. plan for generating energy this week;
6. main unhelpful 'beliefs about sleep' to be aware of;
7. working with nightmares (if applicable).

Confidence Ruler

On a scale from 0 (not confident at all) to 10 (extremely confident), how confident you are that you can improve your sleep?

- Remind yourself of the positive things that you've learned over the week to help motivate your sleep skills training.

References and Further Reading

Aurora, R. N., Zak, R. S., Auerbach, S. H., Casey, K. R., Chowdhuri, S., Karippot, A., Maganti, R. K., Ramar, K., Kristo, D. A., Bista, S. R., Lamm, C. I., Morgenthaler, T. I., and Standards of Practice Committee (2010) "Best practice guide for the treatment of nightmare disorder in adults", *Journal of Clinical Sleep Medicine: Official Publication of the American Academy of Sleep Medicine*, 6(4), pp. 389–401.

Kaplan, K. A., and Harvey, A. G. (2013) "Behavioral treatment of insomnia in bipolar disorder", *American Journal of Psychiatry*, 170(7), pp. 716–720.

Krakow, B. (2002) *Turning nightmares into dreams: The authorized audio series and treatment workbook for New Dream Therapy* [CDs]. USA: The New Sleepy Times.

Morin, C. M., Vallières, A., and Ivers, H. (2007) "Dysfunctional beliefs and attitudes about sleep (DBAS): Validation of a brief version (DBAS-16)", *Sleep*, 30(11), p. 1547.

Ree, M. J., and Harvey, A. G. (2004) "Behavioral experiments in chronic insomnia", in Bennett-Levy, J., Butler, G., Fennell, M., Hackmann, A., Mueller, M., and Westbrook, D. (Eds.) *Oxford guide to behavioral experiments in cognitive therapy*. Oxford, UK: Oxford University Press, pp. 287–308.

Wehr, T. A., Sack, D. A., and Rosenthal, N. E. (1987) "Sleep reduction as a final common pathway in the genesis of mania", *American Journal of Psychiatry*, 144(2), pp. 201–204.

14 Therapist Manual Session 3

Managing Worries and a Busy Mind and Introducing Relaxation

Information for the Therapist

The primary objective of this session is to address the cognitive arousal, or 'busy mind', that so often interferes with sleep. Strategies for managing cognitive arousal include cognitive therapy techniques and relaxation exercises. We suggest that, in this session, the therapist works to maintain hopefulness for change, but is also realistic about what changes may be achievable when forming goals with clients. Of course, be very encouraging of any progress made so far.

Why the Mind Might Be Busy

Common characteristics of cognitive arousal in people with psychotic disorders and Insomnia include unhelpful beliefs about sleep, generalised worry, worry about sleep, catastrophic thinking, intrusive thoughts, rumination, and hallucinations when attempting to sleep. Clients checking the clock to check how much time has passed when unable to sleep is a further trigger for increased cognitive arousal. Clients may also experience cognitive arousal that is not negatively toned, for example, planning, problem-solving, daydreaming, or fantasising.

Working with Distressing Hallucinations and other Psychotic Symptoms

Clients sometimes report distressing experiences that interfere with arousal and night-time sleep. Having an appreciation of psychological interventions designed to assist with positive symptoms of psychosis is useful when embarking on management of cognitive arousal. It is helpful to conduct an assessment to assess the presence of psychotic symptoms and their severity (Chapter 5). We provide some detail regarding cognitive interventions for psychosis in Chapter 2, together with some suggested references for further reading. Clinicians embarking on this work with clients for the first time should seek clinical supervision.

Clients and their families should also be encouraged to increase their understanding of their symptoms and illness via research. This can be done by looking at reputable websites on the Internet (e.g. www.mind.org.uk; www.nimh.nih.gov; www.sane.org) and documents providing information on mental illness (e.g. Cooke, 2014), talking to consumer and carer support groups, and joining networks of individuals with similar experiences ('hearing voices' groups or carer support networks, for example; World Hearing Voices Network, 2012).

Finally, a discussion to uncover factors that increase or decrease hallucinations is helpful, as this can help clients to establish a sense of influence over their hallucinations. Common therapeutic strategies tend to fall into three categories: (1) distraction, (2) focusing on hallucinations, and (3) relaxation and sleep. Note that empirical evidence suggests no advantage of one strategy over another (Haddock et al., 1998), and that clients should be encouraged to use each technique for 1 week at a time to determine what works best for them.

- *Distraction strategies*: Many clients initially report trying to suppress voices (by ignoring them, telling them to be quiet and go away), but evidence suggests this is less effective than distraction (which involves refocusing attention on an engaging task) and does not help with distress (Falloon and Talbot, 1981). Clients should be encouraged to develop a toolbox of strategies that fit most readily into their lives, for both at home and daily activities (work, social occasions, etc.). Behavioural changes may also assist with distraction: for example, increased physical exercise, listening to music, or socialising more with a good friend or family member.
- *Focusing approaches*: Focusing involves clients examining events prior to and after the onset of the hallucination and being aware of patterns (e.g. did a change in mood, a certain environment, or a certain thought precede the hallucination?). For example, people often report that hallucinations occur when surroundings are noisier or completely silent, or during periods of social isolation. Another common antecedent is increased anxiety. Identification of stimuli that precede hallucinations can help clients plan and problem-solve around these situations.
- *Use of relaxation/meditation*: Relaxation and sleep can be effective approaches for managing hallucinations and other intrusive thoughts (Falloon and Talbot, 1981). In this programme, we aim to ensure that there is not an over-reliance on sleep as a management strategy for hallucinations (but accept that there are situations in which this is appropriate).

With regard to anxiety reduction via relaxation and meditation, a minority of clientsmay experience *increased* anxiety when practising meditation or imagery. Being aware of the risk of increased anxiety is important, as well as implementing the following guide-lines: (1) practise in-session relaxation (with careful observation of how the client responds); (2) encourage very short (2-minute) relaxation exercises for clients who are agitated or anxious; (3) prepare for any increases in anxiety with grounding techniques; and, finally, (4) avoid *vipassana* techniques (insight/analytical-based meditation) and instead use relaxation strategies that encourage grounding and focusing on the present moment, such as body scanning and counting breaths (Shonin et al., 2014).

Rare cases of meditation-induced psychosis have been reported (Kuijpers et al., 2007; Dobkin et al., 2012), but most psychological interventions for psychosis that incorporate relaxation components have not reported adverse effects (Chen et al., 2009; Vancampfort et al., 2011; Moritz et al., 2015). You may also encounter clients who are not keen on the idea of meditation or relaxation. In these cases, you can suggest to the client that they simply try it consistently for the week to test out whether it has potential to be helpful. Remind the client that relaxation and meditation can feel uncomfortable or frustrating at first, as can be the case when getting used to most things for the first time, and emphasise that it is a skill that gets easier with continued practice. Also reiterate that there are many different forms of relaxation and meditation available, and that it is about finding the right strategy that works for them.

Session 3 Structure

The structure for Session 3 is as follows:

- weekly review;
- why the mind might be busy at night;

- linking thoughts and feelings;
- managing overly negative thoughts;
- managing a busy mind at night;
- motivation boost;
- summary and weekly plan.

Materials Needed

- Client Resource Pack (Session 3);
- In-Session Feedback (Appendix 6).

Supplementary (Optional) Handouts

- Sleep Diary (Appendix 2);
- Linking Thoughts and Feelings Worksheet (Appendix 11);
- Relaxing and Fun Activities (Appendix 12);
- Additional Relaxation Exercises (Appendix 13).

Session Content: Weekly Review

Aspects of Sleep and Functioning Addressed in this Session

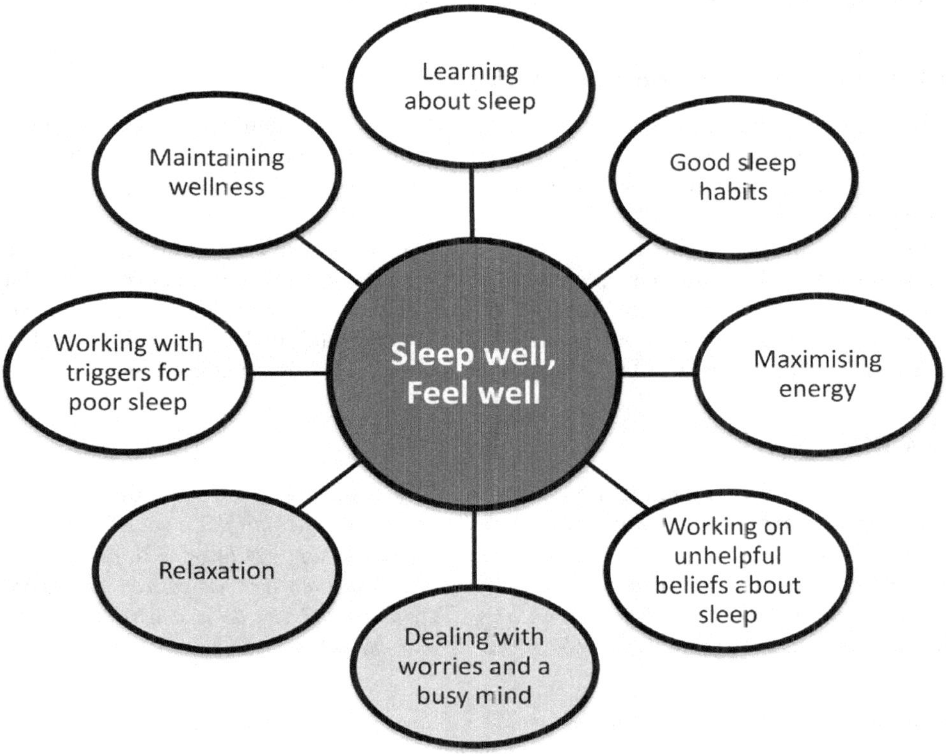

Figure 14.1 Topics Addressed this Week (Session 3)

Activity 21: A Review of Skills We Have Been Learning

In the last session, we learned about:

- maximising daytime energy;
- establishing helpful beliefs and attitudes about sleep;
- managing nightmares.

In the previous sessions, other sleep skills we learned about were:

- sleep hygiene (everyday habits to help us sleep better at night);
- winding down before bed (to help fall asleep);
- getting out of bed if you can't sleep (GOOBICS);
- regular wake-up time (not oversleeping and limiting naps);
- winding up into the day.

Did you put any new sleep skills to the test? How did you find it?

- What went well?
- Did you try some activities to generate more energy for the day? Was it helpful?
- Have you been more mindful about unhelpful beliefs about sleep this week?
- Did you try the TNID strategies? Were they helpful?
- What was challenging?
- Let's brainstorm some ways to get around these challenges.

Why Might the Mind Be Busy at Night?

Many people with Insomnia comment that they have a 'busy mind' when trying to sleep. They might feel that their mind is racing and/or that they have negative thoughts and worries. This can come from low mood, stress, anxiety, psychotic symptoms, or even lack of sleep.

Sometimes, people might not be having negative or worrying thoughts; it's just that their mind is very busy, perhaps planning the next day, or replaying a conversation, for example. When the mind is very busy, it can be difficult to sleep. So, learning to calm the mind can be an important part of Insomnia treatment. We can't make the mind go blank—this just isn't what minds do—but it is possible to work towards it being calmer.

Clock Watching

One more reason that the mind can be busy at night is related to checking the clock.

Therapist notes: *Not all clients watch the clock overnight. Skip over this if it is not relevant. There is evidence that checking the clock overnight contributes to cognitive arousal and longer SOL (Tang et al., 2007). Checking the time tends to lead to a calculation to see how much time has passed while awake, how much sleep has been lost, and how much sleep is likely to be gained for the remainder of the night. These calculations then trigger predictions about what the next day will be like.*

Why Might It Be Unhelpful to Look at the Clock?

Clock watching often leads to anxiety and staying awake. When we are anxious about falling asleep, we naturally tend to check the time to see how long we have been lying

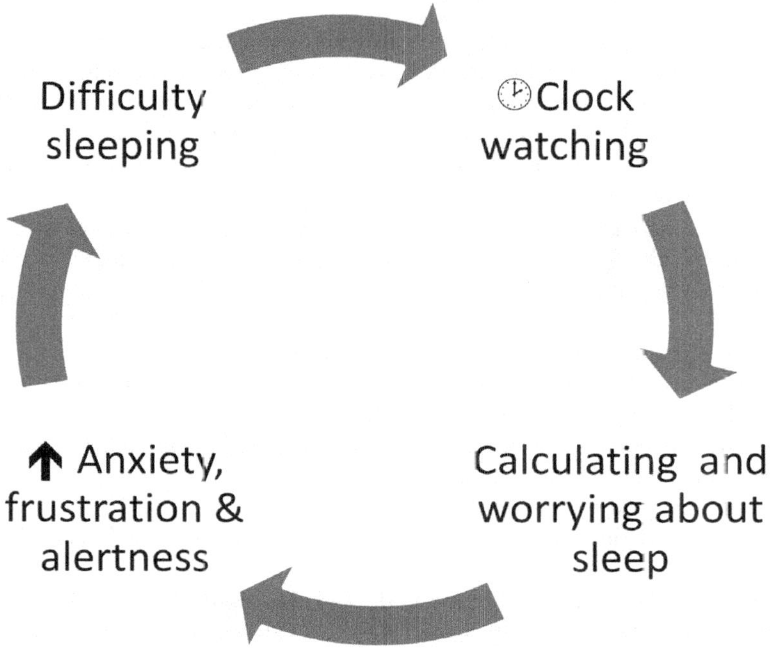

Figure 14.2 The Cycle of Clock Watching at Night

awake and how much time there is left to sleep. This can lead to worry about not getting enough sleep and how we will feel the following day. This increases anxiety, frustration, and alertness, which further leads to difficulties sleeping (see Figure 14.2).

Activity 22: The Clock Watching Experiment

If you watch the clock at all overnight, try this experiment to test whether clock watching is helpful or unhelpful:

- One night, watch the clock as normal.
- The next night, put the clock/phone under your bed or cover it somehow, so that you won't be able to look at it (but can still hear the alarm).
- In the morning, note down whether you looked at the clock or not, and how you slept.

Most people find that it is not helpful to look at the clock over the night.

Whether it is 11 p.m., 2 a.m., or 4 a.m., we want you to do the same thing. Knowing the time should not change your strategy. Relax and let sleep happen.

Low Mood and Anxiety

Therapist notes: *Discuss the list of suggested strategies with each client. Emphasise that they will not find all of these strategies useful and should use the list as a starting point for generating strategies that they will find useful. Responses to the same strategy will vary between clients. Ensuring that each client has at least one strategy to experiment with is important.*

Activity 23: How the Mind Affects Sleep (1): Low Mood and Anxiety

Insomnia is very common in people who have problems with depression or anxiety. Sometimes, people may find it hard to sleep because they are having many sad thoughts and memories, or they are feeling very anxious in bed (e.g. feeling of dry mouth, racing heart, and panic). Sometimes, people have thoughts that make them feel paranoid or scared to go to sleep at night. It is important to recognise when this is happening, so that they can find ways of managing low mood or anxiety before it ruins their sleep.

It can be challenging to manage these uncomfortable feelings, but practice and patience can help to achieve good results. The activity sheet lists strategies for coping with low mood and anxiety. Tick any that you think may be helpful for you to use:

- ❒ Don't be too hard on yourself. Everyone has bad days.
- ❒ Give yourself permission to write this off as one bad day and look to have a better day tomorrow. What might you be able to put in place to help make tomorrow better?
- ❒ Speak to people who make you feel positive. This could involve contacting family, friends, a helpline, or online forum members.
- ❒ Make a list of the things you're grateful for.
- ❒ Concentrate on the here and now (what can you see, hear, touch, smell?) and just breathe.
- ❒ Do something that comforts and relaxes the body and the mind. This can include cooking a favourite meal, taking a warm bath, lighting a candle, cuddling a soft toy, wearing your favourite pyjamas, stretching gently, listening to music, or reading a good book.
- ❒ Organise your problems. Spend a few minutes problem-solving, then make a point of setting problems aside for today and coming back to them tomorrow. Give yourself permission to let them go.
- ❒ Try and take your mind off things by doing an activity you don't do often: rearrange your furniture, get some flowers in the house, change the bedsheets, visit a neighbour.
- ❒ Compile a 'Happy Box' of different possessions and trinkets that make you feel relaxed or happy or bring positive memories. Some examples of what could go into the box include a favourite DVD, nail polish, magazine, photo album, scented candles, relaxation CD, or puzzle book.
- ❒ Do a fun activity (see Appendix 12).

What else could you do when feeling down and depressed or anxious?

Intrusive Thoughts (Thoughts that Go Endlessly Round and Round)

Activity 24: How the Mind Affects Sleep (2): Intrusive Thoughts that Go Endlessly Round and Round

***Therapist notes**: Many clients experience negative, intrusive, or recurrent thoughts at night (including hallucinations and delusions). Clients may use unhelpful strategies such as engaging in further worry or becoming angry that they cannot suppress the thoughts. The use of control strategies can be assessed with the TCQI-R (Ree et al., 2005). Encouraging clients to explore more helpful strategies is the focus of this section.*

Many people experience negative, intrusive, or recurrent thoughts at night that are hard to switch off. These thoughts can make it hard to get to sleep.

Some helpful suggestions for managing intrusive thoughts are listed here on the activity sheet. Tick the strategies that you may like to try:

- ❐ Label the thoughts as 'intrusive thoughts'. For example, say to yourself, 'I'm having an intrusive thought'.
- ❐ Remind yourself that you can practise choosing not to engage with the thought (e.g. 'I don't have to change, argue with, or get rid of this thought').
- ❐ Remind yourself that everyone has intrusive thoughts from time to time. It is OK for the thought to be there, even if you don't like it. You can choose to not become tangled up in the thought.
- ❐ Use relaxation and meditation exercises.
- ❐ Take a few slow, deep breaths.
- ❐ Repeat a phrase or 'mantra'—for example, words such as 'calm and relaxed'—over and over.
- ❐ Recite a soothing poem or prayer.
- ❐ Have a poster or a note by your bed with reassuring messages written on it to read when you are woken up (e.g. 'This experience is temporary and will pass').
- ❐ Try using a 'worry box'—write down your worries and place them into a box to deal with in the morning.

What else could you do when intrusive thoughts bother you at night?

Once you have carried out one or two of the strategies chosen, return your attention to whatever you were doing before the thought bothered you. As best you can, fully engage in the activity and pay full attention to it.

Keep trying. This work takes practice and patience.

Voices, Visions or other Unusual Sensations (Hallucinations)

Activity 25: How the Mind Affects Sleep (3): Voices, Visions or other Unusual Sensations

It is common for people with voices, visions, and other sensory experiences (hallucinations) to report that their voices are worse at night, and that they are unable to use their usual coping strategies at night-time, such as going for a walk. People are also often alone at night and lack distractions, and this may bring on the voices when they are trying to wind down for the night. Voices, visions, or other feelings might also wake them up in the middle of the night.

In your resource pack, some strategies are listed for coping with voices, visions, and other unusual sensory experiences. Tick those that you have found helpful, or may like to try:

- ❐ Converse with the voice, explaining that now is not the time to be talking, but that you can talk again tomorrow.
- ❐ Listen to and focus on the calming voice of an audiobook.
- ❐ Listen to the radio or watch the TV on low volume.
- ❐ Listen to 'white noise' (e.g. the sound of a fan).
- ❐ Wear earplugs.

- ❒ Sing a song or read out loud.
- ❒ Get up, go to another room, and start an activity.
- ❒ Try sleeping with a dim light, using a night light or glow-in-the-dark stars.
- ❒ Wear eye shades (e.g. sunglasses, night mask) if visions are disturbing you at night.
- ❒ Use visualisation techniques (e.g. imagining a protective force field to fend off unwanted visions or voices).
- ❒ For bodily sensations (e.g. feeling insects crawling, pain, feeling limbs change shape), try switching the light on so that you can see the affected area or try massaging the affected area gently.

Note: It might also be useful to use a timer on TVs, radios, and other digital devices, so that they will turn themselves off after a set time. This helps to save electricity and prevents them from disturbing your sleep later in the night.

What else could you do about hearing voices or seeing visions when they keep you awake at night?

In the following section, we will talk about *the link between thoughts and feelings*, how this impacts on sleep, and what we can do to minimise their impact.

Becoming aware of our thoughts and managing them make a valuable way to help address clock watching, low mood, anxiety, unwanted intrusive thoughts, and hallucinations in the night.

Linking Thoughts and Feelings

The Role of Negative Thoughts in Insomnia

Most people assume that the events in their everyday lives directly cause their feelings. For example:

- If we're running late for an appointment, we may feel anxious or annoyed.
- If someone gives us a compliment, we may feel happy.

An important part that we usually miss is the *interpretation* of what an event *means* to us (i.e. what thoughts we had about the event). Our thoughts help us to understand our emotional reaction.

Events or situations by themselves do not create emotions. In other words:

Event or situation → Thought → Feelings or emotions

Therapist notes: *In this section, the job of the therapist is to help clients understand that events or situations by themselves do not create emotions; rather, it is thoughts about events or situations that create emotions. Indeed, the interpretation a person makes of an event strongly influences their emotional response to it. Also important is the notion that thoughts are not facts; rather, they are interpretations that are often subjective and idiosyncratic.*

Coming to understand the thoughts that a person has in a given situation is very helpful for understanding why they felt the way they did. Perhaps return to the examples above: Is it possible to have a different feeling when running late (e.g. calm or guilty)? Is it possible to imagine a different feeling after receiving a compliment (e.g. uncomfortable or anxious)? How can we understand these different reactions?

To see how this process happens, look at the following example.

Activity 26: Linking Thoughts and Feelings

Imagine you are at a party and wave at a friend across the room. They don't wave back to you. There are a number of feelings you might feel in this situation. Whereas one person might feel angry, another might feel sad. What kind of thought might make you feel angry in this situation? What about sad? What kind of thought might make you feel unconcerned or calm? (See Table 14.1)

Table 14.1 Linking Thoughts and Feelings

Event/Situation	*Thought: What are the Thoughts that Might Make You Feel . . .*	*Feelings*
Imagine you are at a party and wave at a friend across the room, and they don't respond to you	'My friend ignored me on purpose, how rude.'	Angry?
	'I must look silly, and they don't want to be my friend.'	Embarrassed or sad?
	'My friend is distracted at the moment and didn't see me.'	Calm?

In the example above, there are many different ways of reacting. It is the person's thoughts about the situation that determine how they feel. Thoughts are not facts; they are opinions. Sometimes, they are accurate, and sometimes they are not.

Therefore, thoughts are a clue to understanding mood.

- You can understand your moods better by looking at the thoughts you have had whenever your mood has changed.
- It is helpful to learn to manage unhelpful thoughts during the day and the night, to improve sleep and daytime tiredness.

Let's do another example. We've just been learning about the link between thoughts and feelings. Now, let's see how this link can be applied to poor sleep.

Activity 27: Another Example of the Link between Thoughts and Feelings

What might Mary's thoughts be in the example below? The situation is waking up in the morning after a poor night of sleep and feeling nervous and upset. (See Table 14.2)

Mary: When I noticed my eyes feeling sore and my brain feeling foggy, I remembered that I hadn't slept well last night. That made me feel nervous about whether I would be able to sleep tonight, and if I'd cope the next day. I guess I then worried that there was nothing I could do to feel better and that made me feel upset.

Table 14.2 Another Example of the Link between Thoughts and Feelings

Event/Situation	*Mary's Thoughts*	*Feelings*
Didn't sleep well last night	Noticed eyes feeling sore, and brain feeling foggy. She will be too tired to function today	Nervous
	She won't sleep well tonight There is nothing she can do to help herself feel better	Upset

Most of us would feel nervous and upset if we thought that not getting enough sleep would lead to not coping, sleeping poorly the next night and not being able to do anything about it. Now we can better understand her feelings.

It is helpful to be able to spot thoughts that are *overly* negative, as they can have a big impact on how we feel. These overly negative thoughts are sometimes not very helpful or very accurate, and, if we can catch them, we can question them and change them into something more helpful.

Becoming Aware of Overly Negative Thoughts

Therapist notes*: It is important that clients are not given the impression that they should write down or respond to all negative thoughts, rather just the real troublemakers (the ones that are overly negative and causing significant shifts in mood).*

Encourage clients to consider the particular time of day when they are best placed to engage in this work (e.g. in the morning after going for a walk, after lunch, after dinner—but not after the pre-bed wind-down period, as this should be reserved for relaxing).

Some clients report that writing down overly negative thoughts or images makes them feel worse rather than better. In this case, one suggestion is for clients to write down positive thoughts about the day or positive events instead and observe whether this is helpful. It may also be useful to help clients to select one or two strategies from Activities 23 and 24, to assist them with responding in a new and helpful way when they spot overly negative thinking. A further alternative is the 'catch it, check it, change it' activity (Activity 29) for those clients who can manage more complicated cognitive work. Encourage clients to experiment with strategies and remind them that this programme is about finding what strategy works best for them.

Activity 28: Become More Aware of Negative Thoughts

Thoughts can occur automatically and come in the form of:

- words (e.g. 'I'll never be able to sleep, I can't cope'); or
- images (e.g. seeing yourself tossing and turning in bed).

The following questions can help you catch and resolve negative automatic thoughts:

1. *Situation*: What exactly is happening at this moment?
2. *Feelings*: What am I feeling?
3. *Thoughts*: What is making me feel this way? What do I think might happen? What would be so bad about that? What am I thinking about myself right now?

Ask yourself these questions until you have identified the thoughts that help you understand your emotional reaction. You may need to ask yourself these questions two or three times to uncover the automatic thoughts.

Let's Try a Practice Exercise on this Now

Imagine it's 2 a.m., and you've been awake tossing and turning for 2 hours. If anything, you feel you are getting more awake, more alert, and more frustrated. You're thinking about how tired you'll feel tomorrow:

- How do you feel emotionally?
- What is making you feel this way?
- What do you think might happen?
- What are you thinking about yourself?

Thoughts that are overly negative will have a significant impact on how you feel and may also affect your behaviour and your coping with poor sleep.

See if you can become more aware of negative thoughts this week and notice the impact they have on your mood. Sometimes, catching overly negative thoughts and recognising them as 'overly negative' can help you to feel a bit better.

If you catch overly negative thoughts, remind yourself that this is just a thought, not a fact. You can choose whether or not you listen to the thought. (Also, see Appendix 11: 'Linking Thoughts and Feelings Worksheet'.)

- What thoughts do you have when you haven't slept well?
- What thoughts to do you have when you are having trouble sleeping at night?
- Do you notice the same thing during the day?
- What do you feel like doing after experiencing these thoughts and feelings?

Managing Overly Negative Thoughts

This section suggests how to change overly negative thoughts that get in the way of sleep and contribute to tiredness during the day.

Activity 29: Managing Negative Thoughts

How can we change the thoughts and feelings that interfere with sleep and getting activated during the day?

The benefit of learning that thoughts, not situations, create feelings is that *it is possible to manage our feelings by changing our thoughts.*

To address unhelpful thoughts, we need to apply the **3 Cs** (adapted from Holden and Granholm, 2012) See Table 14.3.

Table 14.3 The 3 Cs

The 3 Cs	*Action*
Catch it	Identify the unhelpful, overly negative or intrusive thought
Check it	Identify evidence that supports and disputes the thought
Change it	Change the thought so that it is more accurate and helpful

Having Trouble with the 3 Cs?

***Therapist notes**: Challenging overly negative thoughts may be too complicated for some clients. In this case, encourage clients to write about what is bothering them on a piece of paper or in a journal, write down positive thoughts or events about the day instead, or encourage clients to select one or two strategies from Activities 23 and 24 to assist them with responding in a new and helpful way when they spot overly negative thinking.*

Writing down or drawing thoughts and feelings can have a positive effect, as it may help you to:

- become aware of the link between thoughts and feelings
- detach from the thought/image, get some distance, and experience the thought less intensely;
- manage the negative thought/image by developing a new perspective that could be more helpful.

***Therapist notes**: For clients who are able, use the 'Negative Thoughts Record' and 'Managing Unhelpful Thoughts' worksheets. Work through an example in session with clients and assist them in developing more helpful alternatives.*

Worksheets: You can also try using the next two worksheets on the following pages to help you manage negative thoughts:

- The *Negative Thoughts Record* (*Catch It*) can be used to help identify overly negative thoughts and feelings.
- The *Managing Unhelpful Thoughts* (*Check It and Change It*) worksheet can help you *check* and *change* unhelpful thoughts related to sleep.

Activity 30: Negative Thoughts Records (Catch It)

The Negative Thoughts Record is used to catch overly negative thoughts. Use the worksheet to note down the thoughts or images you are having when you are experiencing difficult emotions (e.g. feeling down, guilty, scared, frustrated, or anxious). (See Table 14.4)

Table 14.4 Negative Thoughts Record Worksheet

Thoughts and Images	***Feelings***
Write Down the Unhelpful Thought or Image that Is Going through Your Mind	*Tick how the Thought/Image Makes You Feel*
	Positive feelings: ❐ Happy ❐ Content ❐ Excited Negative feelings: ❐ Weak/useless ❐ Guilty/ashamed ❐ Angry/frustrated ❐ Anxious/scared ❐ Sad/depressed Others: ❐ ______________ ❐ ______________ ❐ ______________ Rate how strong the feeling(s) you've ticked is from 0 to 10 (circle below): 0 1 2 3 4 5 6 7 8 9 10 Not strong at all Extremely strong

Now that you've caught the overly negative thought that's bothering you, use this next sheet to help you examine, question, and change it into something more helpful.

Activity 31: Managing Unhelpful Thoughts Worksheet (Check It and Change It)

This activity is about starting to feel like you have a little more influence over your feelings and responses. Try it when your thoughts are bothering you, and you can't seem to wind down. Use the sheet at night, or during the day if too difficult at night-time.

Catch it:

- Write down the unhelpful, overly negative or intrusive thought you are working on (e.g. 'If I don't get enough sleep, I am going to relapse and get hospitalised again').

Check it: Let's look closer at this thought:

- How much do you believe this thought, from 0 to 100 per cent? (Colour in how much on the thermometer.)
- How does this thought make you feel?
- Is it a helpful thought?
- Thinking of your calmest, most rational, and most supportive friend, carer, or family member, what advice would they give?
- Would you feel better if you chose not to listen to this thought?
- If a good friend was in this situation, what would you tell him/her?

Change it:

- What is a more helpful thought? (e.g. 'I have felt this way before, and did not relapse from having a bad night's sleep. I'm doing lots of helpful things and won't get hospitalised just because I'm not sleeping well')
- How much do you believe the *new* thought (from 0 to 100 per cent)?
- How much do you believe the *old* thought (from 0 to 100 per cent)?

Managing a Busy Mind at Night

***Therapist notes**: For clients who experience a busy mind at night, discuss with them the strategies listed below and those in Activity 24. Encourage clients to try one or more of these skills during the week, before they go to bed, to help manage a busy mind. It is important to emphasise that the client should go to bed only once they feel sleepy (not just tired or low in energy, but sleepy, with eyelids drooping, etc.).*

Activity 32: Managing a Busy Mind at Night

Try these skills before going to bed to help manage a busy mind:

Winding Down before Bed

***Therapist notes**: A good way to manage a busy mind is by winding down each night, as it helps to calm the mind, so that sleep comes more easily. Engaging in wind-down activities each night should help break the 'cycle' in which a busy mind gets in the way of sleep, which makes the mind busier, and so on.*

Clients may find a reasonably fixed routine before bed is helpful. Refer the client back to activities they may have chosen for their wind-down in Session 1 (Activity 6).

Remember the wind-down activities discussed in the first session. Doing your wind-down activities each night may help break the 'circuit' of a busy mind getting in the way of sleep.

Winding down involves doing relaxing activities 1 hour before bed and having a fixed bedtime routine right before bed, where you might have a warm drink (e.g. cup of cocoa or milk), brush your teeth, and do a relaxation exercise.

To-Do Lists and Prioritising

Therapist notes*: This exercise can be performed on a daily basis or when required. To-do lists mean that the client is no longer needing to hold information to be remembered in their head and can assist in the process of reducing cognitive arousal. Encourage the client to think of what they need to do and what they would like to do the next day.*

- *Encourage your client to be specific—for example, help them to generate a to-do list in session and to consider what time of day might work best for them to do their list. If they have a reminder function on their phone, this can be a useful tool for reminding the client to compile their to-do list.*
- *Once the to-do list has been compiled, ask the client to consider which the top two or three most important tasks are. These are the tasks that may be urgent owing to an external demand (e.g. needing to pay a bill by the due date) or may be important because they are tasks that may help the client to feel energised, motivated, relaxed, or brighter in mood.*
- *More complicated tasks may need breaking down into smaller steps, and clients that tend to be disorganised may need some assistance here.*
- *Some people like to keep their list by their bed so that they can jot down more items if they come to mind while they are in bed (no need to even turn on the light).*

To-do lists are a way of putting the 'day to bed' and busy thoughts out of mind, so that you can go to sleep.

- The list can be done before you leave work at the end of the day, after dinner, or any other time you feel it would be handy.
- Some people like to keep their list by their bed so that they can jot down any items that come to mind while they are in bed (no need to even turn on the light).
- When would be the best time for you to make a to-do list?
- Can you set a reminder on your phone to make sure you do this?

Avoid Watching the Clock Overnight

It is hard to put the mind to rest if you are always checking the time to see how long you have been lying awake or calculate whether you will get enough sleep for the night.

If you find that you often check the time when you are having trouble falling back to sleep, try the clock watching experiment we talked about for Activity 22.

How will I avoid watching the clock at night? ______________________________

You can also try setting your alarm for the morning to help you worry less about whether you will wake up on time for the next day.

Relaxation Exercises

Activity 33: Relaxation Exercises

Relaxation strategies can help you to wind down and avoid worry keeping you up at night. There are many relaxation exercises available. Let's practise a few simple relaxation strategies you can try out before bed.

- *Shoulder shrugs*: Raise your shoulders as if trying to touch your ears with them, and breathe in while doing this. Feel the muscles in your neck and shoulders tense. Then, all at once, let your shoulders drop while breathing out. Feel the tension leaving the muscles of your neck and shoulders. Repeat the shrug a few times, inhaling on the shrug and exhaling on the release. Keep your jaw relaxed as you do this.
- *Releasing tension*: Become aware of the difference between holding tension in your body and letting go of this tension. Bend your toes up as if to touch your shins. Hold them there while you tighten your thighs, buttocks, and fists. Take a deep breath and hold it while you clench your jaw and close your eyes. Hold all that tension for 5 seconds. Then, as you exhale, let it go all at once and feel the tension draining from your body.
- *Cued relaxation response*: Pick a word or phrase that has either positive or neutral connotations for you (for example, 'Easy', 'I am relaxed', or 'Sparkle'). Sit quietly in a comfortable position and begin breathing slowly and naturally. As you exhale, say to yourself your cue word or phrase. If your mind starts to wander, that's OK; just come back to your breathing and to repeating your cue word or phrase.
- *Equalising breathing*: Take 4 seconds to breathe in and 4 seconds to breathe out. That is, as you inhale count '1 . . . 2 . . . 3 . . . 4' and do the same as you breathe out. Do this four or five times. Avoid holding your breath after the inhalation or the exhalation; just smoothly transition from one phase to the other.
- *Your relaxation place*: Begin with a few slow relaxation breaths. Then, with your eyes closed, take a moment to create, in your mind's eye, an ideal spot to relax. You can make it any place you'd like, such as the mountains, beach, lake, prairie, or park. It can be either a real or made-up place. See yourself comfortably enjoying this place. Now, once you have created it, go and use it for 15 seconds or so whenever you feel the need to relax.

Remember that relaxation requires practice. It may take many tries before it is found useful. There are also many different types of relaxation and meditation exercise out there. Find one that you feel comfortable learning.

Try giving one or two of these relaxation exercises a go during the week, and see if it helps with your sleep (*also see Appendix 13 for more relaxation exercises*). You can also check out App downloads on topics related to meditation, relaxation, and breathing.

The Motivation Boost: Helpful Thoughts about Sleep

Therapist notes: *By way of a summary, emphasise to clients that sleep is important, but it is not the end of the world to have a few poor nights. There are lots of things that can be done to help clients function better during the day, even if they haven't slept well the night before. This way of thinking can help clients to negotiate a healthy balance when they worry excessively about sleep.*

Remember that sleep is important, but it is not the end of the world if it goes pear-shaped. There are lots of things you can do to help yourselves function better during the day, even if you haven't slept well the night before.

Summary

Summary of Key Points

Activity 34: The Main Things I Learned Today

Let's write down today's key points on your worksheet.

Take home messages:

- There are lots of strategies that may assist you in managing low mood, anxiety, intrusive thoughts, and hallucinations.
- Your thoughts affect how you feel.
- Overly negative thoughts = more anxiety/stress/low mood/frustration, which can affect your sleep and daytime energy.
- Catching overly negative thoughts can be helpful, as it helps us to take a step back from them.
- Changing overly negative thoughts can help to make strong emotions less intense.
- There are many ways to manage a busy mind at night—which were most important for you?
- Relaxation takes practice but can be very helpful for calming the mind and the body.

Action Plan for the Week

Activity 35: My Action Plan for the Week

On the activity sheet, you should write down your planned sleep strategies for the week, including:

1. My regular rising time for *each* morning is: ______.
2. Some energy-generating activities and changes to my sleep hygiene that I will keep working on: ____________________ (See point 1.)
3. Start to manage overly negative thoughts:
    - Watch out for overly negative thoughts and the impact that they have on my sleep and energy—*How and when will I do this?* (e.g. after dinner; with my morning coffee; after taking my medications; whenever I notice a strong negative change in my mood (feeling very anxious/depressed); set up a reminder alarm on my phone).
    - When thoughts/images are distracting me from winding down or falling asleep at night, I must write them down on a piece of paper/journal.
    - Remember the 3 Cs—catch it, check it, change it (challenge the unhelpful thoughts using the worksheets provided).
4. Use strategies for dealing with a busy mind:
    - Experiment with strategies for managing:
        - low mood and/or anxiety (see *Activity 23*);
        - intrusive thoughts (see *Activity 24*);
        - voices, visions, other unusual sensations (see *Activity 25*);
    - Continue with winding down before bed: *Think about what I might try.*

- To-do list: *Think about when and how I might do this.*
- Avoid watching the clock when you can't sleep: Try the clock watching experiment.
- Relaxation or imagery: Practise this during the day for short periods at first. When I become more skilled, I will be able to use it more effectively at night.

References and Further Reading

Chen, W.-C., Chu, H., Lu, R.-B., Chou, Y.-H., Chen, C.-H., Chang, Y.-C., O'Brien, A. P., and Chou, K.-R. (2009) "Efficacy of progressive muscle relaxation training in reducing anxiety in patients with acute schizophrenia", *Journal of Clinical Nursing*, 18(15), pp. 2187–2196.

Cooke, A. (2014) *Understanding psychosis and schizophrenia: Why people sometimes hear voices, believe things that others find strange, or appear out of touch with reality, and what can help*. Leicester, UK: British Psychological Society Division of Clinical Psychology. Available at: www.bps.org.uk/system/files/Public%20files/rep03_understanding_psychosis.pdf (accessed December 2, 2016).

Dobkin, P., Irving, J., and Amar, S. (2012) "For whom may participation in a mindfulness-based stress reduction program be contraindicated?", *Mindfulness*, 3(1), pp. 44–50.

Falloon, I. R. H., and Talbot, R. E. (1981) "Persistent auditory hallucinations: Coping mechanisms and implications for management", *Psychological Medicine*, 11(2), pp. 329–339.

Haddock, G., Slade, P. D., Bentall, R. P., Reid, D., and Faragher, E. B. (1998) "A comparison of the long-term effectiveness of distraction and focusing in the treatment of auditory hallucinations", *British Journal of Medical Psychology*, 71(3), pp. 339–349.

Holden, J., and Granholm, E. (2012) "Group cognitive behavioural social skills training for schizophrenia", in Steel, C. (Ed.) *CBT for schizophrenia: Evidence-based interventions and future directions*. Oxford, UK: John Wiley, pp. 169–190.

Kansas State University (2005) "Quick relaxation strategies", Personal Assessment Challenge-Choosing Activities for Today's Success (PAC-CATS): Counselling Services. Available at: www.k-state.edu/paccats/Contents/Stress/Quick%20Relaxation%20Strategies.pdf (accessed December 2, 2016).

Kuijpers, H. J. H., van der Heijden, F. M. M. A., Tuinier, S., and Verhoeven, W. M. A. (2007) "Meditation-induced psychosis", *Psychopathology*, 40(6), pp. 461–464.

Moritz, S., Cludius, B., Hottenrott, B., Schneider, B. C., Saathoff, K., Kuelz, A. K., and Gallinat, J. (2015) "Mindfulness and relaxation treatment reduce depressive symptoms in individuals with psychosis", *European Psychiatry*, 30(6), pp. 709–714.

Ree, M. J., Harvey, A. G., Blake, R., Tang, N. K. Y., and Shawe-Taylor, M. (2005) "Attempts to control unwanted thoughts in the night: development of the thought control questionnaire-insomnia revised (TCQI-R)", *Behaviour Research & Therapy*, 43, pp. 985–993.

Shonin, E., Van Gordon, W., and Griffiths, M. D. (2014) "Do mindfulness-based therapies have a role in the treatment of psychosis?", *Australian & New Zealand Journal of Psychiatry*, 48(2), pp. 124–127.

Tang, N. K. Y., Anne Schmidt, D., and Harvey, A. G. (2007) 'Sleeping with the enemy: Clock monitoring in the maintenance of insomnia', *Journal of Behavior Therapy & Experimental Psychiatry*, 38(1), pp. 40–55.

Vancampfort, D., De Hert, M., Knapen, J., Maurissen, K., Raepsaet, J., Deckx, S., Remans, S., and Probst, M. (2011) "Effects of progressive muscle relaxation on state anxiety and subjective well-being in people with schizophrenia: A randomized controlled trial", *Clinical Rehabilitation*, 25(6), pp. 567–575.

World Hearing Voices Network (2012) "Better sleep for voice hearers." Available at: www.hearing-voices.org/resources/free-downloads/ (accessed December 2, 2016).

15 Therapist Manual Session 4

Maintaining Wellness and Working with Triggers for Poor Sleep

Information for the Therapist

This final session focuses on:

1. emphasising the impact of substances on sleep and energy;
2. stress management (life balance); and
3. relapse prevention.

In this last session, praise clients for their progress so far (attending sessions, making even small changes) and encourage continued work to implement new sleep skills wherever needed.

Effect of Substances on Sleep and Energy

The first section in Session 4 considers the effects of substance use on sleep and daytime energy. Some discussion of and planning for substance use may have occurred in previous sessions, but, if not, this session aims to develop a personalised action plan for managing substance use where appropriate. This could best be described as a harm minimisation approach for substance use as it relates to the client's sleep problems. The use of alcohol, caffeine, cigarettes, and illicit drugs is much higher in people with psychosis than in the general population (Barrowclough et al., 2007; Gregg et al., 2007; Galletly, 2012), with some research finding that about 50 per cent of patients meet criteria for drug or alcohol abuse or dependence. Substances can have a significant impact on energy during the day and sleep at night. It is important to think about how best to maximise the benefits of substances while minimising any negative consequences.

It is also important to work to understand what makes your client reach for substances (other than their prescribed medications), both day and night. Is it a physical dependence, a habit, a strategy for escaping low mood or anxiety, a way to avoid or induce sleep, a form of fun and self-nurturing, a way to mitigate medication side effects, or a combination of these?

- In the case of physiological dependence, encourage gradual reduction of intake. Discuss having alternatives at the ready—for example, decaffeinated and non-alcoholic drinks, nicotine patches or gum, a healthy snack, or an engaging activity. Ask the client to experiment with delaying substance use when cravings arise by increasing the amount of time each day before they use the substance (e.g. waiting 5 minutes, then half an hour, by which time the craving may well have passed). Other options include medications for assisting smoking cessation, such as champix (varenicline).

- If the substance use is a habit, the client might set up some reminders to make a different choice in the moment—for example, a note on the kettle, alcohol container, biscuit tin, cigarette packet, or lighter.
- If the substance use is because of desire to stay awake in the evening (because of fears about going to bed), discuss the client's fears and make a plan for making sleep feel less threatening—for example, winding down, relaxation techniques, gentle challenging of any unhelpful thoughts and predictions, and desensitisation to the fear (graduated exposure).
- If the substance use is a form of self-nurturing, encourage the client to think about other, healthier ways to nurture (see Appendix 12 for suggestions).

In most cases, consideration of the costs and benefits of current use patterns is an important motivational tool. We suggest discussing costs and benefits of substance use in general, but making sure that sleep- and energy-related consequences are emphasised. Written goals and plans for change are also important. Do check how confident the client is in making changes to their substance use, and work to simplify and break down goals if confidence is low.

Most commonly, abrupt cessation of substances should be avoided, with gradual reduction being favoured. Withdrawal effects are common. Withdrawal effects from caffeine include headache, fatigue, dysphoric mood, irritability, anxiety, difficulty concentrating, and flu-like symptoms. Common withdrawal effects from nicotine include irritability, fatigue, dysphonic mood, difficulty concentrating, increased appetite, restlessness, and low mood.

Medications

The great majority of people with a diagnosis of a psychotic disorder take psychotropic medications. The clinical assessment will have revealed information regarding the type and dosage of medication prescribed, as well as medication adherence, but it is useful to check this again.

Sometimes, medications can have side effects that impact on sleep without the client realising these are due to their medications. For example, some medications can cause bad dreams or drowsiness in the day. Others can make clients feel too alert at night. If you suspect these side effects are present, a discussion with the prescribing doctor may be warranted. Sometimes, the type, dose, or timing of medication can be altered to good effect.

Working towards Balance

Life stress and poor life balance can impact on sleep and mental health symptoms. For clients with psychotic disorders, even a seemingly mild stressor (a date, usual doctor or health worker being away, a job interview) can have a large impact. Stress is most likely to impact negatively if the client has low self-efficacy, that is, if they believe they cannot cope well with the stress. Further, it is often the case that clients with psychosis have more stress in their lives—for example, managing their symptoms, previous trauma, financial strain, social isolation, and lack of occupational opportunity.

The presence of psychosis and comorbid conditions can result in clients' lives becoming 'illness-centric'. A large part of life for many clients involves attending health and medical appointments, worrying about symptoms, taking medications, and coping with side effects. Clients may feel defined by their illness and lose sight of who they are as a person, aside from their mental health problems. In this way, their lives become unbalanced. Although this is understandable, it is beneficial to assist clients in considering how they might be able to achieve a better balance and periods of time devoted to non-illness-related activity.

This section of the programme aims to help the client to clearly identify sources of stress and areas where life lacks balance. An important therapeutic aim is to validate, on the one hand, that dealing with symptoms of psychosis is hard and involves a lot of time, energy, and resources. On the other hand, however, it is important to consciously plan to have periods of 'time out' from the illness to focus on and establish other interests and to pursue valued activities. What would the client like to do if the illness wasn't in charge? Ideally, a balance between periods of conscious focus, problem-solving, goal setting, and proactivity around the psychosis are balanced with periods of engaging in activities that are independent of their illness. Emphasise the value of taking small steps on a daily basis and breaking a big task into smaller tasks, so that is it more manageable and less daunting.

Keeping Progress Going: Relapse Prevention

Aims are to assist clients in maintaining improvements gained over the programme, identify triggers for relapse, and equip them to manage future recurrences of worsening sleep early on. It is important to remind clients that many things can temporarily trigger poor sleep or daytime energy (e.g. stress, physical or mental illness symptoms, change of personal circumstance, etc.), but that they can act to prevent poor sleep from becoming a chronic issue again.

In relapse prevention, the following actions are important:

- Revise the most pertinent skills for each client.
- Emphasise that transient periods of poor sleep are to be expected in the future, but that an acute exacerbation in symptoms does not have to lead to a full relapse.
- Help clients to identify controllable contributing factors in the face of worsening symptoms.
- Frame a bad night's sleep, not as a disaster, but as an opportunity to test their mastery of the sleep knowledge and skills that they have learned.
- Look out for unhelpful beliefs concerning self, illness, and the future that may act as barriers to further progress. For example, if the client holds a belief that they will slip back into their bad sleep habits when the programme concludes, you may highlight that, as the therapist, you have simply been there to supply them with information about how to achieve better sleep, but that the client was the one who put in all the hard work to make the positive changes seen happen. If workable, offer follow-up sessions to support continued progress.
- Revisit the client's personal motivation to engage in sleep treatment in order to encourage continued use of their new sleep strategies and knowledge.

We echo Dr. Perlis (National Sleep Foundation, 2014) in emphasising two main strategies for protection against relapse of Insomnia in the context of an acute bout of poor sleep:

1. Don't compensate for sleep loss (e.g. avoid (extra) napping or sleeping longer the next day). Trust that a poor sleep will serve to increase sleep drive the next night. Sleeping in, napping, or going to bed early will reduce sleep drive and may start a cycle of poor sleep at night.
2. Start stimulus control procedures immediately (i.e. GOOBICS).

Follow-up Sessions

Lastly, it is valuable to offer clients at least one follow-up session (1–6 months post-treatment) to review progress, offer support, and boost motivation to continue practising skills. Many clients will benefit from more than one follow-up. Follow-up sessions do not introduce new content but are an important opportunity to revise concepts and troubleshoot areas of difficulty.

Appendix 16 presents a worksheet called 'Evaluating My Progress' that can be used to review the client's success with the treatment programme. The 'Change Plan Worksheet' in Appendix 17 may then be used to plan the next steps towards maintaining their sleep management. Worksheets on 'Things to Consider to Create Better Balance' (Activity 43) and 'Planning for Setbacks' (Activity 48) from the Client Resource Pack (Session 4) may also be used in follow-up appointments.

Session 4 Structure

The structure for Session 4 is as follows:

- weekly review;
- the impact of medication, alcohol, caffeine, smoking, and drugs on sleep and energy;
- stress management;
- keeping your progress going—relapse prevention;
- motivational boost;
- action plan and goal setting.

Materials Needed

- Client Resource Pack (Session 4);
- In-session feedback (Appendix 6).

Supplementary (Optional) Handouts

- Sleep Diary (Appendix 2);
- Information on Sleeping Tablets (Appendix 14);
- Reducing Your Usage of Sleeping Tablets (Appendix 15): This handout contains advice on how to go about reducing the use of sleeping tablets, which may be a future goal for some of your clients. It is important that any changes are discussed with the client's treating doctor.

Session Content: Weekly Review

Aspects of Sleep and Functioning Addressed in this Session

Activity 36: A Review of Skills We Have Been Learning

In the last session, we learned about:

- dealing with a busy mind: managing intrusive thoughts and voices, winding down, not clock watching, journal writing, to-do lists and relaxation;
- working with overly negative thoughts—catch it, check it, change it (the 3 Cs).

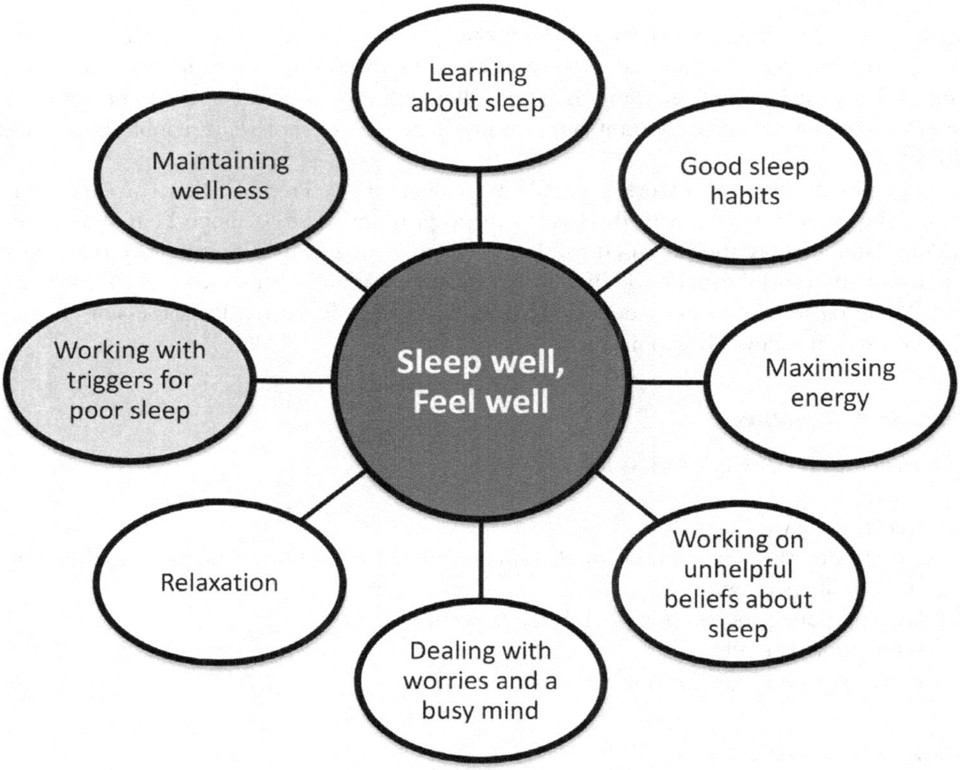

Figure 15.1 Topics Addressed this Week (Session 4)

In previous sessions, the other sleep skills we learned about were:

- sleep hygiene (everyday habits to help us sleep better at night);
- winding down before bed (to help fall asleep);
- getting out of bed if you can't sleep (GOOBICS);
- regular rising time (not oversleeping, and limiting naps);
- winding up into the day in the morning;
- maximising daytime energy;
- establishing helpful beliefs and attitudes about sleep;
- managing nightmares.

Did you put your sleep skills to the test? How did you find it?

- What went well?
- Have you been winding down every night?
- Did you use the negative thoughts worksheets?
- Did you find relaxation exercises helpful for you this week?
- Did you make to-do lists to help with sleep?
- What was challenging? Let's brainstorm some ways to get around these challenges.

The Impact of Medication, Alcohol, Caffeine, Smoking, and Drugs on Sleep and Energy

Medication

***Therapist notes**: See Chapter 6, which discusses side effects of common medications.*

Many people who experience mental illness take prescribed medications, such as antipsychotics and antidepressants. These medications work very well for symptoms such as racing thoughts, hearing voices, low mood, or anxiety. It is important to take prescribed medications according to the doctor's instructions and at a regular time.

It is helpful to understand the side effects of common medications. Common side effects may include daytime sleepiness, night-time alertness, nightmares, sleep-walking, and night-eating.

Activity 37: Effects of Medications on Sleep

***Therapist notes**: Strategies for dealing with **drowsiness** will largely draw on the energy-generating activities discussed in Session 2 and may include: exercise, exposure to sunlight, social contact, mood-lifting activity, accomplishing a task, healthy snacks and meals, and looking at the timing of medications (e.g. perhaps take earlier in the evening).*

*With respect to **sleep-walking**, it is important to ensure that the home environment is safe (that the doors are locked, and that there are no objects on the ground that could be tripped over). Furthermore, a good sleep routine and reduced stress are known to help reduce the severity and frequency of sleep-walking episodes.*

***Bad dreams** may be addressed with reference back to the seven strategies for dealing with nightmares, covered in Session 2.*

***Night-eating** is more common with certain antipsychotics, such as seroquel. Many people who experience night-eating may also be binging on sweets, chips, or a heavy meal before bed. Suggest healthier food options that are lower in sugar and not too large in quantity (e.g. crackers, fruit, a slice of bread, handful of nuts). Other strategies include seeing a dietician, replacing night-eating with another activity (e.g. crossword books or a craft), and accessing a self-help book on night-eating disorders (see Allison et al., 2004).*

Let's now talk about the benefits and disadvantages that your medications have for your sleep, and some strategies to manage the side effects. Use the worksheet and write the following:

- What are the benefits and disadvantages of medications for your sleep? For example, have there ever been any particular side effects from medications that have disrupted your sleep quality, sleep routine, or morning energy levels?
  - *Common advantages* of medication include coping with stress, fewer psychotic symptoms (e.g. racing mind, voices, visions, paranoia), improved mood, and improved sleep routine if medications are taken at a regular time.
  - *Common disadvantages* of medications include side effects such as heart palpitations, agitation, weight gain (and distress about weight gain at night), difficulty sleeping (Insomnia) or over-drowsiness, sweating, dry throat or increased thirst, nocturia (having to go to the toilet in the night), and bad or intense dreams. Other problems may include sleep-walking and night-eating from certain medications taken for sleep. Other disadvantages include dependency on the medication to get to sleep and 'rebound' Insomnia if you stop taking the medication.

- What strategies can you use to reduce the side effects of medications when they make you too sleepy or when they worsen sleep problems (e.g. too alert, nightmares, sleep-walking, night-eating)?
- On a scale of 0–10, how confident do you feel about applying these strategies?

General Guidelines for Sleep

- Take prescribed medications only as directed (correct time, correct dose).
- Be proactive in managing side effects and discuss any ongoing problematic side effects with your doctor

Caffeine and Smoking (Stimulants)

How might smoking and caffeine affect winding down or staying asleep at night?

Caffeine and nicotine in cigarettes have a stimulant effect on your brain and body. Stimulants cause you to feel more alert and awake. Caffeine is a relatively long-acting stimulant with a half-life of about 4–5 hours. Nicotine has a shorter half-life of about 2 hours. Both caffeine and nicotine can cause difficulty falling asleep and increased sleep fragmentation (i.e. more wake-ups) during the night.

Although caffeine and smoking may be enjoyable and help increase alertness in the daytime, it is unhelpful to drink caffeine or smoke during the evening. The disrupted sleep that may result from caffeine or nicotine can lead to increased tiredness, low mood, and anxiety the next day. These consequences may lead to more caffeine and nicotine use, becoming a vicious cycle.

***Therapist notes**: Through discussion of the benefits and disadvantages of caffeine and smoking, highlight that these substances are addictive and can be expensive. Cigarettes are also very unhealthy. The disadvantage of the expense of smoking resonated with some of our clients, who noted that it becomes harder to save up for things such as a favourite food, new clothes, a car, or a holiday. In line with motivational interviewing principles, it is important to base any discussion of benefits and costs around factors that are important for each individual client.*

Activity 38: Effects of Caffeine and Smoking

Use the worksheet and write down the following:

- What are the benefits and disadvantages of caffeine and smoking?
  - *Common advantages* of caffeine and smoking include coping with stress, boredom, tiredness, and low mood, and enjoyment of the taste.
  - *Common disadvantages of caffeine* include poor sleep, diuretic effect overnight, anxiety symptoms (heart palpitations), agitation and cravings, greater daytime energy fluctuations, increased risk of diabetes and weight gain if caffeine is ingested in sugary drinks, and the belief that it is not possible to cope without caffeine. Caffeine can also cause reflux.
  - *Common disadvantages of nicotine* include poor sleep; expense (makes it harder to save for things such as your favourite food, a car, or a holiday); yellow skin and fingers; the smell; cravings; increased risk of serious health problems, such as cancer, heart disease, stroke, and breathing problems (chronic obstructive pulmonary disease); and the belief that it is not possible to cope without nicotine, and so you miss out on learning other coping strategies.

- What strategies can you use to reduce your use of caffeine and cigarettes at night? (You could try gradually delaying your intake each night, or switch to having nicotine gum or a nicotine patch, and decaffeinated coffee, milk, or some other drink at night instead.)
- On a scale of 0–10, how confident do you feel about applying these strategies?

General Guidelines for Sleep

- Avoid caffeine 5 hours before bed.
- Avoid nicotine 2 hours before bed: Work towards quitting smoking or reducing the number of cigarettes you smoke over the day.

Alcohol

***Therapist notes**: In our work with clients, most had tried alcohol to help with getting to sleep at some point in their lives, but stopped after advice from their treating doctor or discovering that it had negative interactions with their prescribed medications. For those who showed persistent alcohol use in the evening, this was heavily tied to depression, boredom, socialising, and, for those with trauma, trying to block out distressing flashbacks. We also encountered some clients whose social circle would celebrate disability/pension 'pay day' with a heavy night of drinking and drug use. Work with the client to devise alternative strategies that can be used to tackle these driving factors. For example, managing overly negative thoughts (as addressed in Session 3), behavioural activation, relaxation and grounding techniques, or suggesting alternative fun activities to do with friends (e.g. board games, watching a movie, having a picnic), which are also more cost-effective. Clients are also often largely unaware of the effect of alcohol on increased wakefulness during the night and difficulties attaining deep sleep, and in any of these cases benefit from the information provided. An additional consideration is that, for some clients, smoking and alcohol may have become associated with one another (e.g. the client habitually has a smoke after a beer), and so working on reducing these two factors together is often helpful.*

Another lifestyle and health factor that could be affecting your sleep is alcohol.

Alcohol can interfere with mood and the quality of sleep. People often think that drinking alcohol will help sleep. But, in fact, as the body digests alcohol overnight, it can cause fragmented sleep (i.e. more wake-ups). So, although alcohol may shorten the time you take to fall asleep at the start of the night, it gets in the way of achieving a good deep sleep for the rest of the night. It can also lead to you feeling dehydrated, nauseous, headachy, tired, low in mood, and unrefreshed in the morning.

Let's now talk about the benefits and disadvantages of alcohol for sleep, and some strategies to help reduce usage of alcohol at night.

Activity 39: Effects of Alcohol on Sleep

Use the worksheet and write down:

- What makes you reach for alcohol in the evening?
- What are the benefits and disadvantages of alcohol for you?
  - *Common advantages* include it being fun; relaxing; a way to cope with stress, boredom, tiredness, and low mood; enjoyment of the taste; helps you get to sleep.
  - *Common disadvantages* include that it is expensive and that it leads to poor sleep; waking to go to the toilet overnight; hangover in the morning; inability to make progress on goals; reduced productivity and energy; poor decision-making; poor

concentration and memory; aggression; irritability; cravings; withdrawal symptoms; increased snoring or OSA symptoms; weight gain; increased risk of liver problems, cancer, and high blood pressure; the belief that it is not possible to cope without alcohol; and negative interaction with medications.

- What could you do to reduce reliance on alcohol for getting to sleep?
- On a scale of 0–10, how confident do you feel about applying these strategies?

General Guidelines for Sleep

- Avoid alcohol for 4 hours before bed.
- Drink plenty of water after heavy drinking.

Illicit Drugs

Therapist notes*: Assess illicit drug use openly with your client in the clinical intake session (see Chapter 8). We focus here on cannabis use, as this is the illicit drug most commonly used in psychotic populations. Cannabis use is more common in younger clients and is associated with psychotic relapse. In terms of sleep and daytime function, cannabis use can facilitate sleep onset, and some research shows that it can lead to deeper sleep. However, cannabis also leads to reduced motivation and increased fatigue. This can lead to reduced motivation to get up at a regular time, keep up with appointments, socialise, or exercise in the day. Additionally, clients may become reliant on cannabis to get to sleep. For clients who have problems with cannabis use, you may consider using the self-help manual by Helen Mentha (2001).*

Many drugs can cause either sleepiness (sedatives such as marijuana and heroin) or increased alertness (stimulants such as meth, speed, and ecstasy), and impact on mood and sleep patterns.

Let's take the example of marijuana and discuss the benefits for sleep, and the disadvantages.

- Benefits of marijuana may be that it can help people fall asleep faster and get a deeper sleep.
- However, some disadvantages of marijuana use include:
  - difficulties waking up at a regular time;
  - less motivation during the day to study, work, exercise; and socialise;
  - possibility of becoming reliant on marijuana to go to sleep.

So, although marijuana may help deal with sleep problems in the short term, it can make sleep worse in the long term and make it harder to follow good sleep habits.

Activity 40: Effects of Drugs on Sleep

Do you use recreational drugs such as marijuana, meth, speed, heroin, or ecstasy? Let's now talk about the other drugs you are taking, and let's use the worksheet to write down some notes on their benefits and disadvantages.

- What are the benefits and disadvantage of drugs for you?
  - *Common advantages* to drugs can include having fun, a way to socialise, relaxing, a way to cope with stress, boredom, tiredness and low mood, can help with sleep onset.

- *Common disadvantages*, however, include expense, hangover in the morning, clumsiness, inability to make progress on valued goals, reduced productivity and energy, poor decision-making, poor concentration and memory, cravings, withdrawal symptoms, increased depressive symptoms, anxiety and paranoia, belief that it is not possible to cope without the drug.

- What may be some *strategies* to help reduce your use of these substances, so that you can start to sleep and feel better?
- On a scale of 0–10, how confident do you feel about applying these strategies?

Stress Management

Life Balance

A *balanced lifestyle* can have a very positive impact on sleep and fatigue. A balanced lifestyle involves 'everything in moderation'. This means not focusing on only one part of your life, to the detriment of other areas. It is also about making yourself a priority by doing things that bring you joy or satisfaction, and looking after your health with your diet and exercise. Stress management involves a balanced approach to life.

How satisfied are you with your life balance? In what ways do you feel it is out of balance?

In order to live a balanced lifestyle, it is important know what is important to you—what would be helpful to prioritise. Creating a balanced lifestyle involves being aware of what's important to you, what you value. If you're not living a life that reflects your values, it's more likely that it will feel stressful. We tend to be able to cope with difficulties better when they occur in pursuit of something that we truly value.

Activity 41: Stress Management: Values Exercise

This exercise aims to give you a better idea of what is important to you (in addition to managing your mental health). Considering what you value can be a helpful step in setting goals and focusing on aspects of life that can bring you happiness, peace, and/or satisfaction.

Close your eyes and say the first answer that pops into your mind for the following questions:

- What's important to me?
- What do I value?
- When do I feel happy or relaxed?
- I spend too much time worrying about . . .
- I spend too little time doing things such as . . .
- What I would like to do differently from today is . . .

Working towards Balance

Activity 42: Working towards Balance

With your answers to the above exercise in mind, identify any areas of your life that you feel are out of balance. These areas might include:

- health—physical or mental;
- hobbies, leisure;
- family, carers, friends;
- employment, study;
- money, finances;
- creativity;
- other.

Rate each of the above life areas according to whether you feel it is lacking, about right, or overpowering.

Can you select a top 2 from the list in your resource pack?

If you feel that one of the above areas is lacking or overpowering, think about what changes might be made and work towards small goals for change. It is helpful to check in with yourself regularly to think about your life balance, direction, and stress levels. If you're not living a life that reflects your values, it's more likely that it will feel stressful.

Activity 43: Things to Consider to Create Better Balance

On your worksheet, circle the areas on the table that you would like to make a change to and write about your possible changes/goals. (See Table 15.1).

Motivational prompts: If your illness was impacting on you less, what would you be doing differently? What could you do to move one step forward in that direction?

Table 15.1 Life Balance Plan

Area	*Immediate (Today)*	*Short term (Next Week)*	*Mid term (Next Month)*
Health			
Hobbies, leisure, holidays			
Family, carers, friends			
Work, study			
Money, finances			
Creativity			
Other:			

Coping with Demands

Activity 44: Coping with Demands

Did you know that there is both good stress and bad stress?

When demands seem too big to cope with, we feel overstressed. For example, people can become 'burnt out' and stressed by managing their illness. In contrast, too little stress, and inactivity lead to boredom and reduced interest and motivation. This can be referred to as 'rust-out' or 'couch potato' mode.

Did you know that not all stress is bad?

We all live with different amounts of stress in our lives and need a certain amount of stress to be motivated to function. We function best when we care about what we are doing. The optimal amount of stress varies from person to person. It can depend on personality, coping style, and the way our bodies respond to stress. Also, if we are working towards something that we really care about, we tend to be able to tolerate more stress.

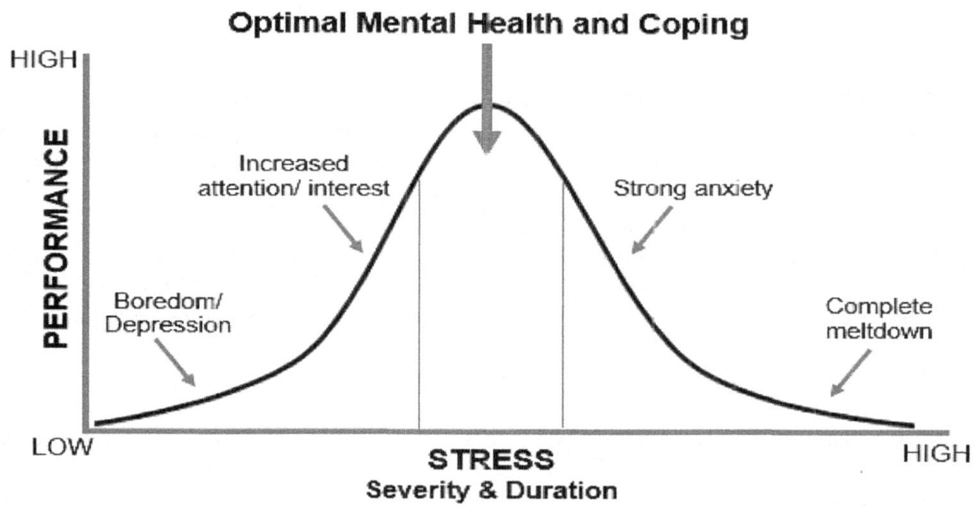

Figure 15.2 Not All Stress Is Bad

Looking at the graph in Figure 15.2, remember that it's OK to have some stress in your life. In fact, you need it to be active and engaged and to perform well, but you also need to make sure you have the coping skills to deal with stress.

Which best describes you? (See Table 15.3)

A person will feel distressed when the demands placed on them seem too big to cope with. So, stress can happen when there are too many demands, or when we feel that we don't have the right coping skills and assistance to deal with the demand.

Too many demands and expectations from others	➪	Demands *exceed* coping skills	➪	Burnt out/ Meltdown ("Overstressed")
Feeling productive and able to meet the tasks placed on me	➪	Demands are *equal* to coping skills	➪	Balance ("Good stress")
Having little to do and nothing to look forward to	➪	Demands are *too low* so coping skills are not challenged	➪	Couch Potato/ Bored ("Under-stressed")

Figure 15.3 Which Describes You Best?

Activity 45: My Coping Resources

What coping resources do you have for managing the following?

Managing overstress:

- How can you relax, problem-solve, get organised, worry less, seek support?
- What are your strengths? How can you make use of these?

- What are your main difficulties when it comes to dealing with stress? How can you manage these?

Therapist notes*: *Examples of internal coping resources *include relaxation or meditation skills; engaging in enjoyable activities such as craft; communication skills; time-management skills; managing worry; problem-solving; prioritising your health and happiness; setting limits and boundaries (e.g. saying 'no' when you need to); taking a daily break from technology (setting aside a time each day to disconnect from the phone, laptop, and emails); stress journal; taking up a new/old hobby.*

Examples of external coping resources *include support from family, housemates, friends, and recreational activities; talking to someone from the mental health team (e.g. psychiatrist, nurse, psychologist, occupational therapist, case manager); church or other community groups; choosing job opportunities where there is a positive, balanced work culture.*

Managing under-stress:

- How can you engage in activities and have something to look forward to? Hobbies (new or old)? Causes you care about (or used to care about)? Are there skills that you would like to do better in? Are there people you care about that you have not seen or caught up with for a long time?
- See Appendix 12 for ideas.

Therapist notes: *Under-stress, or 'couch potato mode', happens when clients have disengaged from major life areas. Clients often have problems with low motivation and negative affect, and this makes it harder for them to engage. Furthermore, some may have social anxiety that precludes them from engaging in community activities. It is important to tailor suggestions to the client's situation. After listing some ideas with the client, we suggest asking them to also rank which of the ideas they would be most likely to put into practice, and make a plan with steps to achieve this if they feel it would be helpful (e.g. scheduling activities in their diary, or having a support worker come visit them). Examples of ways in which some of our clients chose to re-engage include: volunteering at an animal shelter, joining a walking group, joining the church choir, learning guitar at a community drop-in centre, and taking up crocheting to make gifts for family and friends.*

Examples of internal resources *include prioritising your health and happiness; starting the day with a relaxing ritual (spend at least 15 minutes doing something that inspires you); taking up a new/old hobby; use activity scheduling (plan activities to do each day in a diary); employment or volunteering; learning something new (taking an online course or going to an information session).*

Examples of external resources *include visiting/calling/texting family and friends for a catch-up; taking pets for a walk or grooming them; joining the gym or a sports club; going out for a recreational activity (with a friend, peer support worker, or case manager); cleaning or reorganising an area of the house; participating in a group programme where you can learn new skills (e.g. computer course, stress management, cooking, language).*

Keeping Your Progress Going: Relapse Prevention

Well done on your progress through this programme! It's hard to make changes and takes guts to give it a go, so be proud of your effort!

It is so important now to keeping your progress going. Don't see this final session as the end of your sleep skills training; rather, see it as a springboard to the rest of your life where you can continue to learn and improve.

By now, you understand what was keeping your poor sleep and energy going, and you will also have practised some strategies to improve your sleep and reduce worry about sleep. It's now very important to spend time putting your new skills into practice on your own.

You can help keep progressing by making a plan for using the sleep skills you have learned. We will also consider what might get in the way of progress and make a plan for these setbacks.

Activity 46: Keeping Your Progress Going: Relapse Prevention

It's important to:

- read over what you have learned at least once a month, or if you notice your sleep deteriorating;
- plan for any setbacks that may happen;
- set goals to guide what you will do over the coming months;
- keep using the skills you learned in therapy;
- come back to your workbooks regularly to think of what you need to do to get your sleep back on track.

Knowing the difference between a bad night and a relapse: It is important to understand the difference between the odd bad night of sleep (or two or three), which everyone gets every now and then, and the signs that Insomnia may be coming back (e.g. ongoing poor sleep with no clear cause, together with unhelpful thoughts and behaviours creeping back in).

Planning for setbacks: It is very normal to have ups and downs in the quality and amount of your sleep. Recovery from Insomnia is a gradual process over time, and there will be ups and downs (see to Figure 15.4). Planning for triggers for poor sleep and energy can increase confidence moving forward and can prevent a short bout of poor sleep turning into a long-term problem again (see Activity 48).

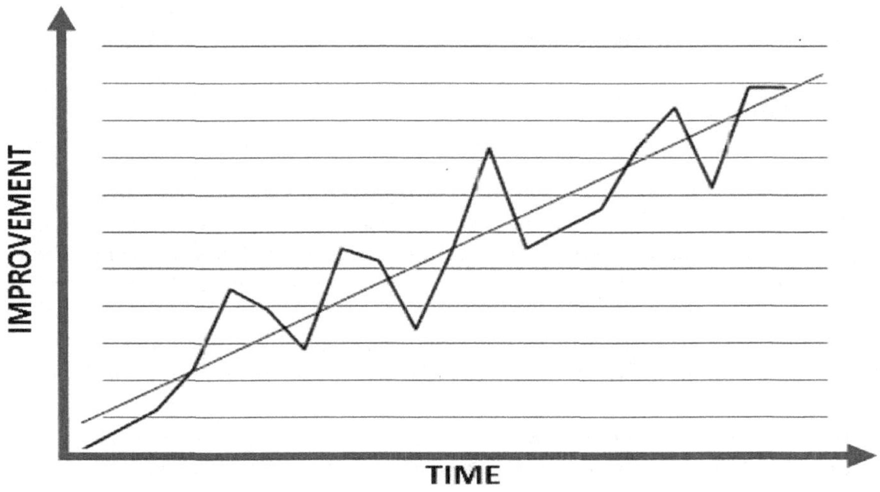

Figure 15.4 The Pattern of Recovery

Be realistic: Remember that it is unrealistic to expect to sleep well every single night. It is much more realistic to expect that you will have some periods of feeling like you are sleeping very well, and other phases where you feel that your sleep is more unstable. So, when you go through a period of more unsteady sleep, try not to become discouraged or concerned, and remember to stick to your sleep routine.

Activity 47: Blueprint Summary

Insomnia is like a weed. It can slowly grow from a trigger (the seed), then take hold and grow roots over time. When you leave it growing for long enough, it becomes difficult to uproot and can affect other areas of your life (the whole garden). One way of getting rid of the weed is to run over it with a lawn mower, which may provide a short-term fix (in the case of poor sleep and fatigue, this might be napping, sleeping in, or using cannabis or a sleeping pill to assist sleep). The problem is that the root of the problem is still there, and so the weed (poor sleep or tiredness) keeps growing. Until you get to the root of the problem, it will be there. The strategies in this programme help you to pull the problem out by its roots.

We have looked into the factors that have kept the sleep problem alive and have begun work on addressing each of these factors to provide a long-term solution. The strategies we have been learning over the sessions are much like pulling the weed out with its roots, to reduce its chance of coming back in the future. Use the Blueprint Summary worksheet to tie together what you have learned.

- How did the problem develop? (*What was the precipitating factor or trigger?*)
- What kept it going? (*The perpetuating factor: Draw on the barriers to sleep identified in the formulation.*)
- What did you learn during the programme about sleep and what is important in managing it?
- What were your most unhelpful habits and thoughts about sleep? (*If unsure, look back to answers on the DBAS scale in Activity 16 from the Client Resource Pack for Session 2.*)
- What are the alternatives to these?
- How will you build on what you have learned? What are the most important things to remember to keep your progress going?

Planning for Setbacks

Activity 48: Planning for Setbacks

Sleep and tiredness can worsen for a variety of reasons. It is normal to have some days when you feel tired and some nights when you don't sleep well. The odd night of poor sleep or the odd off day does not have to turn into a long-term problem if you know how to respond to it.

If you expect possible setbacks, then it becomes easier to prepare for them. Let's look at some 'high-risk' situations for you—i.e. factors that made your sleep and tiredness worse in the past.

There's no need for a setback to lead to a complete tumble back into Insomnia (i.e. relapse). A good way to reduce the impact of setbacks is to have a back-up plan of strategies to use when they occur. Setbacks remind you to use the skills that you have learned in therapy.

Let's talk about your triggers for poor sleep and tiredness:

- For example, 'after not sleeping well for a few nights, I've started to sleep in, get worried about my sleep and I'm feeling very tired during the day'.
- What can you do to plan ahead?

***Therapist notes**: Common triggers for poor sleep in this population include psychotic relapse, reduced mood, withdrawal effects from ceasing psychiatric or sleep medications, and temporary side effects of a new medication or recent depot injection (leading to severe daytime tiredness). Planning for excessive tiredness from medications (e.g. after monthly depot injection) may entail strategies for getting one's sleep routine and activity levels gradually back on track after a couple of days of increased sleep, and having regular check-up calls with the therapist or staff from the mental health team.*

The Motivational Boost: Facing Challenges

Activity 49: The Motivation Boost

If you're faced with a high-risk time with your sleep and tiredness, what do you plan to do? These ideas have been helpful to others in this situation:

- Remind yourself why you wanted to tackle your Insomnia in the first place—the reasons are probably just as relevant now as they were then.
- Talk to someone supportive (who would this be for you?).
- Think of what helped with improving your Insomnia in the past—chances are that whatever worked then will help you now too.

Action Plan and Goal Setting

Activity 50: Action Plan and Goal Setting

For the month ahead, set some goals (perhaps three at most) for your sleep and/or daytime energy and plan how you will go about this:

1. The changes I want to make (or continue making) are . . .
2. The reasons why I want to make these changes are . . .
3. I will know that my plan is working if . . .

Each day ask yourself: What can I do ***today*** *that will take me towards better sleep and away from Insomnia?*

Consider what things to do and what things to avoid or watch out for that will help you continue to sleep better.

References and Further Reading

Allison, K. C., Stunkard, A. J., and Thier, S. L. (2004) *Overcoming night eating syndrome: A step-by-step guide to breaking the cycle*. Oakland, CA: New Harbinger.

Barrowclough, C., Haddock, G., Lowens, I., Allot, R., Earnshaw, P., Fitzsimmons, M., and Nothard, S. (2007) 'Psychosis and drug and alcohol problems', in Baker, A., and Velleman, R. (Eds.) *Clinical handbook of co-existing mental health and drug and alcohol problems*. Hove, UK: Routledge, pp. 241–265.

Chan, S., and Yu, I. W. (2004) 'Quality of life of clients with schizophrenia', *Journal of Advanced Nursing*, 45(1), pp. 72–83.

Galletly, C. (2012) 'People living with psychosis: The good news and the bad news', *Australian & New Zealand Journal of Psychiatry*, 46(9), pp. 803–807.

Gregg, L., Barrowclough, C., and Haddock, G. (2007) 'Reasons for increased substance use in psychosis', *Clinical Psychology Review*, 27(4), pp. 494–510.

Gumley, A. I. (2013) 'CBT for relapse in schizophrenia: A treatment protocol', in Steel, C. (Ed.) *CBT for schizophrenia: Evidence-based interventions and future directions*. Chichester, UK: John Wiley, pp. 127–142.

Mentha, H. (2001) *Getting out of it: How to cut down or quit cannabis use*. Victoria, Australia: Inner East Community Health Service. Available at: www.menthaconsulting.com.au/images/pdfs/getting%20out%20of%20it.pdf (accessed December 2, 2016).

National Sleep Foundation (2014) *Cognitive behavioral therapy for insomnia*. Available at: http://sleepfoundation.org/sleep-news/cognitive-behavioral-therapy-insomnia (accessed July 15, 2014).

Part III

Client Resource Packs

16 Client Resource Pack Session 1

Learning about Sleep and Good Sleep Habits

Topics addressed this week:

- Activity 1: Identifying Goals and Motivations
- Activity 2: What Happens in Normal Sleep, and Common Sleep Complaints
- Activity 3: How Our Choices Affect Tiredness
- Activity 4: What Factors May Be Impacting on Your Sleep?
- Activity 5: Sleep Hygiene Checklist
- Activity 6: Winding Down Before Bed
- Activity 7: Getting Out of Bed if You Can't Sleep (GOOBICS)
- Activity 8: Which Stage Do You Think You're at Right Now in Terms of Treating Your Insomnia?
- Activity 9: The Main Things I Learned Today
- Activity 10: My Action Plan for the Week

Session 1: Learning about Sleep and Good Sleep Habits

Welcome!

Thank you for taking part in the sleep skills programme. We are confident that your sleep will improve as the treatment progresses.

Clients who have completed the programme have reported dramatic improvements in their sleep since starting the programme:

> 'I had a good night of sleep—I haven't had that for a long time.'
>
> 'I know that when I go to bed, I will eventually go to sleep.'
>
> 'I have more energy during the day.'
>
> 'I get a lot more time in my day.'
>
> 'I can cope better with my symptoms.'

What you should do to get the most out of this programme:

1. *Attend all the sessions*: The programme is here to help you achieve your goals. It is normal to have times when you don't feel like coming, but you will find that you often feel worse, rather than better, for not attending.
2. *Contribute*: Be willing to speak in an open and honest manner. Put your own issues forward and ask questions if you don't understand or you disagree with something that was said.
3. *Listen*: Some topics discussed may seem irrelevant to you now, but become useful later. The information that other people share in the sessions could also be helpful to you.
4. *Don't compare*: Remember that no two people are exactly the same. Even if two people have the same goals, what works for you might not work for them, and vice versa—so, develop some strategies that work for you.
5. *Maintain confidentiality in group sessions*: People must feel relaxed that what they say will remain confidential.
6. *Take responsibility*: Remember that, in therapy, 'What you put in is what you get out'. Being non-active in the programme tends to create little or no positive change.
7. *Review the sleep resources*: It is helpful to read over the material at home each week.
8. *Other*: ____

Topics Addressed this Week

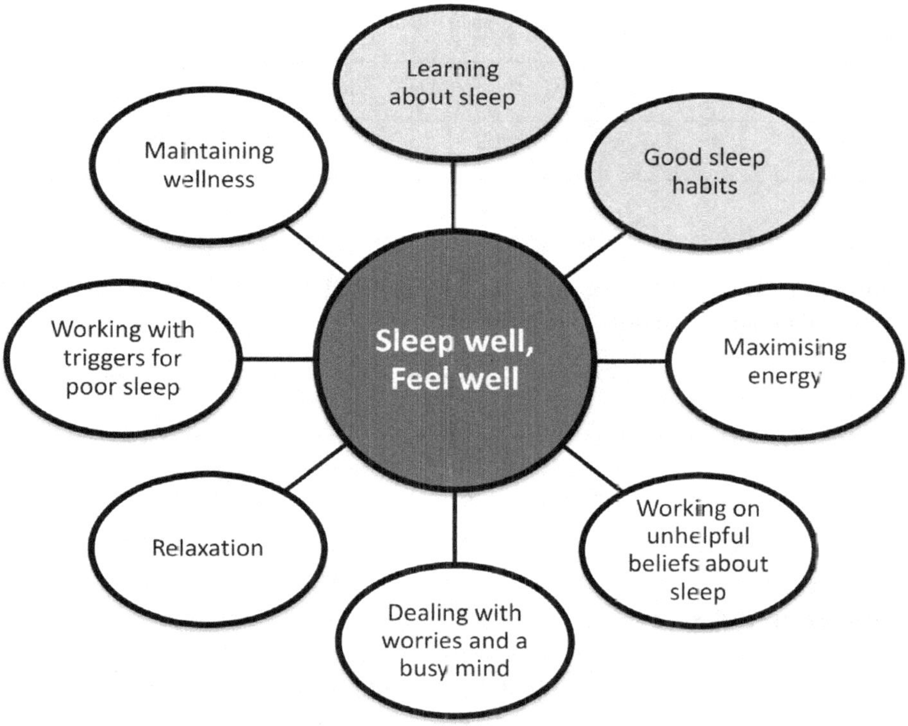

Activity 1: Identifying Goals and Motivations

My GOALS for the programme:

____

____

____

____

Why am I MOTIVATED to treat my Insomnia? How might sleeping better and having more energy improve things for me?

____

____

____

____

Importance Ruler

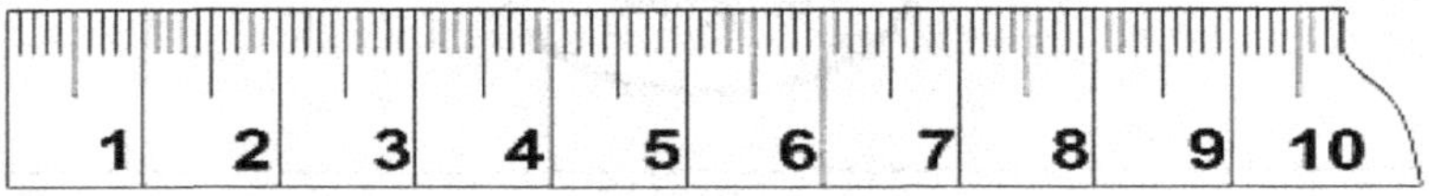

Not Important at all *Extremely Important*

On this scale of 0–10, how important it is for you to treat your poor sleep? _____

Activity 2: What Happens in Normal Sleep, and Common Sleep Complaints

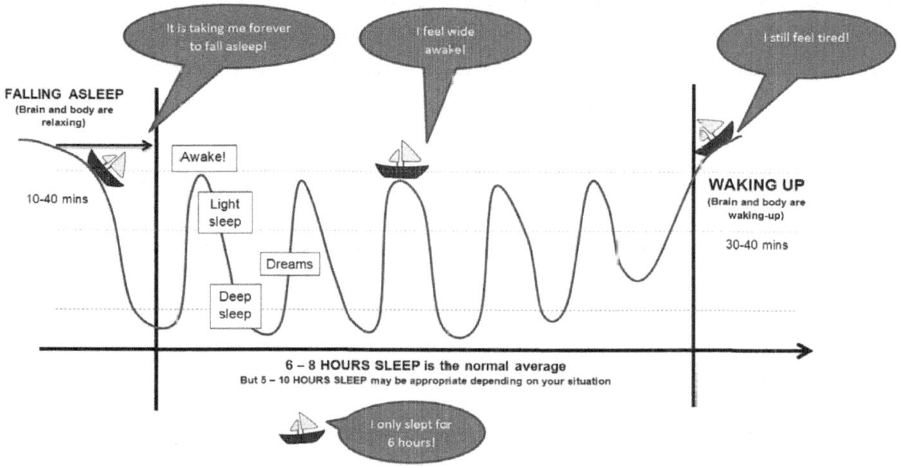

Activity 3: How Our Choices Affect Tiredness

How tired or sleepy (or lacking in energy) are you feeling, on a scale of 0–10?

<table>
<tr><th colspan="2">NO FATIGUE AT ALL</th><th colspan="2">MILD</th><th colspan="3">MODERATE</th><th colspan="2">EXTREME</th><th colspan="2">THE WORST FATIGUE</th></tr>
<tr><td>0</td><td>1</td><td>2</td><td>3</td><td>4</td><td>5</td><td>6</td><td>7</td><td>8</td><td>9</td><td>10</td></tr>
</table>

- *Right now?* Rating = _____
- How do you rate your tiredness after doing a bit of *reading*? Rating = _____
- How do you rate your tiredness after *a short walk or other increase in activity*? Rating = _____

As we can see from this short activity, energy levels and sleepiness change over the course of the day. Lots of factors bring this about and can be affected by the choices we make.

Activity 4: What Factors May Be Impacting on Your Sleep?

What do you notice might help you to sleep better?

- ______________________________
- ______________________________
- ______________________________
- ______________________________

When do you sleep worse?

- ______________________________
- ______________________________
- ______________________________
- ______________________________

What do you think leads to better daytime energy?

- ______________________________
- ______________________________
- ______________________________

What do you think leads to less daytime energy?

- ______________________________
- ______________________________
- ______________________________

Activity 5: Sleep Hygiene Checklist

Complete the checklist below to see what sleep hygiene factors you may need to work on.

Things that Can Make Sleep Worse

About the bedroom and environment:

- ❒ Noise late at night or early in the morning (pets, street noise).
- ❒ Not having a set place that is just for sleeping (e.g. sleeping on the couch).
- ❒ Untidy, cluttered, or unclean sleeping space that makes you feel restless.

During the day:

- ❒ Staying inside your living accommodation all day (no real daylight).
- ❒ Staying in bed long after waking up.
- ❒ Taking long naps.
- ❒ Limited daytime activity.

One to two hours before bed:

- ❒ Watching TV in bed.
- ❒ Using computer or electronic device (phone, iPhone, iPad).
- ❒ Having drinks that contain caffeine (tea, coffee, energy drinks).
- ❒ Having a cigarette before sleep.
- ❒ Drinking alcohol.
- ❒ Eating a heavy meal.
- ❒ Taking illicit drugs.

During the night:

- ❒ Watching the clock! (Turn the clock face away so that you cannot see it.)

Things that Can Make Sleep Better

About the bedroom and environment:

- ❒ Comfortable bed and pillow with appropriate covers (light in summer, heavy in winter).

continued . . .

Activity 5: Continued

- ❒ Warm bed, dark room (or only low light).
- ❒ Quiet.

During the day:

- ❒ Getting in some bright light each day (being outdoors).
- ❒ Increased activity—walking, running, cycling, sports, tidying, cleaning, hobbies, cooking.
- ❒ Social contact (friends family, carers, or just saying hello to the cashier at the shops).
- ❒ Set aside 'worry time' to put any issues that are bothering you to rest until the next day (write about the worries or make a to-do list of what needs to be done tomorrow).

At least 1 hour before bed:

- ❒ Have a relaxing bedtime routine (e.g. read, brush teeth, shower, do a puzzle).
- ❒ Set your alarm clock for the next day.
- ❒ Relaxation (breathing exercises, imagery, soothing music).

Activity 6: Winding Down Before Bed

Making a Bedtime Routine

	Example of Wind-Down Activities	*My Wind-Down Activities Will Be:*
1 hour before bed	Reading	______
	Listening to music	______
	Sewing/knitting	______
	Shower	______
	Drawing	______
	Doing a puzzle	______
	Relaxation exercise	______
	Warm bath	______
	Light snack	______
	Gentle stretching	______
At bedtime	Brush teeth	______
	Go to the toilet	______
	Relaxation exercise	______
	Switch on alarm clock	______

Barriers to Bedtime Routine

What Might Get in the Way of My Routine?	*How Can I Address this?*
______	______
______	______
______	______

Activity 7: Getting Out of Bed if You Can't Sleep (GOOBICS)

GOOBICS is very useful if you have trouble falling asleep. It teaches your mind to make the bed and bedroom positive triggers for sleep, so that you can expect to fall asleep easily when you go to bed or wake up in the night. To learn this skill, follow these five Steps:

Step 1. Only use the bedroom for sleep	Do not use your bedroom for activities such as eating, watching TV, smoking, talking on the phone, working, or arguing
Step 2. Only go to bed when sleepy	Only go to bed when you feel sleepy, not because of a set routine. You take much longer to get to sleep if you go to bed before feeling sleepy or drowsy
Step 3. Get out of bed when you can't sleep	If you do not fall asleep within about 30 minutes after going to bed and turning off the lights, *and* you are feeling restless, frustrated, or anxious: Get out of bed, go to another room, and do something relaxing. When you feel sleepy, go back to bed and try again to fall asleep. If you do not fall asleep quickly, repeat this step again. You should not try hard to fall asleep

What should I do while I'm out of bed?

____

____

Step 4. Get out of bed at the same time each day	This includes weekends, even when you stay up at night later than usual. If you set your alarm for a regular wake-up time, you will be more likely to get sleepy at about the right time each night to allow yourself to get the sleep you need. Choose a rising time that suits your usual situation

My chosen rising time *will be between* _____ *and* _____

What will I do when I first wake up to help me wind up into the day?

____

____

Step 5. Avoid or reduce daytime napping	Sleeping in the day weakens your need for sleep at night. Aim to reduce daytime naps. Ideally, naps should be 30 minutes or less and before 2 p.m. Set an alarm to help you not oversleep. Discuss with your therapist what might be realistic for you

Activity 8: Which Stage Do You Think You're at Right Now in Terms of Treating Your Insomnia?

Show this on this diagram:

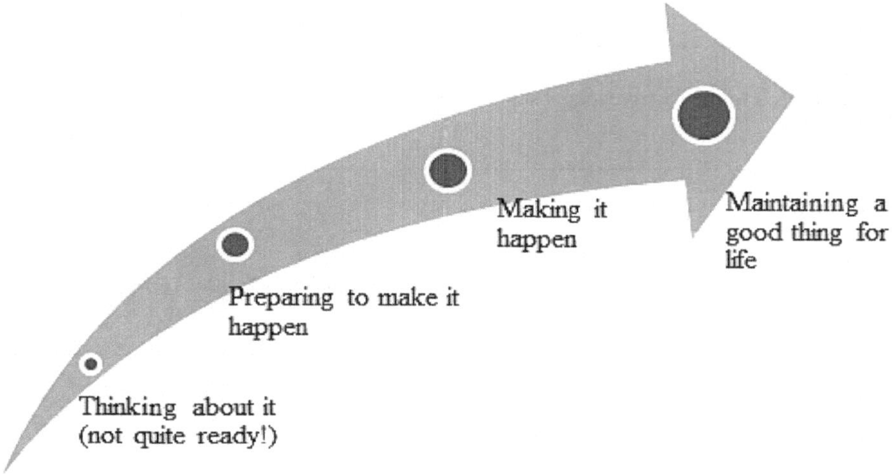

Making changes to improve your sleep may be hard, but we will be here to help you through this.

Activity 9: The Main Things I Learned Today

- ____
- ____
- ____
- ____
- ____
- ____

Activity 10: My Action Plan for the Week

1. What I will do for wind-down before bed?

   ____

   ____

2. Some changes to my sleep hygiene or environment that I may start making:

   ____

   ____

3. What will I do when I get up because I can't fall asleep/get back to sleep quickly?

   ____

   ____

4. My regular wake-up time for *each* morning will be: ______

5. My goal for napping this week is to nap for ______ (hours/minutes), no later than ______ (time of day).

6. Activities I can engage in instead of napping include:

   ____

   ____

Confidence Ruler

On this scale of 0–10, how confident are you about trying out your action plan for the week? _____

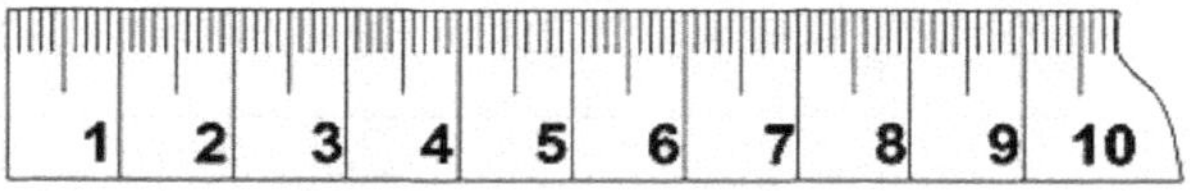

Not Confident at all *Extremely Confident*

17 Client Resource Pack Session 2

Maximising Energy and Working with Unhelpful Beliefs about Sleep

Topics addressed this week:

- Activity 11: A Review of Skills We Have Been Learning
- Activity 12: Sources of Daytime Tiredness
- Activity 13: How Behaviour and Activity Affect Energy Levels
- Activity 14: How Can We Generate Energy during the Day?
- Activity 15: Use of Bright Light during the Day
- Activity 16: Beliefs about Sleep
- Activity 17: Seven Strategies to Manage Unpleasant Images and Nightmares
- Activity 18: Sleep and Mental Health
- Activity 19: The Main Things I Learned today
- Activity 20: My Action Plan for the Week

Session 2: Maximising Energy and Working with Unhelpful Beliefs about Sleep

Topics Addressed this Week

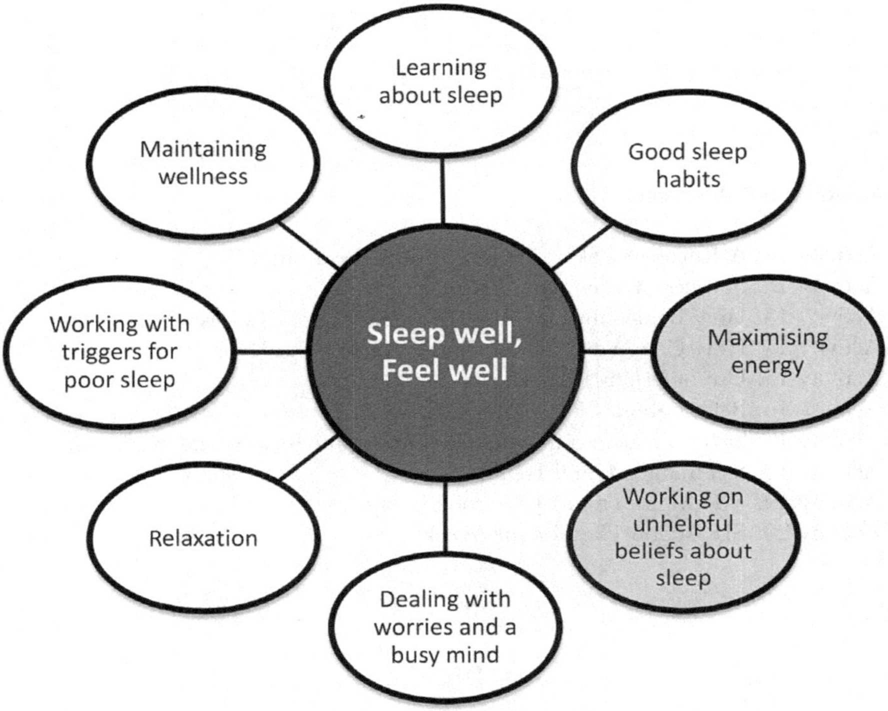

Activity 11: A Review of Skills We Have Been Learning

Last week we learned about:

- facts about sleep;
- sleep hygiene (everyday habits to improve sleep at night);
- winding down before bed (to help fall asleep);
- getting out of bed if you can't sleep (GOOBICS);
- having a regular wake-up time (not oversleeping and limiting naps);
- winding up into the day.

What went well?

____

____

____

What was challenging?

____

____

____

Let's brainstorm ways to get around these challenges:

____

____

____

Activity 12: Sources of Daytime Tiredness

Sources of tiredness and low energy levels

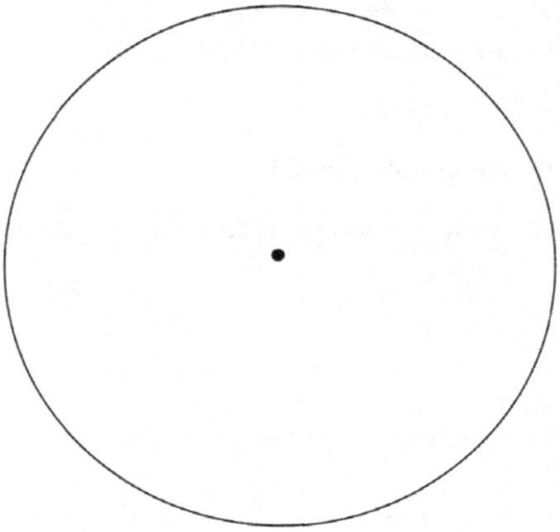

☐ ____________________
☐ ____________________
☐ ____________________
☐ ____________________
☐ ____________________
☐ ____________________
☐ ____________________
☐ ____________________
☐ ____________________
☐ ____________________

Activity 13: How Behaviour and Activity Affect Energy Levels

First, how energised are you feeling *now*, on a scale of 0–10 (please circle)?

NO ENERGY AT ALL					MODERATELY ENERGETIC					EXTREMELY ENERGETIC
0	1	2	3	4	5	6	7	8	9	10

Try a couple of these quick activities:

- Go for a short walk around the building or do some star jumps.
- Have a small, healthy snack (e.g. a piece of fruit).
- Tell some jokes.
- Stretch your neck, arm, legs.
- Have a cold drink.
- Get into some light.
- Listen to some music that makes you feel happy or energised.
- Watch a video that makes you laugh.

Now, how do you rate your energy levels after trying these activities? Was one activity more effective than another (please circle)?

NO ENERGY AT ALL					MODERATELY ENERGETIC					EXTREMELY ENERGETIC
0	1	2	3	4	5	6	7	8	9	10

We should find that tiredness levels decrease as activity increases.

Activity 14: How Can We Generate Energy during the Day?

That's right: It is possible to *generate* energy during the day! Often, people think that doing activity will take energy away and make them feel more tired, but actually there are many forms of activity that you can do to help you feel more energised.

Energy-**generating** activities and strategies to **try out during the week** (*what I should do*):

- ______________________________
- ______________________________
- ______________________________
- ______________________________

Energy-**depleting** activities and behaviours to **minimise** (*what I should avoid*):

- ______________________________
- ______________________________
- ______________________________
- ______________________________

Activity 15: Use of Bright Light during the Day

Exposure to bright light during the day has many benefits, including:

- aligning your body clock with the time of the day;
- improved mood;
- improved alertness and concentration.

For good, natural sleep, it is important to have both a healthy sleep routine and a body clock that works at the right time. Morning exposure to bright light (i.e. 30 minutes of natural sunlight) helps to reduce drowsiness and increase alertness for the day by reducing the level of hormones that usually make our bodies feel sleepy at night (e.g. melatonin).

To help your body clock, make sure you get in some bright light (sunlight or a light box) each day. You may even find that getting more sunlight during the day improves your mood.

If you feel very tired most mornings, try getting some sunlight after waking up to help start your day (e.g. take a walk or have breakfast outside, in the sun).

What things can I do to get more light during the day?

- ____
- ____
- ____
- ____

What things can I do to reduce bright lights at night?

- ____
- ____
- ____
- ____

Activity 16: Beliefs about Sleep

The statements below reflect some beliefs and attitudes that people may have about sleep. Show how much you agree or disagree with these statements by placing a mark (/) along the line to reflect your answer for each.

1. When I don't get a proper amount of sleep on a given night, I need to catch up on the next day by napping or by sleeping longer the next night.

Strongly Disagree ⟵⟶ Strongly Agree

2. I am worried that, if I go for one or two nights without sleep, I may have a nervous breakdown.

Strongly Disagree ⟵⟶ Strongly Agree

3. I have little ability to manage the negative consequences of disturbed sleep.

Strongly Disagree ⟵⟶ Strongly Agree

4. When I feel tired, have no energy, or just seem not to function well during the day, it is generally because I did not sleep well the night before.

Strongly Disagree ⟵⟶ Strongly Agree

5. Medication is probably the only solution to sleeplessness.

Strongly Disagree ⟵⟶ Strongly Agree

6. The only way to improve my energy is to rest or sleep more.

Strongly Disagree ⟵⟶ Strongly Agree

7. I believe Insomnia is essentially the result of a *chemical imbalance.*

Strongly Disagree ⟵⟶ Strongly Agree

Establishing Helpful Beliefs about Sleep

Unhelpful Belief	***Helpful Thoughts and Strategies to Try Instead***
When I don't get a proper amount of sleep on a given night, I need to catch up the next day by napping or by sleeping longer the next night	If we always try to catch up on lost sleep by napping or sleeping longer the next night, this may actually make it harder for us to get into a good sleep pattern. A good sleep pattern is important for helping to relieve Insomnia Try generating energy by going for a walk or eating something healthy instead If you do need to nap, keep it short (less than 30 minutes, ideally) and more than 8 hours before you go to bed that night
I am worried that if I go for one or two nights without sleep, I may have a nervous breakdown	Worrying about not having enough sleep can make it even harder to get to sleep at night Winding down each night will help you start feeling more relaxed again and sleep better Although short-term lack of sleep can make mood and anxiety worse, it generally won't lead to a nervous breakdown. Remember that, if you can stay relaxed, poor sleep on one night will make it more likely you will sleep better the next night (as your body will want to catch up) There are things you can do during the day to help prevent worse mood and anxiety. For example, talk to someone about worries, get some light exercise, or try relaxation strategies
The only way to improve my energy is to rest or sleep more	There are actually lots of ways to improve your energy, aside from sleep, such as doing some exercise or eating a healthy snack (e.g. apple, banana, celery, carrots, oats, nuts, and dried fruit)
I have little ability to manage the negative consequences of disturbed sleep	We can't force sleep to happen, but there are many things we can do to set up good conditions for sleep and lessen the impact of poor sleep on health Research shows that people with Insomnia *can* successfully learn to manage their sleep using various skills and coping strategies. This programme aims to teach you these skills. Can you tell me a couple of ideas?

continued . . .

Establishing Helpful Beliefs about Sleep . . . Continued

Unhelpful Belief	***Helpful Thoughts and Strategies to Try Instead***
When I feel tired, have no energy, or just seem not to function well during the day, it is generally because I did not sleep well the night before	Poor sleep can lead to feeling more tired and less energetic during the day, but is not always the main culprit Think about what other factors could also be making you feel tired and less energetic, such as: exercise levels, diet, hormones, medications, or boredom, etc.
Medication is probably the only solution to sleeplessness	Medications are not the only solution to sleeplessness. Making some healthy changes to our thinking and lifestyle is often just as useful. Remind yourself that sometimes other good solutions just take a bit more time and practice
I believe Insomnia is essentially the result of a chemical imbalance	It is not helpful to focus solely on external causes for your sleep problem, as they are not in your control Regardless of the initial cause of your Insomnia, there are likely to be things that you could change about your thinking and daily habits to improve your sleep and daytime energy

Activity 17: Seven Strategies to Manage Unpleasant Images and Nightmares

1. *Stop*: Clap hands while saying 'Stop!'.

2. *Breathe*: Breathe in deeply, and exhale the image away.

3. *Ground yourself*: Open your eyes, put your feet on the floor, and focus on your immediate environment. Perhaps turn on a dim light. What can you see, feel, hear, and smell?

4. *Talk it out*: Talk to a friend or family member about the images or nightmares.

5. *Write it down*: Write down images or nightmares in a diary.

6. *Acknowledge and move on*: Without accepting or denying, *acknowledge* the unpleasant image and then *return to the pleasant ones*.

7. *Choose*: Consciously *choose* to return to the pleasant images without feeling that it is a struggle to do so.

What are some pleasant images that you can think of?

- ______________________________
- ______________________________
- ______________________________

Reference

Krakow, B. (2002) *Turning nightmares into dreams: The authorized audio series and treatment workbook for New Dream Therapy* [CDs]. USA: The New Sleepy Times.

Activity 18: Sleep and Mental Health

Many people believe that their sleep problem cannot get better because of their mental health problems. This belief can leave people feeling powerless and reduce motivation to be active in searching for solutions to tackle the sleep problem.

- *On a scale of 0–10, how much do you believe that having a mental illness makes your sleep unchangeable?* _____

If you scored 6 or above, let's think about how this belief may be unhelpful, and whether it forms part of your cycle of Insomnia.

Mental health problems are often linked to difficulties with sleep. However, this does not mean that your Insomnia will not get better. It is important to know that your sleep can be improved—you just need a little time and the right tools to help you with it!

Symptom Safety Plan

What do I do if I notice my symptoms (voices, visions, etc.) getting worse as a result of the sleep skills I'm trying?

1. Let the group facilitator know as soon as you can.
2. Talk to a family member, friend, or case manager about it.
3. Write about it in the comments section of your sleep diary for the week.

Activity 19: The Main Things I Learned Today

- ______________________________
- ______________________________
- ______________________________
- ______________________________
- ______________________________
- ______________________________

Activity 20: My Action Plan for the Week

1. Continue winding down before bed.

2. Continue with GOOBICS.

3. My regular rising time for *each* morning is: __________

4. Changes to my sleep hygiene that I will work towards:

    ____

    ____

5. Plan for generating energy this week:

    ____

    ____

6. Main unhelpful 'beliefs about sleep' to be aware of:

    ____

    ____

7. Work with nightmares (if applicable).

Confidence Ruler

Imagine that this ruler shows how confident you are that you can improve your sleep. On this scale of 0–10, where are you at now?

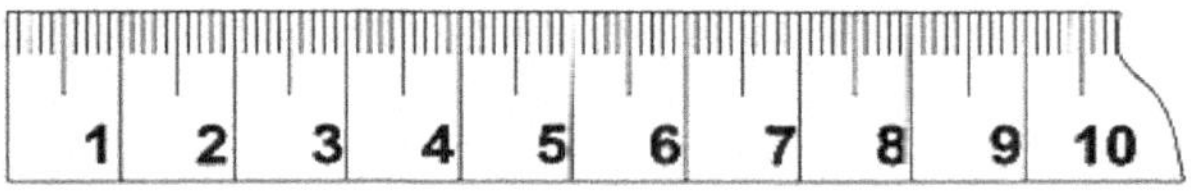

Not Confident at all *Extremely Confident*

Remind yourself of the positive things that you've learned over the week to help motivate your sleep skills training.

18 Client Resource Pack Session 3

Managing Worries and a Busy Mind and Introducing Relaxation

Topics addressed this week:

- Activity 21: A Review of Skills We Have Been Learning
- Activity 22: The Clock Watching Experiment
- Activity 23: How the Mind Affects Sleep (1): Low Mood and Anxiety
- Activity 24: How the Mind Affects Sleep (2): Intrusive Thoughts that Go Endlessly Round and Round
- Activity 25: How the Mind Affects Sleep (3): Voices, Visions, or other Unusual Sensations
- Activity 26: Linking Thoughts and Feelings
- Activity 27: Another Example of the Link between Thoughts and Feelings
- Activity 28: Becoming Aware of Negative Thoughts
- Activity 29: Managing Negative Thoughts
- Activity 30: Negative Thoughts Record (Catch It)
- Activity 31: Managing Unhelpful Thoughts Worksheet (Check It and Change It)
- Activity 32: Managing a Busy Mind at Night
- Activity 33: Relaxation Exercises
- Activity 34: The Main Things I Learned Today
- Activity 35: My Action Plan for the Week

Session 3: Managing Worries and a Busy Mind and Introducing Relaxation

Topics Addressed this Week

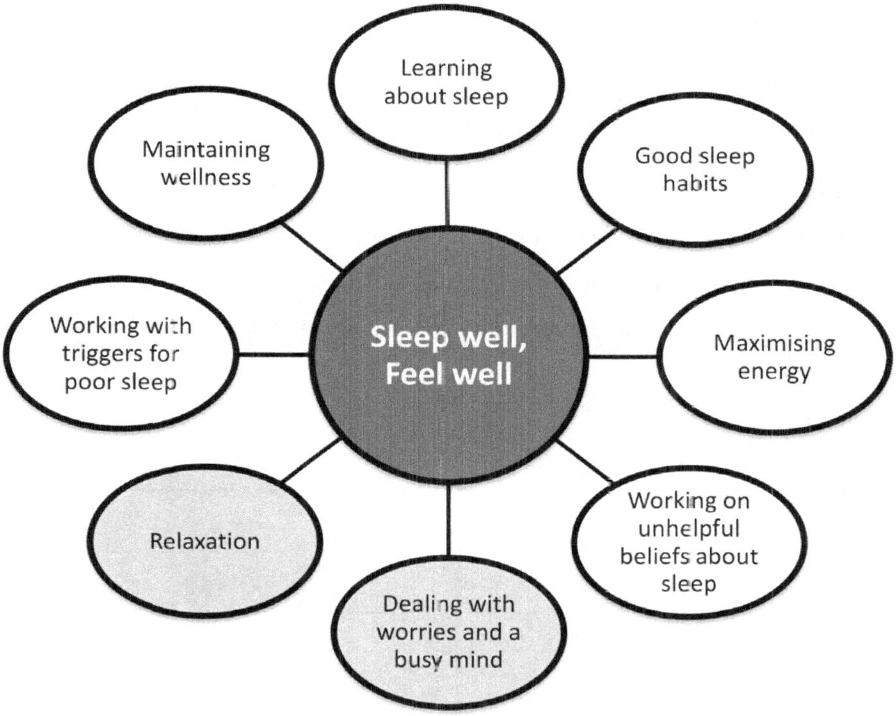

Activity 21: A Review of Skills We Have Been Learning

Last week we learned about:

- maximising daytime energy;
- establishing helpful beliefs and attitudes about sleep;
- managing nightmares.

The other sleep skills we have also been learning are:

- sleep hygiene (everyday habits to help us sleep better at night);
- winding down before bed (to help fall asleep);
- getting out of bed if you can't sleep (GOOBICS);
- having a regular wake-up time (not oversleeping and limiting naps) and winding up into the day.

What went well?

____

____

____

What was challenging?

____

____

____

Let's brainstorm ways to get around these challenges:

____

____

____

Activity 22: The Clock Watching Experiment

When we are anxious about falling asleep, we naturally tend to check the time to see how long we have been awake for, and how much sleep we are likely to get. This can lead to predictions and worries about what the following day will be like.

The Cycle of Clock Watching at Night

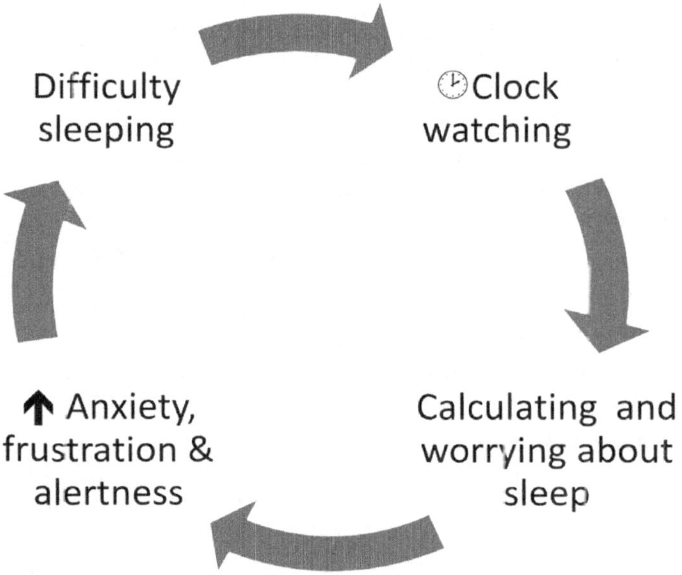

The Clock Watching Experiment

If you watch the clock at all overnight, try this experiment to test whether clock watching is helpful or unhelpful:

1. One night, watch the clock as normal.
2. The next night, put the clock/phone under your bed or cover it somehow so that you won't be able to look at it (but can still hear the alarm).
3. In the morning, note down whether you looked at the clock or not, and how you slept.

Most people find that it is not helpful to look at the clock over the night!

Whether it is 11 p.m., 2 a.m., or 4 a.m., we want you to do the same thing. Knowing the time should not change your strategy. Relax and let sleep happen.

Activity 23: How the Mind Affects Sleep (1): Low Mood and Anxiety

Sometimes, people may find it hard to sleep because of many sad thoughts and memories, or they are feeling very anxious in bed (e.g. feeling of dry mouth, heart racing, and feeling panicky). Sometimes, people have thoughts that make them feel paranoid or scared to go to sleep at night.

It is important to recognise when this is happening, so that you can find ways of managing low mood or anxiety before it ruins your sleep.

Here are some tips for how to help lighten your mood at night, so that you can get into bed feeling more relaxed and peaceful (*tick those you may like to use*):

- ❐ Don't be too hard on yourself. Everyone has bad days.
- ❐ Give yourself permission to write this off as one bad day and look to have a better day tomorrow. What might you be able to put in place to help make tomorrow better?
- ❐ Speak to people who make you feel positive. This could be family, friends, a helpline, or online forum members.
- ❐ Make a list of the things you're grateful for.
- ❐ Concentrate on the here and now (what can you see, hear, touch, smell?) and just breathe.
- ❐ Do something that comforts and relaxes the body and the mind. This can be cooking a favourite meal, taking a warm bath, lighting a candle, cuddling a soft toy, wearing your favourite pyjamas, gently stretching, listening to music, or reading a book.
- ❐ Organise your problems. Spend a few minutes problem-solving and then make a point of putting the problems aside for today and coming back to them tomorrow. Give yourself permission to let them go.
- ❐ Try and take your mind off things by doing an activity you don't do often—rearrange your furniture, get some flowers in the house, change the bedsheets, or visit a neighbour.
- ❐ Compile a 'happy box' of different possessions and trinkets that make you feel relaxed and happy or bring positive memories—for example, a favourite DVD, nail polish, magazine, photo album, scented candles, relaxation CD, or puzzle book.
- ❐ Do a fun activity (see Appendix 12).

What else can you do when you start feeling down and depressed or anxious at night?

____

____

Activity 24: How the Mind Affects Sleep (2): Intrusive Thoughts that Go Endlessly Round and Round

Many people also experience negative, intrusive, or recurrent thoughts at night that are hard to switch off. These thoughts can make it hard to get to sleep.

Here are some tips for dealing with intrusive thoughts (*tick those you may like to use*):

- ❑ Label the thoughts as 'intrusive thoughts'. For example, say to yourself, 'I'm having an intrusive thought'.
- ❑ Remind yourself that you can practise choosing not to engage with the thought (e.g. 'I don't have to change, argue with, or get rid of this thought').
- ❑ Remind yourself that everyone has intrusive thoughts from time to time. It is OK for the thought to be there, even if you don't like it. You can choose not to become tangled up in the thought.
- ❑ Use relaxation and meditation exercises.
- ❑ Take a few slow, deep breaths.
- ❑ Repeat a phrase or 'mantra'—for example, words such as 'calm and relaxed', over and over.
- ❑ Recite a soothing poem or prayer.
- ❑ Have a poster or a note by your bed with reassuring messages written on it to read when you are woken up (e.g. 'This experience is temporary and will pass').
- ❑ Try using a 'worry box'—write down your worries and place them into a box to deal with in the morning.

What else can you do about negative and intrusive thoughts at night?

Once you have carried out one or two of the above strategies, return your attention to whatever you were doing before the thought bothered you. As best you can, fully engage in the activity and pay full attention to it.

Keep trying. This work takes practice and patience.

Activity 25: How the Mind Affects Sleep (3): Voices, Visions, or Other Unusual Sensations

It is common for people with voices, visions, and other experiences to report that their voices are worse at night, and that they are unable to use their usual coping strategies at night-time, such as going for a walk. Some people may even find that voices, visions, or other feelings wake them up in the middle of the night.

Here are a few tips from the *Hearing Voices Network* on what to do about voices, visions, and other experiences that disturb sleep (*tick those you may like to use*):

- ❒ Converse with the voice, explaining that now is not the time to be talking, but that you can talk again tomorrow.
- ❒ Listen to and focus on the calming voice of an audiobook.
- ❒ Listen to the radio or watch TV on low volume.
- ❒ Listen to 'white noise' (e.g. the sound of a fan).
- ❒ Wear earplugs.
- ❒ Sing a song or read out loud.
- ❒ Get up, go to another room, and start an activity.
- ❒ Try sleeping with a dim light, using a night light or glow-in-the-dark stars.
- ❒ Wear eye shades (e.g. sunglasses, night mask) if visions are disturbing you at night.
- ❒ Use visualisation techniques (e.g. imagining a protective force field to fend off unwanted visions or voices).
- ❒ For bodily sensations (e.g. feeling insects crawling, pain, feeling your limbs change shape), try switching the light on so that you can see the affected area or try massaging the affected area gently.

Note: It might also be useful to get a time switch on TVs, radios, and other digital devices, so that they will turn themselves off after a set time. This helps to save electricity and prevents them from disturbing your sleep later in the night.

What else can you do about hearing voices or seeing visions when they keep you awake at night?

____

____

Activity 26: Linking Thoughts and Feelings

Most people assume that the events in their everyday lives directly cause their feelings. For example:

- If we're running late for an appointment, we may feel anxious or annoyed.
- If someone gives us a compliment, we may feel happy.

An important part that we usually miss is the *interpretation* of what an event *means* to us (i.e. what thoughts we had about the event). Our thoughts help us to understand our emotional reaction.

Events or situations by themselves do not create emotions. In other words:

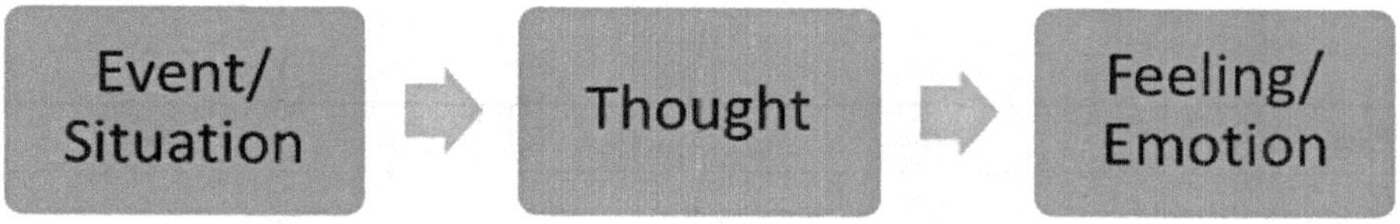

To see how this process happens, look at the following example:

Event/Situation	*Thought: What Are the Thoughts that Might Make You Feel . . .*	*Feelings*
Imagine you are at a party and wave at a friend across the room. They don't respond to you.	. . . ________________	Angry?
	. . . ________________	Embarrassed or sad.
	. . . ________________	Calm?

In the example in the table, there are many different ways of reacting, because the situation is unclear. It is the person's thoughts about the situation that determine how they feel. Therefore:

Thoughts are a clue to understanding emotions.

- You can understand your moods better by looking at the thoughts you have had whenever your mood has changed.

It is helpful to learn to manage unhelpful thoughts during the day and the night to improve sleep and daytime tiredness.

Activity 27: Another Example of the Link between Thoughts and Feelings

We've just been learning about the link between thoughts and feelings. Now, let's see how this link can be applied to poor sleep.

What might Mary's thoughts be in the example below? The situation is waking up in the morning after a poor night of sleep and feeling nervous and upset.

Mary: When I noticed my eyes feeling sore and my brain feeling foggy, I remembered that I hadn't slept well last night. That made me feel nervous about whether I would be able to sleep tonight, and if I'd cope the next day. I guess I then worried that there was nothing I could do to feel better and that made me feel upset.

Event/Situation	*Thought*	*Feelings*
Didn't sleep well last night	Mary thought that:	
	• ______________________	Nervous
	• ______________________	
Noticed eyes feeling sore, and brain feeling foggy	• ______________________	Upset

Most of us would feel nervous and upset if we thought that not getting enough sleep would lead to not coping, sleeping poorly the next night, and not being able to do anything about it. Now we can better understand her feelings.

It is helpful to be able to spot thoughts that are *overly* negative, as they can have a big impact on how we feel.

Activity 28: Becoming Aware of Negative Thoughts

Thoughts can occur automatically and come in the form of:

- words (e.g. 'I'll never be able to sleep, I can't cope');
- images (e.g. seeing yourself tossing and turning in bed).

The questions in the figure can help you catch and resolve negative automatic thoughts.

SITUATION

What exactly is happening at this moment?

⇩

FEELINGS

What am/was I feeling?

⇩

THOUGHTS

What is/was making me feel this way?	*What do I think might happen?*	*What would be so bad about that?*	*What am I thinking about myself right now?*

Ask yourself these questions until you have identified the thoughts that help you understand your emotional reaction. You may need to ask yourself these questions two or three times to uncover the automatic thoughts.

See if you can become more aware of negative thoughts this week and notice the impact they have on your mood.

If you notice an overly negative thought, remind yourself that this is just a thought or opinion, not a fact. You can choose whether or not you listen to the thought.

- What thoughts do you have when you haven't slept well?
- What thoughts to do you have when you are having trouble sleeping at night?
- Do you notice the same thing during the day?
- What do you feel like doing after experiencing these thoughts and feelings?

Activity 29: Managing Negative Thoughts

How can we change the thoughts and feelings that interfere with sleep and getting activated during the day?

The benefit of learning that thoughts, not situations, create feelings is that *it is then possible to manage feelings by changing thoughts.*

To address unhelpful thoughts, we need to apply **the 3 Cs**.

The 3 Cs	
Catch it	Identify the unhelpful, overly negative or intrusive thought
Check it	Identify evidence that supports and disputes the thought
Change it	Change the thought so that it is more accurate and helpful

Having Trouble with the 3 Cs?

Try writing down what is bothering you on a piece of paper or in a journal, or try one of the strategies already discussed today. Writing down or drawing your thoughts and feelings can often have a positive effect on dealing with negative thoughts.

Writing down or drawing thoughts and feelings can have a positive effect, as it may you help to:

- become aware of the link between thoughts and feelings;
- detach from the thought/image, get some distance, and assist in making the thought feel less intense;
- manage the negative thought/image by developing a new perspective that could be more helpful.

Worksheets

You can also try using the next two worksheets on the following pages to help you manage negative thoughts.

- The *Negative Thoughts Record* (Catch It) can be used to help identify overly negative thoughts and feelings.
- The *Managing Unhelpful Thoughts* (Check It and Change It) worksheet can help you check and change unhelpful thoughts related to sleep.

Activity 30: Negative Thoughts Record (Catch It)

The Negative Thoughts Record is used to catch overly negative thoughts. Use it by noting down the thoughts/images you are having when you are experiencing difficult emotions (e.g. feeling down, guilty, scared, or anxious).

Thoughts and Images	***Feelings***
Write Down the Unhelpful Thought or Image that Is Going through Your Mind	*Tick how the Thought/Image Makes You Feel*
	Positive feelings: ❒ Happy ❒ Content ❒ Excited Negative feelings: ❒ Weak/useless ❒ Guilty/ashamed ❒ Angry/frustrated ❒ Anxious/scared ❒ Sad/depressed Others: ❒ ______________ ❒ ______________ ❒ ______________ Rate how strong the feeling(s) you've ticked is from 0 to 10 (circle below): 0 1 2 3 4 5 6 7 8 9 10 Not strong at all Extremely strong

Activity 31: Managing Unhelpful Thoughts Worksheet (Check It and Change It)

Now that you've identified the overly negative/unhelpful thought that's bothering you, use this sheet to help you question and change it.

Catch it: The unhelpful thought I'm working on:

- ______________________________

Check it: Should I listen to this thought?

- How much do I believe this thought, from 0 to 100 per cent? *Colour in how much on the thermometer.*

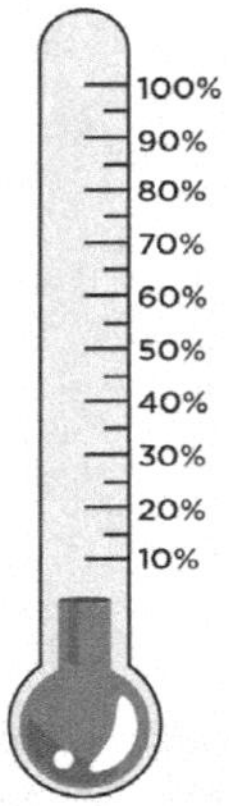

Source: Created by John Lim, www.sightstage.wix.com/home

- How does this thought make me *feel*? ______________________
- Is it a helpful thought? ❐ Yes ❐ No
- Thinking of my *calmest*, *most rational*, and *most supportive* friend, carer, or family member, what advice would they give?
- Would I feel better if I chose to not listen to this thought? ❐ Yes ❐ No
- If a good friend was in this situation, what would I tell him/her?

Change it: What is a more helpful thought?

- ______________________________
- How much do I believe the *new* thought (0–100 per cent)? _______ per cent
- How much do I believe the *old* thought (0–100 per cent)? _______ per cent

Activity 32: Managing a Busy Mind at Night

Try these skills before going to bed to help manage a busy mind.

Winding Down before Bed

Remember the wind-down activities discussed in the first session. Doing your wind-down activities each night may help break the 'circuit' of a busy mind getting in the way of sleep.

Winding down involves relaxing activities 1 hour before bed and a fixed bedtime routine right before bed, where you might have a warm drink (e.g. cup of cocoa or milk), brush your teeth, and do a relaxation exercise.

To-Do Lists and Prioritising

To-do lists are a way of putting the 'day to bed' and busy thoughts out of mind, so that you can go to sleep.

- The list may be done before leaving work at the end of the day, after dinner, or any other time you feel it would be handy.
- Some people like to keep their list by their bed, so that they can jot down more items if they come to mind while they are in bed (no need to even turn on the light).
- When would be the best time for you to make a to-do list? ________________
- Can you set a reminder on your phone to make sure you do this?

Avoid Watching the Clock Overnight

It is hard to put the mind to rest if you are always checking the time to see how long you have been lying awake or calculate whether you will get enough sleep for the night.

If you find that you often check the time when you are having trouble falling back to sleep, try the clock watching experiment we talked about for Activity 22.

- How will I avoid watching the clock at night? ____________________________

Setting your alarm for the morning can help you worry less about whether you will wake up on time for the next day.

Activity 33: Relaxation Exercises

Let's practise a couple of simple relaxation strategies you can try out before bed:

- **Shoulder shrugs**: Raise your shoulders as if trying to touch your ears with them and breathe in while doing this. Feel the muscles in your neck and shoulders tense. Then, all at once, let your shoulders drop while you breathe out. Feel the tension leaving the muscles of your neck and shoulders. Repeat the shrug a few times, inhaling on the shrug and exhaling on the release. Keep your jaw relaxed as you do this.
- **Releasing tension**: Become aware of the difference between holding tension in your body and letting go of this tension. Bend your toes up as if to touch your shins. Hold them there while you tighten your thighs, buttocks, and fists. Take a deep breath and hold it while you clench your jaw and close your eyes. Hold all that tension for 5 seconds. As you exhale, let it go all at once, feeling the tension drain from your body.
- **Cued relaxation response**: Pick a word or phrase that has a positive or neutral meaning ('Easy', 'I am relaxed', or 'Sparkle'). Sit quietly, in a comfortable position, and begin breathing slowly and naturally. On the exhale, say to yourself your word or phrase. If your mind starts to wander, that's OK; just come back to your breathing and to repeating your cue word or phrase.
- **Equalising breathing**: Take 4 seconds to breathe in and 4 seconds to breathe out. That is, as you inhale, count '1 . . . 2 . . . 3 . . . 4', and do the same as you breathe out. Do this four or five times. Avoid holding your breath after the inhalation or the exhalation; just smoothly transition from one phase to the other.
- **Your relaxation place**: Begin with a few, slow relaxation breaths. Then, with your eyes closed, take a moment to create, in your mind's eye, an ideal spot to relax. You can make it any place you'd like, such as the mountains, beach, lake, prairie, or park. It can be either a real or a made-up place. See yourself comfortably enjoying this place. Now, once you have created it, go use it for 15 seconds or so, whenever you feel the need to relax.

Remember that relaxation requires practice. It may take many tries before it is found useful. There are also many different types of relaxation and meditation exercise out there. Find one that you feel comfortable learning.

Try giving one or two of these relaxation exercises a go during the week, and see if it helps with your sleep.

You can also check out App downloads on topics related to meditation, relaxation, and breathing.

See www.k-state.edu/paccats/Contents/Stress/Quick%20Relaxation%20Strategies.pdf

Activity 34: The Main Things I Learned Today

- ____
- ____
- ____
- ____
- ____
- ____

Activity 35: My Action Plan for the Week

1. My regular rising time for *each* morning is: ____________________
2. Some energy-generating activities and changes to my sleep routine and hygiene that I will keep working on:
   - ____
   - ____
   - ____
3. Start to manage overly negative thoughts:
   - ❒ Watch out for overly negative thoughts and the impact that they have on my sleep and energy.

   How and when will I do this? ________________________________

   - ❒ When thoughts/images are disturbing me from winding down or falling asleep at night, write them down on a piece of paper/journal.
   - ❒ Remember the 3 Cs—**C**atch it, **C**heck it, **C**hange it (I can challenge the unhelpful thoughts by using the worksheets provided).
4. Strategies for dealing with a busy mind:
   - Experiment with strategies for managing:
     - ❒ low mood and/or anxiety (see *Activity 23*);
     - ❒ intrusive thoughts (see *Activity 24*);
     - ❒ voices, visions, other unusual sensations (see *Activity 25*).
   - ❒ Continue with winding down before bed.
   - ❒ To-do list: *How and when will I do this?* ____________________
   - ❒ Avoid watching the clock when I can't sleep: Try the clock watching experiment.
   - ❒ Relaxation or imagery: Practise this during the day for short periods at first. When I become more skilled, I will be able to use it more effectively at night.

19 Client Resource Pack Session 4

Maintaining Wellness and Working with Triggers for Poor Sleep

Topics addressed this week:

- Activity 36: A Review of the Skills We Have Been Learning
- Activity 37: Effects of Medications on Sleep and Energy
- Activity 38: Effects of Caffeine or Smoking
- Activity 39: Effects of Alcohol on Sleep
- Activity 40: Effects of Drugs on Sleep
- Activity 41: Stress Management—Values Exercise
- Activity 42: Working towards Balance
- Activity 43: Things to Consider to Create Better Balance
- Activity 44: Coping with Demands
- Activity 45: My Coping Resources
- Activity 46: Keeping Your Progress Going—Relapse Prevention
- Activity 47: Blueprint Summary
- Activity 48: Planning for Setbacks
- Activity 49: The Motivation Boost
- Activity 50: Action Plan and Goal Setting

Session 4: Maintaining Wellness and Working with Triggers for Poor Sleep

Topics Addressed this Week

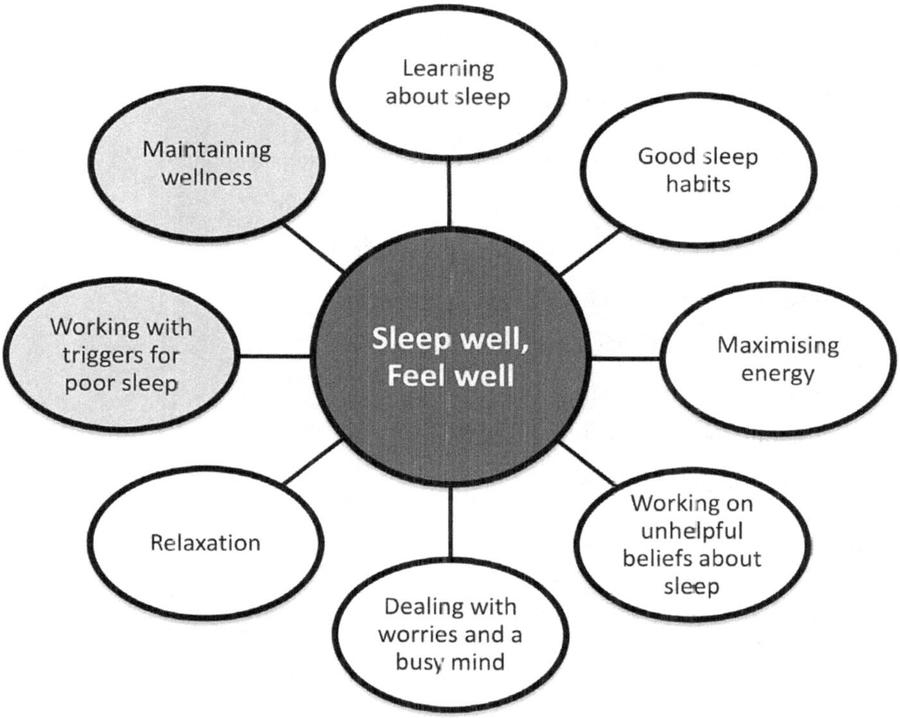

Activity 36: A Review of the Skills We Have Been Learning

Last week, we learned about:

- dealing with a busy mind (managing intrusive thoughts and voices, winding down, not clock watching, journal writing, to-do lists, and relaxation);
- working with overly negative thoughts—**C**atch it, **C**heck it, **C**hange it!

The other sleep skills we have also been learning are:

- sleep hygiene (everyday habits to help us sleep better at night);
- winding down before bed (to help fall asleep);
- getting out of bed if you can't sleep (GOOBICS);
- regular rising time (not oversleeping and limiting naps);
- winding up into the day in the morning;
- maximising daytime energy;
- establishing helpful beliefs and attitudes about sleep;
- managing nightmares.

What went well?

____

____

____

What was challenging?

____

____

____

Let's brainstorm ways to get around these challenges:

____

____

____

Activity 37: Effects of Medications on Sleep and Energy

It is important to take prescribed medications according to your doctor's instructions and at a regular time. Sometimes, however, these medications can have side effects that impact on sleep. For example, some medications can cause bad dreams or drowsiness in the day.

If these side effects worry you, let your doctor know about your side effects so that he/she can make good decisions about whether a medication is right for you, and whether the timing of the medications can be changed.

What are the benefits and disadvantages of your medications for Sleep?

Benefits	*Disadvantages*

Coping Strategies to Reduce the Side Effects of My Medications

On a scale of 0–10, how confident do you feel about applying these strategies (circle)?

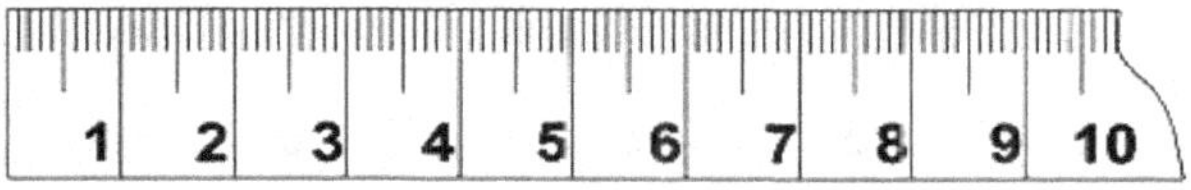

Not confident at all — Very confident

General Guidelines for Sleep

- Take prescribed medications only as directed (correct time, correct dose).
- Be proactive in managing side effects and discuss any ongoing problematic side effects with your doctor

Activity 38: Effects of Caffeine or Smoking

Caffeine and nicotine in cigarettes have a stimulant effect on your brain and body and can cause you to feel more alert and awake.

Do you ever use cigarettes/caffeine to cope with tiredness, stress, or low mood?

Although caffeine and smoking may be enjoyable and help increase alertness in the day, it is unhelpful to drink caffeine or smoke during the evening. Having these at night makes it harder to fall or stay asleep, which can make you feel more tired, low, or anxious the next day. This may lead to more caffeine and nicotine use, becoming a vicious cycle.

What are the benefits and disadvantages of caffeine and smoking for Sleep?

Benefits	*Disadvantages*

Strategies to Reduce the Use of Caffeine or Cigarettes at Night

On a scale of 0–10, how confident do you feel about applying these strategies (circle)?

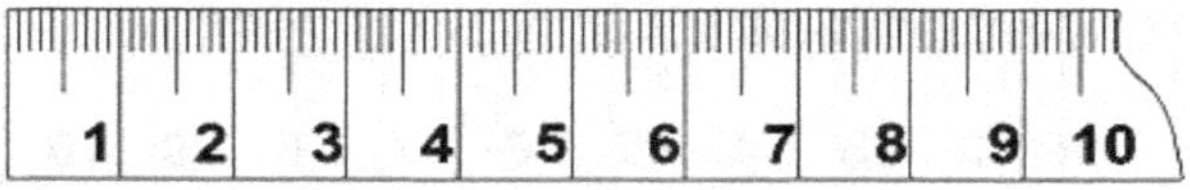

Not confident at all Very confident

General Guidelines for Sleep

- Avoid caffeine 5 hours before bed.
- Avoid nicotine 2 hours before bed: Work towards quitting smoking or reducing the number of cigarettes you smoke over the day.

Activity 39: Effects of Alcohol on Sleep

Another lifestyle and health factor that could be affecting your sleep is alcohol.

Why Shouldn't You Use Alcohol to Get to Sleep at Night?

Alcohol can interfere with your mood and the quality of your sleep. You might think that drinking alcohol would help you sleep. But, in fact:

- Alcohol digestion at night can wake you up.
- Alcohol gets in the way of achieving a deep sleep.
- You would be more likely to wake up feeling tired and unrefreshed in the morning.

What makes you reach for alcohol in the evening?

What Are the Benefits and Disadvantages of Alcohol for Sleep?

Benefits	*Disadvantages*

Strategies to Reduce Reliance on Alcohol for Getting to Sleep

On a scale of 0–10, how confident do you feel about applying these strategies (circle)?

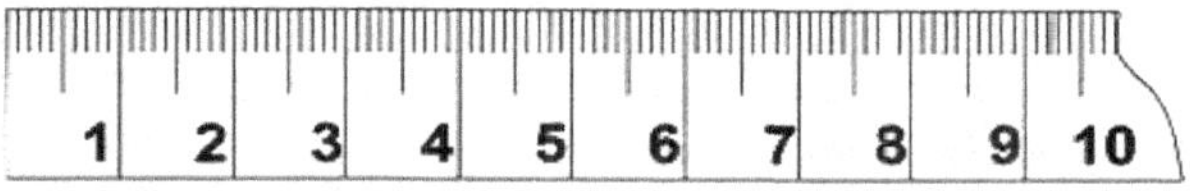

Not confident at all — Very confident

General Guidelines for Sleep

- Avoid alcohol 4 hours before bed.
- Drink plenty of water after heavy drinking.

Activity 40: Effects of Drugs on Sleep

Many drugs can cause either sleepiness (sedatives such as marijuana and heroin) or increased alertness (stimulants such as meth, speed, and ecstasy), and impact on mood and sleep patterns.

Let's take the example of marijuana and discuss the benefits for sleep, and the disadvantages.

Benefits	*Disadvantages*
Can help people fall asleep faster and get a deeper sleep	Difficulties waking up at a regular time Less motivation during the day to study, work, exercise, and socialise May become reliant on marijuana to go to sleep

Overall, marijuana may help deal with sleep problems in the short term, but it can actually make sleep worse in the long term and make it harder to follow good sleep habits.

What Are the Benefits and Disadvantages of Drugs (e.g. Meth, Heroin, Ecstasy) for Sleep?

Benefits	*Disadvantages*

Strategies to Reduce the Use of Drugs that Affect Sleep

On a scale of 0–10, how confident do you feel about applying these strategies (circle)?

1 2 3 4 5 6 7 8 9 10

Not confident at all — Very confident

Activity 41: Stress Management—Values Exercise

An important way to promote good sleep is to have a *balanced lifestyle*. This means not concentrating on only *one* part of your life to the detriment of other areas of your life.

It is also about doing things that bring you happiness or satisfaction, and looking after yourself.

Exercise: Close your eyes and say the first answer that pops into your mind for the following questions:

- What's important to me?
- What do I value?
- When do I feel happy or relaxed?
- I spend too much time worrying about . . .
- I spend too little time doing things such as . . .
- What I would like to do differently from today is . . .

Activity 42: Working towards Balance

Identify areas of your life that you feel are out of balance.

Rate Each of the Life Areas as:	*Lacking*	*About Right*	*Overpowering*
Health (including mental health)	❒	❒	❒
Hobbies, leisure, holidays	❒	❒	❒
Families, carers, friends	❒	❒	❒
Work, study	❒	❒	❒
Money, finances	❒	❒	❒
Creativity	❒	❒	❒
Other	❒	❒	❒

Can you select a top 2 to work on from those that you ticked in the table?

- Think about what changes might be made and work towards small goals for change.
- It is helpful to check in with yourself regularly to think about your life balance.

If you're not living a life that reflects your values, it's more likely that it will feel stressful.

Activity 43: Things to Consider to Create Better Balance

We tend to be able to accept difficulties better when they occur in pursuit of something that we truly value.

In the table, circle the areas that you would like to make a change in and write about possible changes/goals.

Area	*Immediate (Today)*	*Short Term (Next Week)*	*Mid Term (Next Month)*
Health			
Hobbies, leisure, holidays			
Family, carers, friends			
Work, study			
Money, finances			
Creativity			
Other			

Activity 44: Coping with Demands

Did you know that there is both good stress and bad stress?

- *Too little* stress leads to boredom and reduced interest (under-stressed).
- *Too much* stress can cause distress, when there are too many demands, or when we feel that we don't have the right coping skills and assistance to deal with the demand (overstressed).

Not all stress is bad!

- It's OK to have some stress in your life.
- We all need a little bit of stress to give us motivation to function. In fact, we need it to perform well.
- The amount of stress that we can cope with varies from person to person and depends on our personalities, coping styles, and the way our bodies respond to stress.

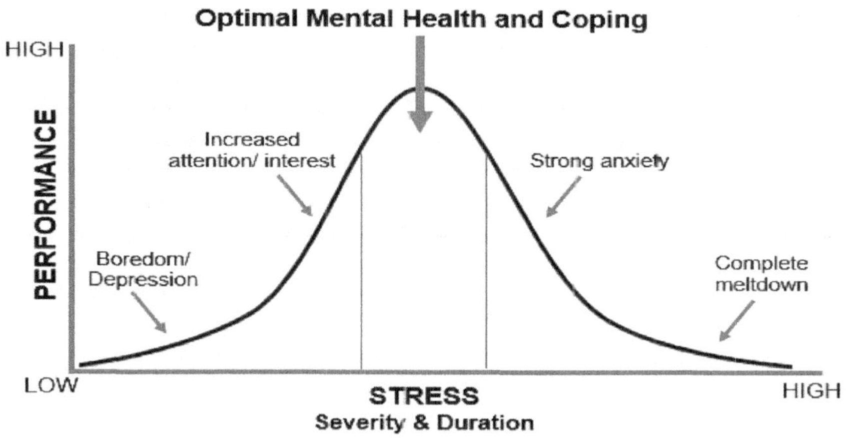

Which describes you best?

Too many demands and expectations from others	⇨	Demands *exceed* coping skills	⇨	Burnt out/ Meltdown ("Overstressed")
Feeling productive and able to meet the tasks placed on me	⇨	Demands are *equal* to coping skills	⇨	Balance ("Good stress")
Having little to do and nothing to look forward to	⇨	Demands are *too low* so coping skills are not challenged	⇨	Couch Potato/ Bored ("Under-stressed")

Activity 45: My Coping Resources

What coping resources do I have for:

- managing *overstress* (how can I relax, problem-solve, get organised, worry less, seek support, use my strengths?):

  ____

  ____

  ____

  ____

- managing *under-stress* (how can I re-engage in life?):

  ____

  ____

  ____

  ____

Activity 46: Keeping Your Progress Going—Relapse Prevention

Well done on your progress through this programme! It is now important keeping your progress going. This can be done by:

- reading over what you have learned at least once a month;
- planning for any setbacks that may happen;
- setting goals to guide what you will do over the coming months;
- keeping using the skills you learned in therapy;
- coming back to this workbook if you need to get your sleep back on track.

People don't plan to fail; they simply fail to plan.

Knowing the Difference between a Bad Night and a Relapse

It is important to understand the difference between the odd bad night's sleep (or two or three), which everyone gets, and the signs that Insomnia may be coming back.

Planning for Setbacks

Setbacks are an inevitable part of progress, but they do not mean that you are relapsing back into Insomnia. Setbacks simply reflect that it is very normal to have ups and downs in the quality and amount of your sleep. Recovery from Insomnia is a gradual process over time that typically follows a pattern with lots of ups and downs, like in the graph below.

Be Realistic

It is unrealistic to expect to sleep well every single night. Instead, you should expect some phases of feeling like you are sleeping very well, and other phases where you feel that your sleep is more unstable. Setbacks are a normal part of overcoming Insomnia, rather than a sign of 'going back to square one'. So, when you go through a period of more unsteady sleep, try not to become discouraged or concerned.

The Pattern of Recovery

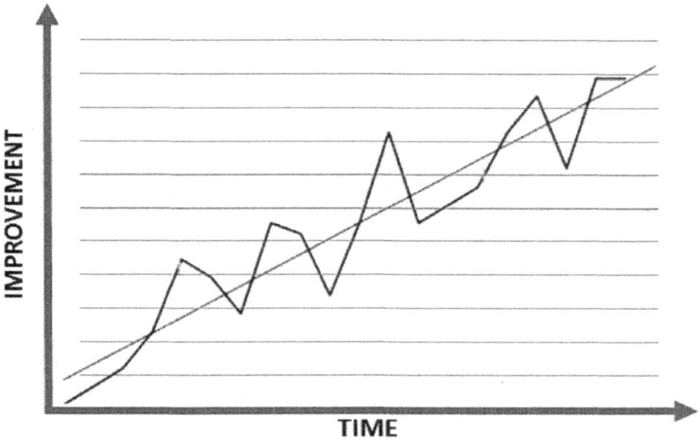

Activity 47: Blueprint Summary

How did the problem develop?

____

____

What kept it going?

____

____

____

____

What did you learn during the programme about sleep, and what is important in managing it?

____

____

____

____

What were your most unhelpful habits and thoughts about sleep?

Habit: ____

Thought: ____

What are the alternatives to these?

____

____

What are the most important things to remember to keep your progress going?

____

____

____

Activity 48: Planning for Setbacks

Be aware of your own 'high-risk' situations.

If you expect possible setbacks, then it becomes easier to prepare for them. Let's look at what are some 'high-risk' situations for you—i.e. factors that made your sleep and tiredness worse in the past.

There's no need for a setback to lead to a complete tumble back into Insomnia (i.e. relapse). A good way to reduce the impact of setbacks is to have a backup plan of strategies to use when they occur. Setbacks remind you to use the skills that you have learned in therapy.

Possible Problem or Setback	*Plan/Strategy*
Example: After not sleeping well for a few nights, I'm getting worried about my sleep. I'm feeling very tired during the day and having longer naps	______
______	______
______	______
______	______
______	______
______	______
______	______
______	______
______	______
______	______
______	______
______	______
______	______
______	______
______	______

Activity 49: The Motivation Boost

If you're faced with a high-risk time for your sleep, try these strategies:

- Remind yourself why you wanted to tackle your Insomnia in the first place—the reasons are probably just as relevant now as they were then.
- Talk to someone supportive.
  Who would this be for you? ______
- Think of what helped with improving your Insomnia in the past—chances are, whatever worked then will help you now too.

Activity 50: Action Plan and Goal Setting

My Plan for the Coming Month

The changes I want to make (or continue making) are:

____

____

____

The reasons why I want to make these changes are:

____

____

____

I will know that my plan is working if:

____

____

____

Each day, ask yourself: What can I do today that will take me towards better sleep and energy and away from poor sleep and tiredness?

Part IV

Appendices

Appendix 1

Clinical Interview for Sleep

Demographic Information

Name: ______________________________ D.O.B (Age): ______________

Country of birth: ______________________ Gender: ________________

Primary language (English fluency): __________ Marital status: ____________

Highest educational level attained (circle):

Primary school *High school* *Vocational certificate* *University degree*

Current employment/study status: ______________________________

Occupation: ____

Accommodation type and who lives with: ___________________________

Psychiatric and Medical Background

Medical problems (physical injuries, physical illness, chronic pain, diabetes, breathing or respiratory problems, any neurologic conditions). Ask whether iron levels and thyroid function have been checked, and whether women over 40 have experienced symptoms of menopause:

____

____

____

Psychiatric history (diagnosis, length of illness, previous hospitalisations, current engagement with treatment and support services):

____

____

____

Current mood (over the last week): ______ 0 = very low; 10 = elevated

Current anxiety (over the last week): ______ 0 = no anxiety; 10 = extreme anxiety

Is mood stable? What are triggers for low or elevated mood, or increased anxiety?

____

Medications (type, dosage, including over-the-counter and prescription drugs):

____

____

____

Relationship between sleep problems and mental illness: Did sleep problems exist prior to psychiatric diagnosis? Do sleep problems make psychiatric symptoms worse, and vice versa? Is there a belief that sleep cannot be improved owing to psychiatric diagnosis?

____

____

Sleep Problem Description

Tell me about your sleep problems (tick those that apply):

____

____

❒ Problem getting to sleep
❒ Problem with waking in the night
❒ Problem with waking too early in the morning
❒ Problem with sleeping in late (difficulty waking on time)
❒ Sleep feels unrefreshing (even when total sleep time is more than 7 hours)
❒ Problem with daytime sleepiness (i.e. can fall asleep easily during the day)
❒ Problem with daytime fatigue/tiredness (lacking in energy)

How long ago did the problem start? ______________________

Has your sleep changed suddenly over the last month? ______________________

(A sudden change or deterioration in sleep, with no clear trigger, can be an indicator of an upcoming psychotic episode.)

Was there a trigger? ______________________

Please tell me about your sleep routine:

Usual bedtime (lights-out time) on weekdays (range): ______________________

Usual wake time on weekdays (range): ______________________

Usual get-out-of-bed time on weekdays (range): ____________________

Same pattern on weekends? ____________________

Daytime and evening naps, including unintentional dozing (e.g. in front of the TV)? How do naps help (e.g. cope with low mood, boredom, anxiety, fatigue)? Length and time of naps (range): ____________________

How many nights a week is sleep a problem? ____________________

Typical sleep onset latency (SOL) after turning lights off (range is OK): ____________________

Typical wake after sleep onset (range is OK): ____________________

Estimate average total sleep time (range is OK): ____________________

If woken in the night—by what (noise, needs the toilet, pain, dreams, anxiety, etc.)? How many wakings and duration of time spent awake?

____

How do you know what time it is when you wake in the night/how long you've been awake? Do you look at the clock? ____________________

How many hours of sleep do you think you need? ____________________

Effects of Substances

Do you take sleeping pills? What type? Dose? How often? How long used? Ever take more than prescribed? Ever take them at a different time than prescribed?

____

____

Which medications:

(a) make you feel sleepy or tired (including depot injections if applicable)?

____

(b) make you feel more awake?

____

Do you take your other prescription medications as directed? Do you ever miss a dose, or take more than is prescribed?

____

Do you drink caffeine? In the evening? ______________________________

Do you smoke cigarettes/roll ups/e-cigarettes? In the evening? ______________

Do you use alcohol during the day? In the evening? How much? ______________

Do you use recreational drugs (e.g. marijuana, speed, meth, cocaine, heroin, ecstasy)?

____

____

Do you take any prescription medications that are not prescribed? ______________

Sleep Environment

Where do you sleep—in a bed or on a couch? Do you have a separate bedroom?

____

Is your bedroom a restful place (do you feel safe and secure in your sleeping space)?

____

Do you sleep with a bed partner? Do they snore/kick/have nightmares? Is there relationship stress?

____

Do you have housemates, children, or pets in the house that disturb your sleep?

____

Is your mattress comfortable? Do you have comfortable bedding? Is your bedroom quiet? What about temperature? Is the bedroom dark?

____

Do you have a TV/radio/phone/desk/papers in the bedroom?

____

Do you watch TV, use the the computer, eat, drink, smoke, or engage in other activities in bed?

____

Fatigue and Sleepiness

Have you suffered with being tired, heavy, foggy, sluggish, low in energy? Rating of fatigue over the last week: _______ (0 = not at all fatigued; 10 = extremely fatigued)

How do your medications affect daytime energy/fatigue (including depot medications, if any)?

How do your psychiatric symptoms affect daytime energy/fatigue (voices, mood)?

When do you feel at your most energetic?

Do you often feel fatigued or sleepy, even after a long night of sleep (more than 8 hours)?

Would you fall asleep in the following situations: reading, watching TV, being a passenger in a car? (Consider administering *Epworth Sleepiness Scale* if sleepiness is a significant problem.)

Other Sleep Disorders

Do you have any previous diagnosis of a sleep disorder? Was there an overnight sleep study conducted? Was any treatment initiated?

Obstructive sleep apnoea: Any snoring, waking up gasping for air or out of breath? (Consider administering Berlin questionnaire if sleep apnoea is suspected.)

Restless legs: Any cramps, aches, or unusual feelings in the legs that make you want to move your legs, especially while in bed at night?

Periodic limb movement disorder: Have you noticed (or others have commented) that parts of your body jerk during sleep?

Nightmares: Do you suffer with nightmares (scary dreams that wake you up, after which you find it hard to get back to sleep)? How frequently? How distressing (scale from 0 = not at all to 10 = extremely)? Are there recurrent themes?

Parasomnias: Do you sleep-walk or talk? Do you eat during your sleep? Frequency and impact?

Narcolepsy: Do you fall asleep very easily during the day or have a sudden urge to sleep at inappropriate times (e.g. when working, eating, or talking with someone)? (If no, don't ask further questions relating to narcolepsy.)

- ❐ Do you experience weakness in your body (legs buckle, or arms feel weak, or jaw drops) when you are happy or sad (cataplexy)?
- ❐ Do you experience vivid dream-like feelings when you wake up or when you fall asleep (hallucinations)?
- ❐ Do you experience sleep paralysis, where you can't move or speak for a short time (under 2 minutes) when waking up or falling asleep (sleep paralysis)?

Sleep–wake dysregulation:

- ❐ For sleep onset problems, check if establishing a later routine (going to bed later and getting up later) would solve the sleep problem (this indicates delayed sleep phase).
- ❐ For early waking problems, check if establishing an earlier routine (going to bed earlier and getting up earlier) would solve the sleep problem (this indicates advanced sleep phase).

Lifestyle

Are you currently working/studying/volunteering? How many days a week? How do you spend your days?

Do you get outside most days? How often would you leave your house? And for how long?

How many times a week do you exercise? What type of exercise? Do you sometimes exercise in the evening?

Do you eat regular meals each day? What foods do you often eat? Do you snack between meals?

Do you have contact with many other people in your week? ____________________

Do you have hobbies? What do you do to relax or have fun?

How satisfied are you with your current life balance? __________ (0 = not at all satisfied; 10 = completely satisfied)

External Stressors, Emotional Contributors

Are there any current significant life events or stressors (accommodation instability or change, relationship, occupational, financial stress, social isolation)?

____

____

Are there any current emotional factors (mood/anxiety) that impact on sleep? How do your psychosis symptoms affect your sleep (e.g. only go to bed once hallucinations subside)?

____

____

Functional Analysis

What is your bedtime routine? (What do you typically do in the 2 hours before bed? Are you exposed to bright light for longer than 60 minutes? Do you engage in activities that make you feel physically or mentally alert?)

____

____

When you have difficulty falling asleep or getting back to sleep, what do you think is getting in the way?

- ❒ Fears (including nightmares, paranoia, and hallucinations)
- ❒ General worry or worry about sleep
- ❒ Mind racing (not necessarily negative themes)
- ❒ Not tired
- ❒ Physically tense
- ❒ Physical discomfort or pain
- ❒ Too hot/cold/uncomfortable
- ❒ Other: ____________________________

What do you do when you can't fall asleep or return to sleep (stay in bed, toss and turn, get up, worry, try to force self to sleep, make mind go blank, have milky drink, go to the toilet, take sleeping pill, have a cigarette, eat, drink alcohol)?

____

What do you do during the day after a poor night of sleep (sleep in, nap, use coffee or other stimulants, worry about feeling tired, go to bed early, avoid outside activities or appointments, stay inside, drink alcohol, take a sleeping pill)?

____

Self-Efficacy and Motivation

How does your sleep difficulty impact on your life? What is the worst thing about your sleep difficulty?

How would your life improve if you were sleeping better and less concerned about your sleep?

Do you believe you can make changes that will improve your sleep?
(0 = don't believe can improve sleep; 10 = certain can improve sleep) ____________

What might be good about attending a programme designed to help you sleep better?

What might be difficult about attending this programme?

Summary—Case Conceptualisation

1. Factors that are increasing arousal:

2. Factors that are reducing sleep drive:

3. Factors that are interfering with the body clock:

Appendix 2

Sleep Diary

	1: Day/date:	*2: Day/date:*	*3: Day/date:*	*4: Day/date:*	*5: Day/date:*	*6: Day/date:*	*7: Day/date:*
Last night, I got into bed at:	____: ____ (hr) (mins)	____: ____ (hr) (mins)	____: ____ (hr) (mins)	____: ____ (hr) (mins)	____: ____ (hr) (mins)	____: ____ (hr) (mins)	____: ____ (hr) (mins)
Last night, I turned the lights off at:	____: ____ (hr) (mins)	____: ____ (hr) (mins)	____: ____ (hr) (mins)	____: ____ (hr) (mins)	____: ____ (hr) (mins)	____: ____ (hr) (mins)	____: ____ (hr) (mins)
Last night, I fell asleep at:	____: ____ (hr) (mins)	____: ____ (hr) (mins)	____: ____ (hr) (mins)	____: ____ (hr) (mins)	____: ____ (hr) (mins)	____: ____ (hr) (mins)	____: ____ (hr) (mins)
During the night (after I fell asleep) I woke up:	__ times (e.g. _2_ times)	____ times	____ times	____ times	____ times	____ times	____ times
Today, I woke up at:	____: ____ (hr) (mins)	____: ____ (hr) (mins)	____: ____ (hr) (mins)	____: ____ (hr) (mins)	____: ____ (hr) (mins)	____: ____ (hr) (mins)	____: ____ (hr) (mins)

My sleep was: (please tick)	Very good	Good	OK	A bit bad	Very bad	(Day 1)
	Very good	Good	OK	A bit bad	Very bad	(Day 2)
	Very good	Good	OK	A bit bad	Very bad	(Day 3)
	Very good	Good	OK	A bit bad	Very bad	(Day 4)
	Very good	Good	OK	A bit bad	Very bad	(Day 5)
	Very good	Good	OK	A bit bad	Very bad	(Day 6)
	Very good	Good	OK	A bit bad	Very bad	(Day 7)
Today, I felt: (please tick)	Very tired	A bit tired	OK	Good	Very good	(Day 1)
	Very tired	A bit tired	OK	Good	Very good	(Day 2)
	Very tired	A bit tired	OK	Good	Very good	(Day 3)
	Very tired	A bit tired	OK	Good	Very good	(Day 4)
	Very tired	A bit tired	OK	Good	Very good	(Day 5)
	Very tired	A bit tired	OK	Good	Very good	(Day 6)
	Very tired	A bit tired	OK	Good	Very good	(Day 7)

Today, I had a nap: (please tick)	No	Yes, from ____ to ____	(Day1)
	No	Yes, from ____ to ____	(Day 2)
	No	Yes, from ____ to ____	(Day 3)
	No	Yes, from ____ to ____	(Day 4)
	No	Yes, from ____ to ____	(Day 5)
	No	Yes, from ____ to ____	(Day 6)
	No	Yes, from ____ to ____	(Day 7)

Appendix 3

Sleep Hygiene Diary

What did you do ONE HOUR before going to sleep? (You can tick more than one activity)	*Is this good for you?*	*Day 1:*	*Day 2:*	*Day 3:*	*Day 4:*	*Day 5:*	*Day 6:*	*Day 7:*
Read a book, e-book, newspaper, or magazine.								
Used the laptop/computer/smart phone/tablet/ games console.								
Listened to the radio, music, or an audio book.								
Watched TV.								
Exercised (eg went for walk, gym, played sport).								
Took a bath/shower.								
Had a soothing drink or small snack.								
Talked to friends/family/partner.								
Went to a bar, pub, nightclub, and/or party,								
Had a caffeinated drink (eg coffee, tea, soda, red bull). If yes, how many?								
Drank alcohol (eg beer, wine, spirits etc).								
If yes, how many glasses/units?								
Smoked cigarettes. If yes, how many?								
Took recreational drugs?								
OTHER:								

Appendix 4

Some Interesting Facts about Dreaming

- We all dream every night.
- Our brains are active throughout the night.
- We dream most vividly during REM sleep.
- Our brains are specially wired not to act out our dreams. During REM sleep, many of our muscles completely relax to stop us from acting out our dreams. If this system doesn't work properly, we may try to act out our dreams, especially if they involve strong emotions.
- Many dreams are bizarre, because part of our brain shuts down. When we are awake, the front part of our brain controls how we make sense of the world. This shuts down during dreaming. Because of this, the dreaming brain puts together ideas that normally do not go together.
- We can learn to control our dreams. Many people have bad dreams or nightmares. These can happen over and over again, but people can change what happens in these dreams so that they are less frightening.
  - To do this, first write down memories of the scary dream, and then think about how it might end differently.
- Scientists disagree about the meaning of dreams.
  - Some people say our dreams mean nothing—they say we have them only because parts of our brain are active when sleep.
  - Other people say dreams have value—they say it is a kind of therapy for when we're feeling down, and that having and remembering vivid dreams about stressful things may help us deal with stress.

Appendix 5

Decision Balance Sheet

This worksheet can be used to help you decide whether you want to make certain changes in your life to help with your sleep (e.g. stopping an old behaviour/thought or doing something new). It is best to complete each section, even if it seems that some of the answers in different sections are similar. Make sure you include both short-term and long-term advantages and disadvantages.

The behaviour or thought I am thinking of changing is:

____

Benefits of STAYING THE SAME	**Costs of STAYING THE SAME**
____________________	____________________
____________________	____________________
____________________	____________________
____________________	____________________
Costs of CHANGING	**Benefits of CHANGING**
____________________	____________________
____________________	____________________
____________________	____________________
____________________	____________________

Compare the costs and benefits of changing and not changing, and ask yourself:

Are the costs worth it? ❒ Yes ❒ No

It's your decision! You are the one who must decide what it will take to tip the scale in favour of changing.

- If someone gave you $1 million to make the change you are thinking about, would you change, and why?

  ____

- What steps would you have to take to achieve the change and receive the $1 million?

  ____

Appendix 6
In-Session Feedback

Session #: ______ Date: ____________ Client: ______________________

1. If you could rate the level of improvement in **your overall sleep quality** over the last 7 days (since I last saw you), from 0 to 10 (0 = none at all; 10 = a huge amount), what would you rate it?

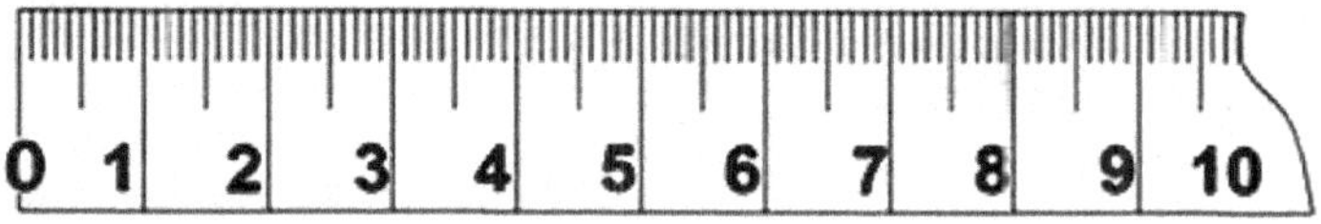

No improvement *Huge Improvement*

2. If you could rate the level of improvement in how you've been **feeling** and how well you have been **coping** since the last session, from 0 to 10 (0 = not at all, 10 = a huge amount), what would you rate it?

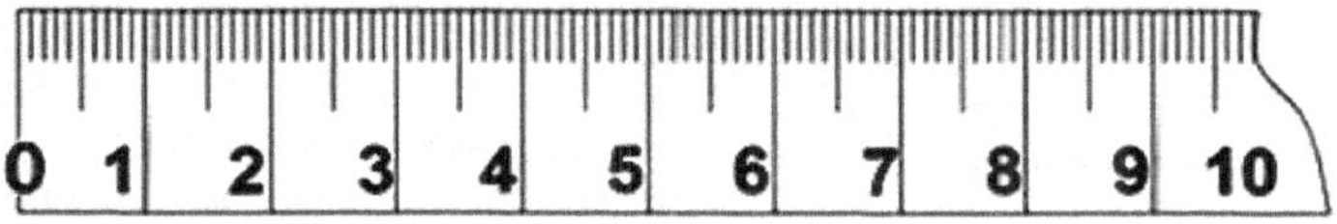

No improvement *Huge Improvement*

3. What personal benefits to your everyday life are you finding from the programme so far?

____

____

____

4. Has last week's session helped with your symptoms in any way (e.g. mood, voices, visions, paranoia)? If yes, how so?

____

____

____

Appendix 7

Time in Bed Restriction Instructions

Time in bed restriction is about *not spending too long in bed.* It can be helpful to reduce the time spent in bed if you are awake for a lot of the time you are in bed (more than an hour or two). If you have trouble staying asleep during the night:

1) Try going to bed 30 minutes or an hour later than you usually would

OR

Try getting up 30 minutes or an hour earlier than you usually would in the morning

With this extra time not sleeping, you can do some wind-down activities at night (eg Arts and crafts, puzzles, reading), or do some winding-up activities in the day (eg Go for morning walk, cook breakfast)

2) After 5 to 7 nights, assess how you are sleeping.

If you are falling asleep and staying asleep more easily than before, you can start sleeping a little longer again.

For example: If you lay awake in bed for less than 40 minutes now, you can start going to bed 15 - 30 minutes earlier.

***Do not** start going to bed earlier if you still wake up and stay awake for more than 30 minutes during the night.*

3) After a few more nights, if you're still falling asleep easily and staying asleep, you can go to bed earlier by another 30 minutes.

You can keep sleeping earlier until you feel less tired in the day or until your sleep starts to get fragmented again (ie. harder to fall/ stay asleep).

If you still feel tired during the day, even though you are falling asleep and staying asleep better, explore some other reasons that may be making you feel tired (medications, illness, diet, depression, lack of activity, vitamin deficiency, sleep apnea etc)

Using time in bed restriction will help you get more solid sleep overnight.

Some tips when using time in bed restriction:

- Even if you have a bad night's sleep, that's OK. You may sleep worse at first, as your body adapts to spending less time in bed. This should improve after a few days.

- It's important to stick to your new routine and minimise naps during the day—otherwise you will find it hard to feel sleepy at night.
- You need to be committed to use this strategy, and it might not suit everyone. If you're unsure about whether it may work for you, discuss this with your therapist.

My plan for time in bed:

- Lights out to go to sleep at: ________ o'clock
- Rise out of bed to start the day at: ________ o'clock
- Plan for napping (time of day and length of nap): ____________________________

Appendix 8

Snacks that Provide Energy throughout the Day

The foods we eat can either boost our energy or slow us down. Here is a list of superfoods that are healthy and that you can try when feeling tired and low on energy. Experiment to see if these will boost your energy levels.

Fruit and Vegetables

- *Apples*: Include them in smoothies too.
- *Avocado*: Try adding avocados to salads or making guacamole.
- *Bananas*: Eat them as is, or drink in a smoothie.
- *Blueberries*: Mix them up in a fruit salad or smoothie, or have them on their own as a snack.
- *Carrots*: Great as a snack, grated in a salad, or in a soup.
- *Celery*: Use it in dips or in smoothies.
- *Cucumber*: Add some slices to your sandwiches and in salads.
- *Pineapple*: Eat it on its own or in a fruit salad.
- *Strawberries*: Perfect on their own, in a fruit salad, or in a smoothie.

Other Healthy Foods

- *Green salad*: Eat with a light dressing that includes lemon and olive oil.
- *Hummus*: Very healthy as a dip and very filling.
- *Oatmeal*: Eat for breakfast, with some fruits added in.
- *Soup*: A vegetable soup is a great way to eat and digest vegetables.
- *Quinoa*: These are very nutritious grains that can be cooked and eaten like rice.
- *Nuts*: A small handful of nuts can make for a filling snack full of energy. There many different types of nut to mix and choose from (e.g. cashews, almonds, pistachios).
- *Pumpkin seeds*: Full of minerals such as magnesium, iron, calcium, vitamin K, and protein. You could have a small handful of these as a light snack.

Healthy Drinks

- *Smoothies*: Try blending lots of fruits into one drink for an easy, nutritious snack.
- *Herbal tea*: This is a good replacement for coffee or other caffeinated drinks.
- *Lemon water*: Lemon juice in hot or cold water is great for rehydration and to provide a zing to the day.

Adapted from: http://kimberlysnyder.net/blog/2011/06/07/25-snacks-that-will-give-you-energy-througout-the-day/

Appendix 9

Challenging Unhelpful Beliefs about Sleep

Here is an example of how an unhelpful belief about sleep can affect us, and how we can go about addressing it:

Belief:
I feel my insomnia is the result of a chemical imbalance (and unless this is corrected by medication, there is nothing I can do to improve my sleep).

Thoughts/ worries/ behaviours/ outcomes that this belief leads to:
- Over-reliance on medications.
- Not feeling motivated to find non-medical solutions to the sleep problem.
- Feeling helpless and powerless.

Evidence for this belief:
- My doctor has told me that certain chemical processes in the brain can make it harder to sleep.
- I only seem to sleep well when I take a sleeping pill.

Evidence against this belief:
- I can see that my worry about sleep makes it harder to sleep.
- I can understand that sleep routines could be helpful in correcting poor sleep.
- Research suggested that CBT for insomnia has more effective treatment outcomes than medication.

What are the benefits of this belief?
- I don't put pressure on myself to change my habits or behaviour.

What are the costs of this belief?
- Reduces the likelihood that a long term solution will be found.

Is there a more helpful or realistic belief?
- It is not helpful to focus solely on external causes for my sleep problem as they are not in my control.
- Regardless of the initial cause of my insomnia, there are likely to be things that I could change about my thinking and daily habits to improve my sleep and daytime energy.

Appendix 10

My Personal Cycle of Insomnia

Therapist notes: *The following worksheet can be completed with clients to help illustrate their individualised cognitive behavioural formulation. A formulation links together the client's situation, thoughts, beliefs, and interpretations in response to the situation, and the emotional and behavioural consequences of their thoughts. We usually observe that the behaviour serves to maintain the problem in the longer term (e.g. a helpless thought such as 'I can't face the day' leads feeling low in mood, and the behavioural response of long daytime naps serves to perpetuate poor sleep at night, which triggers further helpless thoughts the following day, etc.).*

The cycle of Insomnia specifically relates to the client and can be used to guide which strategies are used in therapy. The formulation is continually updated as you learn more about how the client's Insomnia is being maintained, and directs you as to whether the treatment plan needs to be revised during the course of therapy.

Working through this sheet with the client will help them to gain an understanding of how their perceptions, beliefs, and behaviours may relate to their sleeping problem. It also allows the client to recognise the triggers and perpetuating factors for their Insomnia, to encourage a positive change in behaviour and thinking.

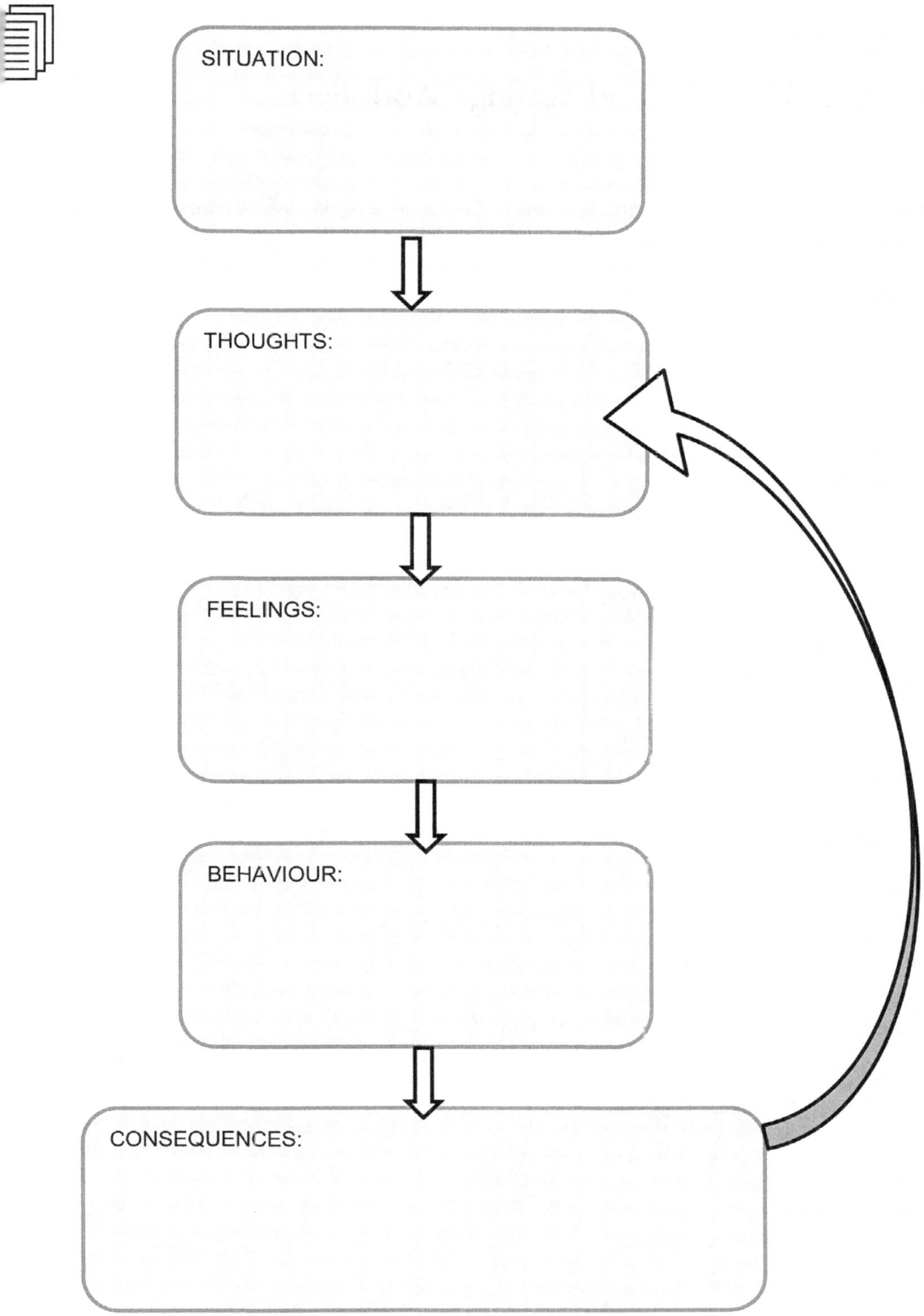
SITUATION:
THOUGHTS:
FEELINGS:
BEHAVIOUR:
CONSEQUENCES:

Appendix 11

Linking Thoughts and Feelings Worksheet

This worksheet explores a recent experience of poor sleep or daytime tiredness. The aim is to learn how thoughts create feelings, and how feelings may lead to certain behaviours.

Let's look at what happened during a recent time when you had a poor night's sleep or felt very tired during the day.

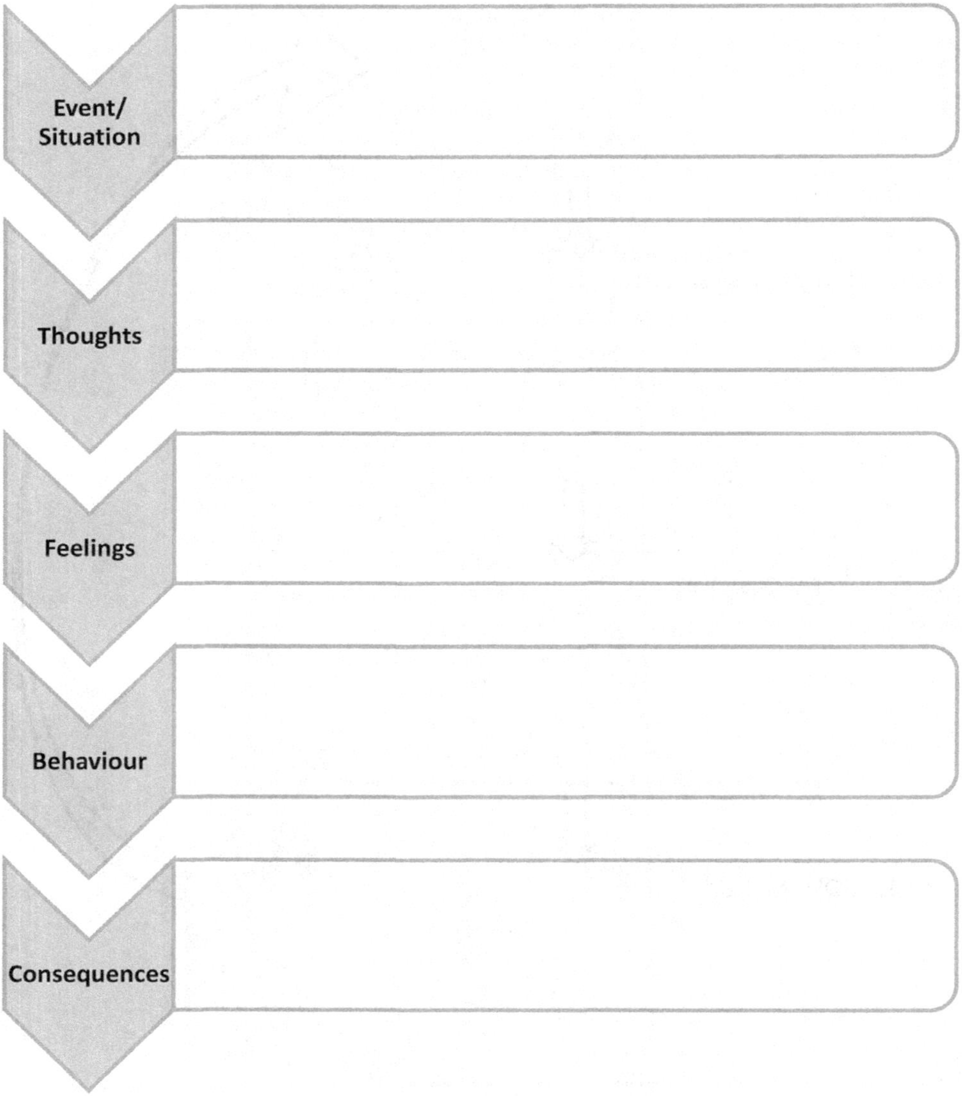

Appendix 12

Relaxing and Fun Activities

Below is a list of activities that you may find fun to do.

Indoors	*Outdoors*
Take a bath with bubble bath or relaxing oils	Sit in the sun
Clear out a cupboard or drawer	Go to the movies
Listen and sing to your favourite music	Jog, walk, hike
Buy and look after some potted plants	Get into nature: local park, river, lake, ocean, forest etc
Read the newspaper, a magazine, a book	Find a walking group
Find and cook up a new recipe	Take a ball to the park
Repair things around the house	Take a walk to the park
Work on your bicycle or car	Go camping
Watch TV, movies, documentaries	Go to church, read more about religion
Make lists of tasks or activities	Plant a vegetable garden
Plan holidays	Go swimming
Write emails	Join the gym
Go on the internet	Take up a martial art (taekwondo, judo)
Do crosswords, Sudoku and other puzzles	Ride a bike
Buy an aquarium and some fish	Go bird-watching
Dance	Watch a game
Do a relaxation or meditation exercise	Do a yoga class (or Pilates or meditation)
Have a cup of herbal tea	
Social activities	*Creative activities*
Visit friends	Make a gift
Play board games	Start a collection (stamps, coins, shells, etc.)
Learn a new card game	Origami
Visit family	Drawing, painting, sketching
Have a barbecue	Embroidery, cross stitching, knitting
Volunteer in community activities	Practice a musical instrument
Go to a party	Arts and crafts
Listen to others talk	Cook, bake
Join a club	Write poetry, letters or keep a journal
Learn a new skill or trade (carpentry, sewing)	Do some woodwork
Join a singing group	Do a puzzle, or take up model building
Go on a picnic	
Have lunch with a friend	
Learn a new language	

Appendix 13

Additional Relaxation Exercises

Steps to Feeling Relaxed and Having a Peaceful Mind

1. Awareness—being aware of when we are feeling tense and stressed: What are your signs?
2. Breathing—take some relaxing breaths or try a short breathing exercise.
3. Calming thoughts—think about something that makes you feel calm.
4. Increased activity—get some exercise to help de-stress and gain a feeling of accomplishment (e.g. go for a walk outside).

Here are two extra relaxation exercises, in addition to those suggested in the client resource packs:

Tense–Relax

Tighten the muscle that you want to relax. Focus on and feel the tension where you tighten. Now let the muscle become loose and limp.

Feel the relaxation flow into the muscle. Feel yourself letting go of all your tensions. Just enjoy that feeling for a minute as your muscles let go more and more.

- Clench fists tightly—hold for 5—relax.
- Pull in stomach muscles tightly—hold for 5—relax.
- Extend fingers—hold for 5—relax.
- Grasp below seat of chair—hold for 5—relax
- Push feet hard into floor—hold for 5—relax
- Imagine a wave of relaxation through your body.

Favourite Place

As you're sitting quietly, recall in your mind the most relaxing image you can. Perhaps it's a favourite place (a holiday spot or favourite retreat of some sort), or it might be a person with whom you feel at peace, or some scene (a waterfall, or the beach, or a mountain). Take a few seconds to get that in mind . . .

Now, see or imagine that in your mind. Be sure to feel those good feelings you have when you are in that place. Just let them take over your whole awareness . . . If your thoughts wander, just take them gently back to that peaceful, relaxing place.

Relaxation Is a Skill that Needs to Be Learned

Relaxation techniques can help reduce the arousal that comes from stress and anxiety. However, without practice, they will not work very well, and it will be easy to get discouraged.

The key is making it part of your routine. Find 15 minutes a day to practise relaxation. Doing a relaxing activity less than once a week is not likely to have a big impact.

Appendix 14

Information about Sleeping Tablets

Common sleeping medications are benzodiazepines such as temazepam (Normison), (Mogadonnitrazepam), Serapax, diazepam (Valium), Xanax, zopiclone, and zolpidem (Stilnox).

Valerian (herbal) and Restavit (antihistamine) are common over-the-counter sleeping aids.

Sleeping tablets are not a cure for Insomnia. They help to treat acute (short-term and severe) sleep difficulties and should only be used as a short-term solution. Sleeping tablets only cover up the symptoms, rather than treating the underlying cause. By contrast, psychological treatments (CBT for Insomnia) focus specifically on the underlying causes of Insomnia.

Sleeping medications can become a problem when they are used every night, or most nights. So, these tablets that started off helping you may become part of the problem.

These common problems may develop:

- **Reduced REM (dreaming) and/or slow-wave (deep) sleep**: Many sleeping tablets reduce dreaming and deep sleep. So, although a sleeping tablet may help you to sleep, it is a different kind of sleep from you would get naturally.
- **Tolerance**: This is when you need to take more of the medication to get the same effect, and, eventually, the medication stops having any good effect at all.
- **Side effects**: The most common side effect is a 'hangover' effect in the morning on waking. Other side effects include nervousness, lack of energy, trembling, sweating, difficulty concentrating, lack of clear thinking, irritability, headaches, and upset stomach.
- **Withdrawal symptoms**: People often report 'rebound Insomnia', which refers to a temporary worsening in Insomnia that usually lasts for between 1 and 3 weeks (but can occasionally last up to 2 months). How long this rebound effect lasts will depend on the type of medication you have been using, the dose, how long you have been taking it, how quickly you come off it, and your normal physical health. The withdrawal that occurs when people decide to come off sleeping pills is one of the main reasons that many people become addicted to, or dependent on, such medication.
- **Nightmares**: Sleeping pills decrease REM sleep. If you suddenly reduce your *regular* use of sleeping pills, it can result in a sudden increase in REM sleep. This may be experienced as unpleasant dreams, or a tendency for sleep to be a little worse for a while.

Please speak with your doctor if you are concerned about your sleeping tablet use.

Appendix 15

Reducing Your Usage of Sleeping Tablets

If you have been taking sleeping medication and you wish to reduce or stop your usage, it is important that you speak to your doctor and reduce the dose of your sleeping medication gradually.

Not everybody has significant problems with reducing their use of sleeping medication, but you may notice that your sleep becomes worse when you reduce your medication. It may be tempting to conclude, 'I was sleeping better before I reduced my medication, so I must need the medication to sleep, and I'd better up my dose again.' If your doctor supports you in reducing your medication, trust that the poorer sleep that you may experience is likely to be part of drug withdrawal symptoms and is most likely temporary. It is important that you are prepared for the possibility that your sleep may get worse temporarily while you are withdrawing from sleep medications.

Tips for Withdrawing

- Reduce your dose gradually, but consistently; **never** suddenly. You can do it slowly, particularly if you are nervous. For example, to cut back from 1 tablet per night, start by taking ¾ of a tablet for a week, then ½ a tablet for the next week, then ¼ for the following week, then none at all. So, it might take around 4 weeks to cut back from one tablet per night. Expect it to take longer if you are taking a larger dose. Make changes in consultation with your doctor. Remember that everyone will have a rate of withdrawal that suits them best, so go at the rate that feels comfortable for you.
- Be structured in your approach. Make a plan and stick to it. Set realistic weekly goals.
- Stay at the same dose for longer, rather than increasing the dose. If you hit a difficult patch, stick at the dose you are on until you feel ready to reduce again. Try not to increase the dose.
- Avoid taking sleeping pills after about midnight to minimise hangover effects the next day.
- Keep a sleep diary while you are withdrawing, as this will help you to keep track of the effects of the withdrawal.
- Talk to your friends and family about how you are feeling, so that they understand your situation and provide you with encouragement and support.
- Remember that withdrawal symptoms are temporary, and they show that you are making a change.
- Withdrawing from sleep medication will allow you to start working towards a longer-term solution to Insomnia.

Further Reading

Trickett, S. (1997) *Free yourself from tranquilizers and sleeping pills: A natural approach*: Berkeley, CA: Ulysses Press.

Neild, L. (1990) *Escape from tranquilisers and sleeping pills: A proven DIY withdrawal plan*. London: Ebury Press.

PubMed Health (2013) *Using medication: What can help when trying to stop taking sleeping pills and sedatives?* www.ncbi.nlm.nih.gov/pubmedhealth/PMH0087084/

Appendix 16

Evaluating My Progress

Where do you feel you are at the moment in terms of keeping on top of your Insomnia? Indicate this on the diagram below?

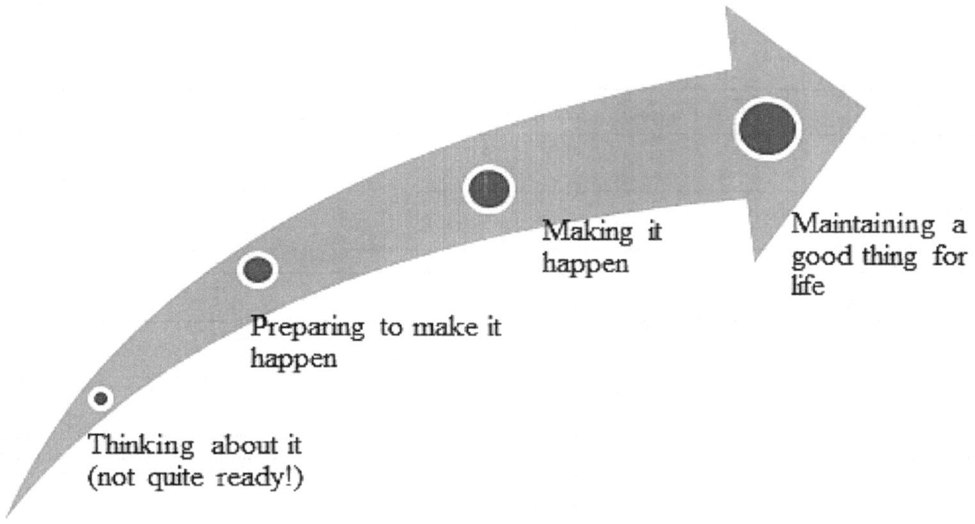

Are you happy and satisfied at the moment in terms of how your sleep is going?

____

____

What would you like to change?

____

____

Appendix 17

Change Plan Worksheet ('My Goals')

My GOALS: The changes I want to make (or continue making) are:

The reasons why I want to make these changes are:

The steps I plan to take to achieve my goals are:

The ways other people can help me are:

Some things that could interfere with my plan are:

What I will do if the plan isn't working:

Index